Global Management of Infectious Disease After Ebola

Global Management of Infectious Disease After Ebola

EDITED BY SAM F. HALABI
LAWRENCE O. GOSTIN
and
JEFFREY S. CROWLEY

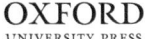

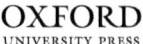
UNIVERSITY PRESS

Oxford University Press is a department of the University of Oxford. It furthers
the University's objective of excellence in research, scholarship, and education
by publishing worldwide. Oxford is a registered trade mark of Oxford University
Press in the UK and certain other countries.

Published in the United States of America by Oxford University Press
198 Madison Avenue, New York, NY 10016, United States of America.

© Oxford University Press 2017

All rights reserved. No part of this publication may be reproduced, stored in
a retrieval system, or transmitted, in any form or by any means, without the
prior permission in writing of Oxford University Press, or as expressly permitted
by law, by license, or under terms agreed with the appropriate reproduction
rights organization. Inquiries concerning reproduction outside the scope of the
above should be sent to the Rights Department, Oxford University Press, at the
address above.

You must not circulate this work in any other form
and you must impose this same condition on any acquirer.

Library of Congress Cataloging-in-Publication Data
Names: Halabi, Sam F., editor. | Gostin, Lawrence O. (Lawrence Ogalthorpe),
editor. | Crowley, Jeffrey S., editor.
Title: Global management of infectious disease after ebola / edited by
Sam F. Halabi, Lawrence O. Gostin, Jeffrey S. Crowley.
Description: Oxford; New York : Oxford University Press, [2016] |
Includes bibliographical references.
Identifiers: LCCN 2016014239 | ISBN 9780190604882 (hardback)
Subjects: | MESH: Hemorrhagic Fever, Ebola—prevention & control |
Epidemics—prevention & control | Communicable Disease
Control—organization & administration | International Cooperation |
Global Health
Classification: LCC RC140.5 | NLM WC 534 | DDC 614.5/ 7— dc23
LC record available at http:// lccn.loc.gov/2016014239

This material is not intended to be, and should not be considered, a substitute for medical or
other professional advice. Treatment for the conditions described in this material is highly
dependent on the individual circumstances. And, while this material is designed to offer
accurate information with respect to the subject matter covered and to be current as of the
time it was written, research and knowledge about medical and health issues are constantly
evolving and dose schedules for medications are being revised continually, with new side
effects recognized and accounted for regularly. Readers must therefore always check the
product information and clinical procedures with the most up-to-date published product
information and data sheets provided by the manufacturers and the most recent codes of
conduct and safety regulation. The publisher and the authors make no representations or
warranties to readers, express or implied, as to the accuracy or completeness of this material.
Without limiting the foregoing, the publisher and the authors make no representations or
warranties as to the accuracy or efficacy of the drug dosages mentioned in the material. The
authors and the publisher do not accept, and expressly disclaim, any responsibility for any
liability, loss, or risk that may be claimed or incurred as a consequence of the use and/or
application of any of the contents of this material.

Global Management of Infectious Disease After Ebola

Global Management of Infectious Disease After Ebola

EDITED BY SAM F. HALABI
LAWRENCE O. GOSTIN
and
JEFFREY S. CROWLEY

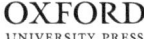

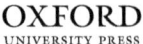

UNIVERSITY PRESS

Oxford University Press is a department of the University of Oxford. It furthers the University's objective of excellence in research, scholarship, and education by publishing worldwide. Oxford is a registered trade mark of Oxford University Press in the UK and certain other countries.

Published in the United States of America by Oxford University Press
198 Madison Avenue, New York, NY 10016, United States of America.

© Oxford University Press 2017

All rights reserved. No part of this publication may be reproduced, stored in a retrieval system, or transmitted, in any form or by any means, without the prior permission in writing of Oxford University Press, or as expressly permitted by law, by license, or under terms agreed with the appropriate reproduction rights organization. Inquiries concerning reproduction outside the scope of the above should be sent to the Rights Department, Oxford University Press, at the address above.

You must not circulate this work in any other form
and you must impose this same condition on any acquirer.

Library of Congress Cataloging-in-Publication Data
Names: Halabi, Sam F., editor. | Gostin, Lawrence O. (Lawrence Ogalthorpe), editor. | Crowley, Jeffrey S., editor.
Title: Global management of infectious disease after ebola / edited by Sam F. Halabi, Lawrence O. Gostin, Jeffrey S. Crowley.
Description: Oxford; New York : Oxford University Press, [2016] | Includes bibliographical references.
Identifiers: LCCN 2016014239 | ISBN 9780190604882 (hardback)
Subjects: | MESH: Hemorrhagic Fever, Ebola—prevention & control | Epidemics—prevention & control | Communicable Disease Control—organization & administration | International Cooperation | Global Health
Classification: LCC RC140.5 | NLM WC 534 | DDC 614.5/ 7— dc23
LC record available at http:// lccn.loc.gov/2016014239

This material is not intended to be, and should not be considered, a substitute for medical or other professional advice. Treatment for the conditions described in this material is highly dependent on the individual circumstances. And, while this material is designed to offer accurate information with respect to the subject matter covered and to be current as of the time it was written, research and knowledge about medical and health issues are constantly evolving and dose schedules for medications are being revised continually, with new side effects recognized and accounted for regularly. Readers must therefore always check the product information and clinical procedures with the most up-to-date published product information and data sheets provided by the manufacturers and the most recent codes of conduct and safety regulation. The publisher and the authors make no representations or warranties to readers, express or implied, as to the accuracy or completeness of this material. Without limiting the foregoing, the publisher and the authors make no representations or warranties as to the accuracy or efficacy of the drug dosages mentioned in the material. The authors and the publisher do not accept, and expressly disclaim, any responsibility for any liability, loss, or risk that may be claimed or incurred as a consequence of the use and/or application of any of the contents of this material.

CONTENTS

Acknowledgments ix
About the Editors xi
Contributors xiii

Introduction 1
SAM F. HALABI, LAWRENCE O. GOSTIN, AND JEFFREY S. CROWLEY

PART I CURRENT AND EMERGING INFECTIOUS DISEASE CHALLENGES

1. The Ebola Epidemic of 2014–2015: A Perfect Storm 21
   ANTHONY S. FAUCI

2. Treating, Containing, Mobilizing: The Role of Médecins Sans Frontières in the West African Ebola Epidemic Response 33
   HEATHER PAGANO AND MARC PONCIN

3. The Effect of Ebola Virus Disease on Health Outcomes and Systems in Guinea, Liberia, and Sierra Leone 55
   JOHN D. KRAEMER AND MARK J. SIEDNER

4. Infectious Disease Threats in High-Resource Settings: The MERS-CoV Outbreak in Korea 75
   SUGY CHOI, JONG-KOO LEE, AND DANIEL R. LUCEY

5. Antibiotic Resistance 87
   GAIL HANSEN

PART II GLOBAL SYSTEMS FOR PREVENTION
AND MANAGEMENT OF INFECTIOUS DISEASE THREATS

6. The International Health Regulations: The Governing Framework for Global Health Security   101
   LAWRENCE O. GOSTIN AND REBECCA KATZ

7. Global Health Diplomacy and the Ebola Outbreak   133
   DAVID P. FIDLER

8. The Future of Global Financing for Infectious Diseases   149
   JENNIFER KATES AND ADAM WEXLER

9. International Public-Private Partnerships as Part of the Solution to Infectious Disease Threats: Operational, Legal, and Governance Considerations   157
   KEVIN A. KLOCK

10. Global Vaccine Access as a Critical Intervention to Fight Infectious Disease, Antibiotic Resistance, and Poverty   179
    SETH BERKLEY

PART III ETHICAL AND HUMAN RIGHTS OBLIGATIONS
IN PUBLIC HEALTH EMERGENCIES

11. Bridging the Gap Between Biomedical Innovation and Access to Treatments to Fight Infectious Disease   193
    VERONICA MILLER

12. Ethical Challenges in the Development and Deployment of Medical Therapies and Vaccines in the Context of Public Health Emergencies   207
    ANNICK ANTIERENS

13. Evidence, Strategies, and Challenges for Assuring Vaccine Availability, Efficacy, and Safety   223
    SAAD B. OMER AND SAM F. HALABI

14. Global Access Considerations for HIV Vaccine Trials   235
    MARY MAROVICH

15. Isolation, Quarantine, and Infectious Disease Threats Arising From Global Migration   245
    MARTIN CETRON

Epilogue   257
    RENÉE C. FOX

Index   275

ACKNOWLEDGMENTS

The authors would like to thank the directors and staff at the O'Neill Institute for National and Global Health Law at Georgetown University who made this project possible: Oscar Cabrera, Mary DeBartolo, Susan Kim, John Monahan, Mike Templeton, Alison Woodworth, and especially Rebecca Reingold. Katherine Dunning, Shaye Guilfoyle, Han-Hsi "Indy" Liu, Lois Sheng Liu, Kyoungho Moon, Sarah Roache, and Tara Williams provided excellent research and editorial assistance. We would also like to thank Chad Zimmerman and Chloe Layman at Oxford University Press for shepherding the project through the publication process and three anonymous reviewers for providing helpful comments. Finally, we would like to express our gratitude to the contributors to this book, as well as our friends and family, for their patience and support throughout the publication process.

ABOUT THE EDITORS

Sam Halabi
Scholar, O'Neill Institute for National and Global Health Law and Associate Professor, The University of Tulsa College of Law

Professor Halabi is a scholar of national and global health law with a specialization in health services and pharmaceutical business organizations. He serves as a Scholar at the O'Neill Institute for National and Global Health Law at Georgetown University, where he has also served as a special advisor to the *Lancet*–Georgetown University Commission on Global Health and Law. He has served as an advisor to the World Health Organization and the National Foundation for the U.S. Centers for Disease Control and Prevention as well as publishing widely on healthcare system design, biomedical innovation, and vaccine safety. Before earning his J.D. from Harvard Law School, Professor Halabi was awarded a British Marshall scholarship to study in the United Kingdom where he earned an M.Phil in International Relations from the University of Oxford (St. Antony's College). He holds a BA and a BS from Kansas State University.

Lawrence Gostin
University Professor and Georgetown University Law Center and Founding Linda D. & Timothy J. O'Neill Professor of Global Health Law; Faculty Director, O'Neill Institute for National & Global Health Law; Director, World Health Organization Collaborating Center on Public Health Law & Human Rights

Prof. Gostin earned his B.A. from the State University of New York, Brockport and his J.D. from Duke University. Prof. Gostin is the Director of the World Health Organization Collaborating Center on Public Health Law & Human Rights as well as on the International Health Regulations (IHR) Roster of Experts and the Expert Advisory Panel on Mental Health. He served on the Director-General's Advisory Committee on Reforming the World Health Organization, as well as numerous WHO expert advisory committees on Pandemic Influenza Preparedness Framework, smallpox, and genomic sequencing data. Prof. Gostin, an elected lifetime Member of the National Academy of Medicine (formerly Institute of Medicine), National Academy of Sciences which has awarded him the Adam Yarmolinsky Medal for distinguished service to further its mission of science and health, as well as a lifetime elected Member of the Council of Foreign Relations and a Fellow of the Hastings Center. Prof. Gostin's latest books are: *Global Health Law* (Harvard University Press, 2014); *Public Health Law: Power, Duty, Restraint* (University of California Press, 3rd ed., 2016); and *Law and the Health System* (Foundation Press, 2014). Professor Gostin is the Health Law and Ethics Editor and a contributing writer and columnist for the *Journal of the American Medical Association*.

Jeffrey Crowley
Program Director of the National HIV/AIDS Initiative at the O'Neill Institute for National and Global Health Law

Mr. Crowley is a widely recognized expert on HIV/AIDS and disability policy. From February 2009 through December 2011, he served as the Director of the White House Office of National AIDS Policy and Senior Advisor on Disability Policy for President Barack Obama. In this capacity, he led the development of the first domestic National HIV/AIDS Strategy for the United States, a five-year plan for aligning the efforts of all stakeholders to reduce the number of new HIV infections, increase access to care, and reduce HIV-related health disparities. He also coordinated disability policy development for the Domestic Policy Council and worked on the policy team that spearheaded the development and implementation of the Patient Protection and Affordable Care Act. He holds an MPH from Johns Hopkins University.

CONTRIBUTORS

Annick Antierens
Deputy Medical Director, Médecins Sans Frontières, Geneva, Switzerland
Annick Antierens is a medical doctor specialized in anaesthesia and emergency medicine. She earned her diploma in these specializations from the Catholic University of Leuven-Belgium as well as a degree in public health from the University of Nancy-France. She started her first humanitarian missions as an anaesthesiologist in Bosnia for Médecins sans Frontières (MSF) in 1995 and in Rwanda for the Belgian Red Cross in 1996. From 1997 to 2007 she served as medical coordinator for MSF in several countries (Mauritania, Kenya, Sudan, and Ethiopia). From 2010 to mid-2014 she was the deputy medical director at the MSF operational centre in Geneva. Since September 2014, she has managed the Ebola Investigational Platform at MSF and from July 2016 she will take the position of Medical Technical Manager at MSF operational centre in Brussels.

Seth Berkley
Chief Executive Officer, Gavi, the Vaccine Alliance
Seth Berkley is the Chief Executive Officer of Gavi, the Vaccine Alliance. Prior to this, he was CEO and Founder of the International AIDS Vaccine Initiative, the first product development public-private partnership. Berkley is a physician who began his public health career as a medical epidemiologist at the US Centers for Disease Control and Prevention. He contributed to the discovery of Brazilian purpuric fever and helped set up Uganda's national AIDS control program. In 2009, Berkley was named one of the "100 Most Influential People in the World" by *Time* magazine. In 2010, *Fortune* magazine named him as one of its "Global Forum Visionaries." He holds an MD from Brown University and trained in internal medicine at Harvard University.

Martin Cetron
Director, Division of Global Migration and Quarantine, US Centers for Disease Control and Prevention

Martin Cetron's primary research interest is international health and global migration. He has led a number of domestic and international outbreak investigations and been involved in domestic and international emergency responses to provide medical screening and disease prevention programs to refugees prior to US resettlement. He played a leadership role in CDC responses to intentional and naturally acquired emerging infectious disease outbreaks, including the anthrax bioterrorism incident, the global SARS epidemic, the US monkeypox outbreak, and the H1N1 pandemic. Dr. Cetron holds faculty appointments in the Division of Infectious Diseases at the Emory University School of Medicine and the Department of Epidemiology at Rollins School of Public Health. Dr. Cetron received his BA from Dartmouth College in 1981 and his MD from Tufts University in 1985. He trained in internal medicine at the University of Virginia and infectious diseases at the University of Washington.

Sugy Choi
Research Associate, J. W. Lee Center for Global Medicine at the Seoul National University College of Medicine

Sugy Choi received her BS in foreign service and MS in global health with a focus on health policy and financing from Georgetown University. She has previously been a consultant to the Malaria, Other Vectorborne, and Parasitic Diseases teams under the Division of Communicable Diseases at the World Health Organization Western Pacific Regional Office in Manila, the Philippines. Her work currently focuses on global health projects and evaluations in Southeast Asia and Africa, especially health equity and vulnerable populations. During the recent MERS outbreak in the Republic of Korea, she served as a volunteer translator and rapporteur for ProMED-mail and received the ProMED-mail Anniversary Award in 2015.

Anthony S. Fauci
Director, US National Institute for Allergy and Infectious Diseases

Anthony Fauci joined NIAID in 1968 and was appointed its Director in 1984. He oversees an extensive portfolio of basic and applied research to prevent, diagnose, and treat infectious diseases such as HIV/AIDS and other sexually transmitted infections, influenza, tuberculosis, malaria, and illness from potential agents of bioterrorism. He has made many contributions to basic and clinical research on the pathogenesis and treatment of immune-mediated and infectious diseases. Dr. Fauci was the world's 10th-most-cited HIV/AIDS researcher in the period from 1996 through 2006 and has received the Presidential Medal of Freedom, the National Medal of Science, and 42 honorary doctoral degrees, among many other honors. He earned an MD from Cornell University Medical College in 1966 before completing an internship and residency at the New York Hospital–Cornell Medical Center.

David P. Fidler

James Louis Calamaras Professor of Law, Indiana University Maurer School of Law

David Fidler is one of the world's leading experts on international law and global health security. He serves as an Associate Fellow with the Centre on Global Health Security at the Royal Institute of International Affairs (Chatham House) and a Fellow with the Pacific and Asia Society. He is also on the Roster of Experts that advises the Director-General of the World Health Organization under the International Health Regulations (2005). Professor Fidler has served as an international legal consultant to the World Health Organization, the US Centers for Disease Control and Prevention, and the US Agency for International Development. He was a member of the Harvard University–London School of Hygiene and Tropical Medicine's Independent Panel on the Global Response to Ebola and a member of the Georgetown University–Lancet Commission on Law and Global Health. Professor Fidler holds a JD from Harvard Law School, a BCL and an MPhil in International Relations from the University of Oxford, and a BA from the University of Kansas.

Renée C. Fox

Annenberg Professor Emerita of the Social Sciences, University of Pennsylvania

Renée C. Fox joined the faculty of the University of Pennsylvania in 1969 after serving as a member of the Columbia University Bureau of Applied Social Research, teaching for 12 years at Barnard College, and then spending 2 years as a Visiting Lecturer in the Department of Social Relations at Harvard. At the University of Pennsylvania, she was a Professor in the Department of Sociology and served as a Fellow of the Center for Bioethics. Her major teaching and research interests—sociology of medicine, medical research, medical education, and medical ethics—have involved her in firsthand, participant observation–based studies in continental Europe (particularly in Belgium), in Central Africa (especially in the Democratic Republic of Congo), and in the People's Republic of China, as well as in the United States. Professor Fox graduated summa cum laude from Smith College in 1949 and earned her PhD in sociology in 1954 from Radcliffe College, Harvard University.

Gail Hansen

Senior Officer, Antibiotic Resistance Project, The Pew Charitable Trusts

Before joining Pew, Gail Hansen served as the State Epidemiologist and State Public Health Veterinarian for the Kansas Department of Health and Environment, where most of her work centered on infectious diseases and public health policy. While there, she led a team of epidemiologists that investigated outbreaks and sporadic cases of infectious disease, evaluated public health prevention measures, and developed disease tracking systems for the state. She has served on or chaired numerous state and federal infectious disease committees and served as a scientific adviser for several national and international conferences. She also served as an adjunct faculty member at the Kansas State University College of Veterinary Medicine. She has authored several peer-reviewed publications on various infectious diseases and public health topics and has provided practical training in applied epidemiology to public health scholars. She received her DVM from the University of Minnesota and her MPH in epidemiology from the University of Washington.

Jennifer Kates
Vice President and Director of Global Health and HIV Policy,
Henry J. Kaiser Family Foundation

Jennifer Kates oversees the Kaiser Family Foundation's policy analysis and research focusing on the US government's role in global health and on the global and domestic HIV epidemics. She regularly publishes and presents on donor government investments in global health; assessing and mapping the US government's global health architecture, programs, and funding; and tracking and analyzing major US HIV programs and financing, and key trends in the HIV epidemic. Prior to joining the foundation, she was a Senior Associate with the Lewin Group. She also directed the Office of Lesbian, Gay, and Bisexual Concerns at Princeton University. Dr. Kates serves on numerous federal and private sector advisory committees on global health and HIV, including the CDC/HRSA Advisory Committee on HIV, Viral Hepatitis and STD Prevention and Treatment (CHACHSPT) and President's Emergency Plan for AIDS Relief's Scientific Advisory Board, and is an Alternate Board Member of the Global Fund to Fight AIDS, Tuberculosis and Malaria. She received her PhD in Health Policy from George Washington University, where she is also a Lecturer.

Rebecca Katz
Associate Professor, Georgetown UniversitySchool of Nursing & Health Studies' (NHS)
Department of International Health

Rebecca Katz is an expert on the intersection of national security and infectious diseases, including the threat posed by the 2014 Ebola epidemic. Her research is focused on public health preparedness, global health diplomacy, biosurveillance, and the relationship between infectious diseases and national security. Her current research projects are focused on implementation of the International Health Regulations (2005). She also works on issues related to food-borne illness surveillance and response, and on biosecurity and biosafety. Since 2004, Dr. Katz has been a consultant to the US Department of State, working on issues related to the Biological Weapons Convention and emerging and pandemic threats.

Kevin A. Klock

Director of Operations/Advisor to the President at the Foundation for the National Institutes of Health

Kevin Klock leads the NIH's Foundation's management and oversight of general policies and procedures, grants and contracts, legal affairs, human resources, office services, and special projects. Prior to joining the FNIH, Director Klock was Head of Governance and Assistant Secretary for Gavi, the Vaccine Alliance, and Company Secretary for the Gavi Campaign. At Gavi, he advised board members, staff, and partners on public sector and corporate governance best practice and was lead staff member on governance for matters that involved Gavi's finance and debt-issuance activities, including the International Finance Facility for Immunisation (IFFIm). Director Klock received his JD, magna cum laude, from Georgetown University Law Center. He is also a graduate of Duke University, received his MA from American University, and attended Oxford University as a Lord Rothermere Scholar.

John D. Kraemer

Assistant Professor, Department of Health Systems Administration, Georgetown University

John Kraemer holds a JD from Georgetown University and an MPH from John Hopkins Bloomberg School of Public Health. His work focuses on the improvement of public health policy through evidence-based and legal approaches, including women's and children's health in sub-Saharan Africa, road safety for vulnerable road users, and constitutional public health law. His current and past projects include work with the Pink Ribbon Red Ribbon initiative against women's cancers, the United Nations Special Envoy for Malaria, and Last Mile Health. At Georgetown, Professor Kraemer teaches about the social and political dimensions of the HIV/AIDS response in the United States and sub-Saharan Africa and the intersection of democracy, rights, and health.

Jong-koo Lee

Director, J. W. Lee Center for Global Medicine and the Office of Policy Development of Healthy Society, and Professor of Family Medicine at Seoul National University College of Medicine

Jong-koo Lee directs undergraduate and postgraduate student education and research for primary health care and public health policies, including global health, at the J. W. Lee Center, as well as infectious disease epidemiology at Seoul National University Graduate School of Public Health. He also acts as Senior Adviser to the Seoul Metropolitan Infectious Disease Control Center and was co-leader of the WHO Joint Mission to the Republic of Korea on MERS-CoV in 2015. He graduated from Seoul National University College of Medicine 1982. He majored in family medicine at Seoul National University Hospital and received his MPH degree in epidemiology from the Seoul National University Graduate School of Public Health in 1985 and his PhD in health policy and management from Seoul National University College of Medicine, Graduate School of Medicine, in 2003.

Daniel R. Lucey
Senior Scholar with the O'Neill Institute for National and Global Health Law and Adjunct Professor, Microbiology and Immunology at Georgetown University Medical Center (GUMC)

Daniel R. Lucey MD, MPH is an infectious disease and public health physician. Between 2003 and 2016, he traveled to work during outbreaks ("panepidemics") including: SARS in China and Canada, H5N1 Avian flu in Thailand, Vietnam, Indonesia, and Egypt, pandemic H1N1 flu in Egypt, MERS across 6 nations in the Middle East and Republic of Korea, Ebola in Sierra Leone, Liberia, and Guinea, and Zika in Brazil. From 1982-2002 he worked on HIV/AIDS from UCSF to Harvard, USAF-Texas, NIH-Bethesda, and in DC as Chief of Infectious Disease Service at the 900-bed Washington Hospital Center. Dr. Lucey graduated from Dartmouth College and Medical School, Harvard School of Public Health, and trained in Medicine at UCSF, and in Infectious Diseases at Harvard.

Mary Marovich
Director of the AIDS Vaccine Research Program at the US National Institute of Allergy and Infectious Diseases

Mary Marovich leads the development and coordination of clinical and preclinical research on HIV vaccines at NIH. She came to NIH from the US Military HIV Research Program (MHRP), where she served as Chief of vaccine research and development since 2005. Additionally, Marovich worked as the Clinic Director for MHRP's Rockville Vaccine Assessment Center, where she led multiple early-stage HIV and non-HIV vaccine clinical trials. She earned bachelor's degrees in biochemistry and chemistry at Illinois State University and a medical degree at Loyola University of Chicago-Maywood. In 1993, she completed a residency in internal medicine and clinical infectious diseases training at the University of Colorado and earned a diploma in tropical medicine and hygiene from the Royal College of Physicians and Surgeons, London School of Tropical Medicine and Hygiene. She is also an Associate Professor of medicine with the Uniformed Services University's Department of Medicine.

Veronica Miller
Senior Researcher and Lecturer, University of California, Berkeley, and Executive Director, Forum for Collaborative HIV Research

Veronica Miller has extensive experience in working with all major global and US organizations and agencies involved in HIV research and policy. Under her leadership the Forum's deliberative process to advance regulatory science applied successfully to HIV was extended to drug development for hepatitis C infection in 2007, and, starting in 2014, to the treatment of liver diseases and human cytomegalovirus disease in solid organ and stem cell transplant patients. Efforts led by Dr. Miller to advance public health policy through stakeholder engagement include the National Summit program, which focuses on the implementation of the National HIV/AIDS Strategy and the Viral Hepatitis Action Plan; and the Bay Area Health Disparities Program. She has published more than 90 peer-reviewed works on HIV treatment strategies and regulatory strategies for HIV and HCV. She joined the Forum in 2001 after having directed the interdisciplinary HIV Research Group at the HIV Outpatient Clinic of the Goethe University in Frankfurt, Germany. Dr. Miller holds a PhD in Immunology from the University of Manitoba.

Saad B. Omer
Professor, Global Health, Epidemiology, and Pediatrics, Emory University, Schools of Public Health and Medicine; Investigator, Emory Center for AIDS Research

Saad Omer is a faculty member at the Emory Vaccine Center. He has conducted multiple studies—including vaccine trials—in Guatemala, Uganda, Ethiopia, India, Pakistan, Bangladesh, South Africa, and the United States. Dr. Omer's research portfolio includes clinical and field trials to estimate efficacy and/or immunogenicity of influenza, polio, measles, and pneumococcal vaccines; studies on the impact of spatial clustering of vaccine refusers; and clinical trials to evaluate drug regimens to reduce mother-to-child transmission of HIV in Africa. He has conducted several studies to evaluate the roles of schools, parents, health care providers, and state-level legislation in relation to immunization coverage and disease incidence. Dr. Omer has published widely in peer-reviewed journals, including the *New England Journal of Medicine*, *JAMA*, the *Lancet*, and the *British Medical Journal*. He is currently a Member of the National Vaccine Advisory Committee.

Heather Pagano
Humanitarian Advisor, Médecins Sans Frontières, Belgium

Heather Pagano is a humanitarian adviser in MSF's Advocacy and Analysis Unit based in Belgium, with a focus on the politics of epidemic response and global health security. She joined Médecins Sans Frontières in 2008, serving as the Ebola Advocacy and Communication Coordinator during the 2014–2015 West African epidemic, after extensive field and operations-level communications experience. She has written widely on public health emergencies such as the Ebola epidemic and the South Sudan conflict, and most recently served as a communications expert analyzing the 2015 bombing of the MSF Kunduz Trauma Center in Afghanistan.

Marc Poncin
Researcher and Humanitarian Expert, Médecins Sans Frontières, Switzerland

Marc Poncin is a researcher and humanitarian expert at the Research Unit on Humanitarian Stakes and Practices (UREPH), Médecins Sans Frontières, Switzerland. He began his career as a researcher in structural biology after obtaining a PhD in Molecular Biophysics from Paris 7 University. He joined MSF in 1995 and in the intervening years has worked extensively in Africa as Emergency Coordinator and Head of various missions. He also served as Deputy Director-General and Head of Programs of the Swiss branch of MSF. During the Ebola crisis, he served as the Coordinator of the MSF response in Guinea from April to December 2014.

Mark J. Siedner
Associate Professor, Harvard Medical School, and Researcher, Division of Infectious Diseases at Massachusetts General Hospital

Mark Siedner is an infectious disease clinician and researcher in the Division of Infectious Diseases at Massachusetts General Hospital. He practices clinical medicine as an internist and general infectious diseases provider at Massachusetts General Hospital. He conducts clinical research, largely focused in sub-Saharan Africa, aimed at mitigating the causes of morbidity and mortality among people living with HIV in low-income countries. Current projects include directing a longitudinal study of aging among HIV-infected persons in Uganda and a randomized trial to evaluate the efficacy and cost-effectiveness of implementing HIV-1 resistance testing into routine care in sub-Saharan Africa. He teaches clinical medicine, epidemiology, and research design both in Boston and in Uganda and serves as a technical consultant to Last Mile Health, a nongovernmental community health partner to the Liberian Ministry of Health. He holds an MD from Johns Hopkins University and an MPH from Johns Hopkins Bloomberg School of Public Health.

Adam Wexler
Director, Global Health Budget Project, Henry J. Kaiser Family Foundation

Adam Wexler focuses on tracking and analyzing the US global health budget, as well as the trends in international donor assistance for HIV and family planning activities. Prior to joining the Kaiser Family Foundation, Adam worked as a policy analyst for the City of San Diego. Director Wexler holds a Bachelor of Science degree in Biology from Gettysburg College and a Master of Public Policy from Georgetown University.

Introduction

SAM F. HALABI, LAWRENCE O. GOSTIN, AND JEFFREY S. CROWLEY

The Ebola virus disease epidemic in West Africa has provided another searing reminder that the fight against emerging and re-emerging infectious diseases is perpetual.[1] Even as this volume was planned, assembled, and finalized, an "explosive pandemic reemergence" of the mosquito-borne Zika virus was spreading throughout the Americas. The most salient concern is that Zika virus infection in pregnant women causes microcephaly and other severe birth defects in their infants, although the virus causes other neurological disorders and severe illness.[2] The World Health Organization (WHO) quickly declared the Zika epidemic a public health emergency of international concern (PHEIC), only the fourth time it has done so since assuming new authority to detect, prevent, and manage infectious diseases under the International Health Regulations (IHR; 2005).[3] The decision to do so was in part a response to the perceived failure of WHO to act with requisite speed and resolve as the Ebola outbreak unfolded. The other two PHEIC designations were for influenza A (H1N1) and polio.

The Ebola epidemic has become a transformative event in global health, with four major commissions devoted to assessing the failures in the global response: WHO,[4]

---

[1] Anthony S. Fauci, *Emerging and reemerging infectious diseases: the perpetual challenge*, 80 (12) Academic Medicine (2005).

[2] CDC, CDC Concludes Zika Causes Microcephaly and Other Birth Defects, Apr. 13, 2016 available at http://www.cdc.gov/media/releases/2016/s0413-zika-microcephaly.html; Anthony S. Fauci and David Morens, *Zika Virus in the Americas—yet another arbovirus threat*, 106 New England Journal of Medicine (Jan. 13, 2016); CB Marcondes and MF Ximenes, *Zika virus in Brazil and the danger of infestation by Aedes(Stegomyia) mosquitoes*, 49(1) Rev Soc Bras Med Trop (Dec. 22, 2015).

[3] World Health Organization, WHO Director-General Summarizes the Outcome of the Emergency Committee Regarding Clusters of Microcephaly and Guillain-Barre Syndrome (Feb. 1, 2016), available at http://www.who.int/mediacentre/news/statements/2016/emergency-committee-zika-microcephaly/en/.

[4] WHO, Report of the Ebola Interim Assessment Panel (July 2015).

the Harvard/London School of Hygiene and Tropical Medicine Independent Panel,[5] the National Academy of Medicine,[6] and the United Nations.[7]

Indeed, it is the general failure of the global community to effectively prioritize and thereby dedicate adequate resources to infectious diseases that has motivated the effort undertaken in this volume. The outbreak of Ebola virus disease beginning in December 2013 and continuing through this writing, typified an all-too-frequent cycle in which outbreaks occur in the countries with the fewest resources available to manage them, and those outbreaks metastasize into international public health emergencies that threaten rich countries as well as poor, followed by inadequate investment in the health system infrastructure in the places that need those resources, giving rise, again, to the conditions that accommodate the outbreak of infectious disease. This volume not only identifies discrete vulnerabilities in the global system for detecting, preventing, and managing infectious disease but also assesses the critical ways in which that global response system has changed, the increasing complexity of the channels between biomedical innovation and patient access to medicines and vaccines, and the reforms necessary for the system to fully reflect the stated international consensus that priority must be given to control of infectious disease and, more broadly, the human right to the highest attainable standard of health.

The Ebola epidemic was pivotal for the worldwide health system.[8] It highlighted the reality that the most important international agreement adopted to address such a threat—the IHR—could not effectively function if the global community generally and individual states specifically were not held accountable for its implementation, including adequate funding for those countries that needed it. The minimal state of healthcare infrastructure in the three most affected states caused the disease to go undetected until March 21, 2014, even though the first case occurred four months earlier.[9] After it was detected, the core public health arms of national governments as well as WHO failed to fully appreciate and respond to the crisis.[10]

Even when the official response was fully mobilized, it failed to factor in the background pressures in Guinea, Liberia, and Sierra Leone, including recent devastating

---

[5] Suerie Moon et al., *Will Ebola change the game? Ten essential reforms before the next pandemic. The report of the Harvard-LSHTM Independent Panel on the Global Response to Ebola*, 386 (10009), Lancet 2204–2221 (Nov. 28, 2015).

[6] Commission on a Global Health Risk Framework for the Future, The Neglected Dimension of Global Security: A Framework to Counter Infectious Disease Crises, National Academy of Medicine (2016).

[7] UN Secretary-General's High-Level Panel on Global Response to Health Crises (Jan. 2016).

[8] Lawrence O. Gostin and Eric A. Friedman, *A retrospective and prospective analysis of the West African Ebola virus disease epidemic: robust national health systems at the foundation and an empowered WHO at the apex*, 385 Lancet 1902–1909 (2015).

[9] Kevin Sack, Sheri Fink, and Adam Nossiter, *Ebola's deadly escape*, New York Times (Dec. 29, 2014).

[10] Gostin and Friedman, *supra* note 8.

conflicts and important cultural practices that caused deep mistrust of governments and healthcare workers. Nongovernmental humanitarian aid organizations like Médecins Sans Frontières (MSF) played unprecedented roles in sounding the global alarm, providing first lines of response, and effectively regulating substantial parts of the response, including the deployment of medicines and candidate vaccines, which necessarily depended on their expertise and facilities.

The loss of healthcare workers and the economic toll will roll back what gains had been made in Guinea, Liberia, and Sierra Leone, which were already among the weakest health systems in the world, by years or decades.[11] Public health officials reported 28,638 cases and 11,316 deaths to WHO, although these numbers are likely conservative.[12] The effect on healthcare systems more generally was severe. In Liberia, more than half of the country's facilities had closed at least temporarily by September 2014.[13] Many facilities closed because they could not control infections, effectively serving as breeding grounds for the virus. Infections occurred because of limited triage and diagnostic capacity, lack of personal protective equipment, and difficulty sterilizing the physical environment in which clinicians worked.[14] The result was the substantially reduced ability of those facilities to care for the large number of population health needs like malaria treatment, childbirth, and prenatal care. Non-facility-based health outreach measures like vaccination campaigns and family planning services were similarly impacted. While the ripple effects of health system disruption are not ultimately quantifiable, Lawrence O. Gostin and Eric A. Friedman placed what numbers could be ascertained in context: "As of March, 2015, Ebola was on track to cost $6 billion in direct expenses and at least $15 billion in economic losses. Recovery plans for Guinea, Liberia, and Sierra Leone developed in April, 2015, total more than $4.5 billion over the next several years. The direct costs alone amount to 3 years of funding for WHO, and is well over 20 times the cost of WHO's emergency response cuts in its 2014–15 budget."[15]

Even as Ebola infections started to decline, new and well-known pathogens threatened both low- and high-income countries, casting further doubt on global preparedness for major infectious disease threats. A 68-year-old Korean businessman contracted the Middle East respiratory syndrome coronavirus

---

[11] Center for Strategic and International Studies, *The road to recovery: rebuilding Liberia's health system*, available at http://csis.org/fi les/ publication/120822_Downie_RoadtoRecovery_web.pdf; WHO, Global Health Observatory data repository, absolute numbers, data by country, available at http://apps.who.int/gho/data/node. main.A1443?lang=e.

[12] World Health Organization, Ebola Situation Report (Jan. 20, 2016).

[13] Kraemer and Siedner, chapter 3, this volume. .

[14] Almea Matanock et al., *Ebola virus disease cases among health care workers not working in Ebola treatment units—Liberia, June–August, 2014*, 63(46) MMWR Morb Mortal Wkly Rep 1077–1081 (Nov. 21, 2014).

[15] Gostin and Friedman, *supra* note 8.

(MERS-CoV)—first identified in Saudi Arabia in 2012—while traveling in the Middle East. Although he was asymptomatic during his arrival, he was not informed about control measures regarding MERS-CoV when he reached Incheon Airport. After he developed a fever, he sought care at a local clinic and three hospitals over the course of nine days before being diagnosed and confirmed to be infected with MERS-CoV, during which time he had direct or indirect contact with dozens of people. Between May 20 and July 4, 2015, the MERS-CoV outbreak caused 38 deaths, yielding a case fatality rate of 20.4%, caused 186 confirmed cases, isolated 16,752 individuals, and resulted in a national economic loss in the tourism industry of 3.4 trillion won.[16] Globally, 1,060 laboratory-confirmed cases of infection with MERS-CoV, including at least 394 related deaths, have been reported to WHO as of March 2015.

Influenza, pandemics of which have killed tens of millions of people over the last century alone, also represents a persistent threat to global health, one for which "the world is ill-prepared."[17] Avian influenza A (H7N9) virus is a subtype of influenza virus that normally infects birds but sometimes infects people. The first human infection was reported in China in March 2013 and was followed by second and third epidemic waves in the winter months of 2014 and 2015. A total of 571 laboratory-confirmed cases of human infection with avian influenza A (H7N9) virus, including 212 deaths, have been reported to WHO. Since November 2014, a rapid increase in human infections with avian influenza A (H5N1) virus was reported in Egypt, with 140 human cases reported between November and March 2015. An unprecedented number of global outbreaks with avian influenza A (H5) viruses are being reported in birds, with subtypes, including H5N1, H5N2, H5N6, and H5N8, in Africa, Asia, Europe, and North America. The avian influenza A (H5N1) and A (H7N9) viruses are the most obvious concern as they continue spreading in birds, reassorting with other avian influenza viruses that are endemic in various parts of the world, and causing infections in humans. The human population is not generally immune to these viruses, which may cause severe disease and death in humans once infection occurs.[18]

Even pathogens for which approved vaccines or medical therapies are available continue to impose a substantial burden on global health and livelihood. On the global scale, it is estimated that 130 to 150 million persons are infected with hepatitis C virus, and around 499,000 persons die every year. The aggregate number of deaths from all forms of viral hepatitis amounts to 1.4 million per year, which is comparable to the

---

[16] See Choi, Koo-Lee, and Lucey, chapter 4, this volume.

[17] World Health Organization, Report of the Review Committee on the Functioning of the International Health Regulations (2005) in Relation to Pandemic (H1N1) (2009), available at http://apps.who.int/gb/ebwha/pdf_files/WHA64/A64_10-en.pdf.

[18] Centers for Disease Control and Prevention, Global Health Security: International Health Regulations, available at http://www.cdc.gov/globalhealth/healthprotection/ghs/ihr/.

number of persons who die of HIV/AIDS.[19] HIV/AIDS continues to inflict substantial burdens on global health, especially in Africa. Globally, 35 million people were living with HIV at the end of 2013. Worldwide, an estimated 0.8% of adults aged 15 to 49 are living with HIV. In sub-Saharan Africa, nearly 1 in every 20 adults lives with HIV, accounting for approximately 71% of the people living with HIV worldwide.[20]

Of even greater concern is that for infectious diseases for which antibiotics and antivirals represent a key intervention, antimicrobial resistance threatens to render many inexpensive and widely available drugs ineffective, therefore shifting the entire fight against infectious diseases to more expensive therapies that are unavailable in many low-income countries. In 2012, WHO reported a gradual increase in resistance to HIV drugs.[21] In 2013, there were about 480,000 new cases of multi-drug-resistant tuberculosis (MDR-TB).[22] Extensively drug-resistant tuberculosis (XDR-TB) has been identified in 100 countries.[23] MDR-TB requires treatment courses that are much longer and less effective than those for nonresistant tuberculosis. In parts of the Greater Mekong Subregion, resistance to the best available treatment for falciparum malaria, artemisinin-based combination therapies (ACTs), has been detected. The spread or emergence of multidrug resistance, including resistance to ACTs, in other regions could jeopardize important recent gains in control of the disease.

The outbreak of Ebola demonstrated how interconnected these disease threats are and how easily failures against one disease may multiply losses against others. The loss of healthcare workers, for example, will interrupt widespread public health efforts that had put all three countries on a positive health trajectory. Before Ebola, the health workforce in all three countries was as sparse as any place on the planet and was distributed toward urban centers. There existed limited capacity to train new workers. Liberia, for example, currently has 40 medical students and 1,200 nursing and midwifery students.[24]

John Kraemer and Mark Siedner describe the widespread ramifications:

> All three countries had pre-Ebola vaccination rates below levels necessary to maintain herd immunity against most vaccine-preventable illnesses. Mathematical models suggest that vaccine disruptions are significantenough to enable large-scale, generalized measles epidemics and increase

---

[19] Rafael Lozano, Mohsen Naghavi, Kyle Foreman, Stephen Lim, Kenji Shibuya et al., *Global and regional mortality from 235 causes of death for 20 age groups in 1990 and 2010: a systematic analysis for the Global Burden of Disease Study 2010*, 380(9859) Lancet (2012).

[20] World Health Organization, Global Health Observatory data, available at http://www.who.int/gho/hiv/en/.

[21] World Health Organization, Antimicrobial Resistance, available at http://www.who.int/mediacentre/factsheets/fs194/en/.

[22] Id.

[23] Id.

[24] Kraemer and Siedner, chapter 3, this volume.

the likelihood that they could affect bordering countries, which also have pockets with vaccination rates below those needed for herd immunity. Similarly, bednet coverage also was well below levels required for substantial community-level effects before the Ebola epidemic. Ceased community bednet distribution is expected to undermine the affected countries' malaria control initiatives, with mathematical models suggesting that an additional 3.5 million malaria cases could be attributed to it in 2014 and 2015.[25]

Global approaches to infectious disease detection, prevention, and control after the experience with Ebola will require reform and rethinking of how global health diplomacy now functions: the relationship between the public and private sectors in planning to prevent the spread of infectious disease as well as coordinating responses when outbreaks occur; the regulatory pathways for biomedical innovation specifically as it applies to vaccines and medical therapies for infectious diseases that afflict low-income countries; and the priorities that should be given to basic public health support programs through aid, development, and other funding channels.

This book is the first to fully assess the meaning of the Ebola epidemic in the context of current and future efforts to combat the threat infectious diseases pose to global public health. While Ebola triggered a flood of reform proposals, including those mentioned at the opening of this introduction, none of the analyses published so far situates the fight to "ensure that this never happens again" within the much broader political, economic, and historical context in which those reforms must take place.[26] To be sure, this volume does provide a straightforward analysis of key diplomatic, logistical, and political failures leading to the world's delayed and preliminarily ineffective response, but it also assesses the relationship between the Ebola outbreak and critical work of public-private partnerships like Gavi, the Vaccine Alliance and the Global Fund to Fight AIDS, Tuberculosis, and Malaria; the novel problems raised by collaborations between private sector vaccine and medical countermeasure developers, public sector regulators and aid personnel, and frontline healthcare facilities; the future of official sources of aid for public health expenditures; and the relationship between public health protection measures and access of medical personnel to areas where a public health emergency is underway.

The book does so by bringing together in a single volume not only the public health leaders at the center of the global response to the outbreak, such as Anthony

---

[25] *Id.*

[26] Commission on Global Health Risk Framework for the Future, Harvard University–London School of Hygiene and Tropical Medicine Independent Panel on the Global Response to Ebola, Review Committee on the Role of the International Health Regulations (2005) in the Ebola Outbreak and Response, UN Secretary-General's High-Level Panel on Global Response to Health Crises; and WHO Ebola Interim Assessment Panel.

Fauci or contributors from MSF, but also analysts from nearly every community now engaged in the fight against infectious diseases: leaders from global public-private partnerships; academic clinicians studying ways to reduce structural barriers to care such as poor roads and communication systems; national and international regulators; scholars of medicine, regulatory science, political science, international relations, and public health; and researchers based at both universities and major nongovernmental organizations.[27] By examining Ebola through a wider lens than existing reform analyses have thus far used, this volume aims not only to provide an effective retrospective on the Ebola episode specifically but also to identify the most important regulatory gaps, public health risks, and promising solutions across the wide range of infectious disease threats now facing humanity.

Following a discussion of the global system for detecting, preventing, and managing infectious disease, as well as the key reform proposals now circulating in the wake of the Ebola outbreak, this introductory chapter presents a conceptual framework with which to examine how those reforms approach systematic change and what aspects of the global system are left unaddressed or marginalized. The topics covered by the contributors to this volume have been selected to allow as comprehensive an understanding as possible of the most significant regulatory challenges facing the widest range of stakeholders and vulnerable populations. They include the very initial approaches to treating patients and containing the outbreak by front-line, nongovernmental healthcare workers while at the same time mobilizing the formal global response; changes in global funding to fight infectious disease; public-private partnership organizations, their governance structures, and their strategies for preventing and treating infectious diseases; regulatory capacity in low- and middle-income countries; and the management of clinical trials that take place both in low-resource countries and in an emergency context. With this comprehensive approach, this book seeks to make significant progress in our understanding of global governance over critical threats to global health and welfare.

A Global System to Fight Infectious Disease, the Human Right to Health, and the Role of Nonstate Actors

The principal reform proposals developed in the wake of Ebola suggest broad changes in international organizations and the States Parties that support them. For example, the members of the Harvard Global Health Institute–London School

---

[27] The editors note that while some contributors to this volume served on the ground in the response to the outbreak, no editor is a national or resident of any one of the most afflicted countries, undoubtedly an important voice missing from a volume of this kind.

of Hygiene and Tropical Medicine Independent Panel on the Global Response to Ebola recommended several reforms affecting WHO, the UN Security Council, and the core capacities of national governments.[28] The final report of the UN Secretary-General's High-Level Panel on the Global Response to Health Crises similarly recommended several steps to enhance the effectiveness of the IHR, establish better preparedness centers and staff at WHO as well as tighten its relationship with official development assistance flowing from wealthy to poorer countries, steepen the role of the United Nations, and adopt a number of government-negotiated measures to increase biomedical innovation and facilitate resulting vaccines and therapies to people who need them most.

To a significant extent, the structural reforms advocated for the global system for detecting, preventing, and managing infectious disease represent a continuation of a trend toward global centralization of infectious disease management dating back to the middle of the nineteenth century. Between 1851 and 1892, predominantly European powers met in an effort to assemble a list of internationally actionable diseases and the appropriate methods by which their spread might be limited.[29] Between 1893 and 1903, four international conventions were convened, steadily expanding diseases deemed appropriate for cooperation and control; international adoption of national policies for surveillance; quarantine of certain items and persons; processes for sterilizing goods suspected of facilitating infection; and notification requirements for other participants.[30] At the 1903 convention, delegates agreed on the need both to codify in the preceding agreements in a single instrument and to establish an international health organization. By 1938, two such organizations were established, and the 1903 International Sanitary Convention was updated to reflect advances in the control of infectious diseases. As historians of the International Sanitary Conferences observed, over time the agenda of the international meetings moved from coordinating European responses to disease threats originating in Asia to serving as the most important forum for clinical researchers, bacteriologists, physicians, and other medical researchers to influence international law and international relations as they affected the spread of disease, changes that were to foreshadow the behavior of WHO upon its establishment in 1948.

Historically, WHO favored its role in developing and communicating technocratic expertise and advising governments and others in the implementation of that expertise. WHO occupied a central coordinating role between governments, researchers, and healthcare providers, rarely exercising the legal authorities

---

[28] Moon *supra* note 5.

[29] Norman Howard-Jones, The Scientific Background of the International Sanitary Conferences, 1851–1938, 9 (1975).

[30] David P. Fidler, *The globalization of public health: the first 100 years of international health diplomacy*, 79 Bulletin of the World Health Organization 842, 843 (2001).

available to it under its constitution. The emergence of new infectious diseases like HIV and the resurgence of older diseases like cholera in the 1980s and 1990s motivated member states to re-examine WHO's role as a legal, political, and technical leader. In 1995, the World Health Assembly instructed WHO's Director- General to revisit the then existing IHR—which at that time covered only three diseases and even at that provided little authority to manage them—because it neglected "the emergence of new infectious agents" and failed to provide for an adequate response of those that were covered.

The IHR (2005) was revised to encompass the detection and prevention of all infectious diseases.[31] Its scope was expanded "to include any event that would constitute a public health emergency of international concern."[32] Acknowledging the importance of communication and cooperation to successful detection and prevention of communicable diseases, States Parties are obligated to "develop the means to detect, report, and respond to public health emergencies . . . [and] establish a National IHR Focal Point (NFP)[33] for communication to and from WHO."[34] The IHR (2005) empowered the WHO Director-General to declare public health emergencies of international concern and to recommend measures to address them. Reforms now proposed after Ebola focus on strengthening this general approach to the global system for managing infectious disease "with national health systems at its foundation and an empowered World Health Organization at its apex."[35]

This book not only analyzes these core aspects of the global system to manage infectious disease (WHO leadership and capable national authorities) in the context of Ebola failures but also highlights two dimensions of the outbreak that are embedded within the global governance system for infectious disease: the human right to the highest attainable standard of health and the role of nongovernmental organizations. Indeed, the Constitution of the World Health Organization established not only that the "highest attainable standard of health is one of the fundamental rights

---

[31] The stated purpose is to "prevent, protect against, control and provide a public health response to the international spread of disease in ways that are commensurate with and restricted to public health risks, and which avoid unnecessary interference with international traffic and trade." World Health Organization, *International Health Regulations (2005)*, 1 (2005).

[32] Rebecca Katz and Julie Fischer, *The Revised International Health Regulations: a framework for global pandemic response*, 3 Global Health Governance, 1, 2 (2010), available at http://blogs.shu.edu/ghg/files/2011/11/Katz-and-Fischer_The-Revised-International-Health-Regulations_Spring-2010.pdf.

[33] The NFP is a "national centre, established or designated by each State Party [and] must be accessible at all times for IHR (2005)-related communications with WHO." *International Health Regulations (2005): toolkit for implementation in national legislation*, World Health Organization 1, 7 (2009), available at http://www.who.int/ihr/NFP_Toolkit.pdf. As of July 2009, 99% of all states have established an NFP.

[34] Katz and Fischer, *supra* note 31, at 4.

[35] Gostin and Friedman, *supra* note 8.

of every human being" but also the importance of communicating with nongovernmental organizations that share WHO's mission, including them in its deliberations and research activities, relying upon their expertise, and understanding their role in promoting the organization's purpose.[36]

In the context of the global system to manage infectious disease in light of the Ebola outbreak, those principles—the human right to the highest attainable standard of health and the importance of nongovernmental organizations—are, however implicitly, central to many of the reform proposals now discussed as principally state-centered measures for coordination and response. The frontline and immediate reaction to Ebola was driven by nongovernmental organizations with mandates related to the right to the highest attainable standard of health such as the right to humanitarian assistance or the obligation to prevent suffering. These organizations similarly played important roles in facilitating clinical trials of promising vaccines and in ensuring that the rights of trial participants were safeguarded. Major nongovernmental organizations like the Global Fund and Gavi contributed crucial resources as part of the global response and more generally provide models of public-private governance in the global system to detect, prevent, and manage infectious disease. Gavi, for example, has adopted a model whereby a large percentage of stakeholders in a specific field—vaccinology—are brought together to address a specific aspect of infectious disease control.

Neither human rights nor the role of nongovernmental organizations has been ignored by current reform proposals, but these influences have occupied surprisingly little space in the reports now circulating. This volume contributes fully half of its chapters toward these dimensions of the global system to manage infectious disease as it restructures and reassesses a number of governance and resource allocation possibilities.

The Plan of This Book

The views presented in this book document the perspectives of clinicians, epidemiologists, humanitarian activists, governments, and scholars who shaped the response to the Ebola outbreak and are now engaged in the retrospective process of identifying and remedying the failures that led to the crisis. The various chapters investigate a wide range of activities by national and international public health leaders; the circumstances prevailing in Guinea, Liberia, and Sierra Leone that made detecting and managing the Ebola outbreak so difficult, as well as inherent weaknesses in the global system for managing infectious disease that led the outbreak there to exact such a substantial toll; the current infectious disease threats

---

[36] Constitution of the World Health Organization, Preamble, articles 18, 33, 41, 71.

most likely to precipitate the next public health emergency; alternative forms of governance to address specific disease threats—especially public-private partnerships; and the human rights implications of various measures taken during times of public health emergency, including isolation, quarantine, and the rights of clinical trial participants and patients.

The book is divided into three parts. Part I outlines current and emerging infectious disease challenges, including cultural, structural, and resource challenges that characterized the Ebola outbreak. Part II then analyzes the global mechanisms for detecting, preventing, and managing the outbreak of infectious disease, including national and international regulatory structures and official development assistance targeted toward minimizing threats of the kind posed by Ebola. Part III identifies the human rights and ethical implications of development and deployment of medical therapies and vaccines in the context of public health emergencies; it also addresses challenges and strategies for assuring vaccine availability, efficacy, and safety outside of emergency contexts, as well as isolation, quarantine, and the balance between public health interests and civil liberties. The chapters in these parts contribute unique insights on coordination, resource, and regulatory problems in global infectious disease governance and implications for debates over the future of assuring the integrity of the global infectious disease management system as it unfolds over the next several years.

In chapter 1, Anthony S. Fauci provides an overview of the complex challenges that led the Ebola outbreak to go relatively undetected and, even after it was better understood, to cause problems for the local, regional, and international responses. Starting with the enzootic and epizootic cycles of the Ebola virus, Fauci explains how key aspects of the virus and the disease in humans remain uncertain. He attributes the rapid spread of the disease to a "perfect storm" of converging and compounding factors: poor countries with histories of conflict, political unrest, and resultant mistrust of government; densely populated cities; severely limited healthcare infrastructure; and long-standing cultural practices that enhanced the potential for contact with infectious bodily fluids. The chapter provides an overview of Ebola viruses, their routes of transmission, and the clinical manifestations of Ebola virus disease. The chapter then assesses the factors facilitating the spread of Ebola from Guinea to Liberia and Sierra Leone and then elsewhere. The chapter concludes by analyzing the lessons the outbreak teaches about prevention, detection, and management of the inevitable future emergences of infectious diseases, including the deployment of military and civilian personnel; the development of diagnostics, medical therapies, and vaccines; and the balance between aid and containment.

In chapter 2, MSF's Heather Pagano and Marc Poncin detail the unique features of the outbreak that made past approaches to filovirus-infection emergencies more difficult to implement—unconnected chains of transmission in multiple locations, epidemiological spread to a major urban center (Guinea's capital, Conakry), and circumstances in neighboring Liberia.[37] Pagano and Poncin describe how the dispersal of small numbers of cases over a wide geographical area multiplied the human resources, logistics, and laboratory capacity required in each individual location to bring the epidemic under control while also presenting communication and coordination difficulties between MSF, healthcare workers, UNICEF, WHO, and the US Centers for Disease Control and Prevention (CDC). They analyze WHO leadership over the period between March and August 2015, when WHO suffered not only from a poor logistical presence in the region but also from a politicized decision-making process that delayed its declaration of a public health emergency of international concern. Under those circumstances, MSF began occupying unconventional roles as (1) technical adviser, particularly in Guinea and Liberia, on control strategies and coordination efforts; (2) principal training organization through centers established in Europe; and (3) partner in the ethical review and implementation of clinical trials for medical therapies and vaccines. The chapter highlights the critical gaps in the formal national and international system for responding to serious infectious disease threats—including facilities and personnel—and the process by which those gaps may be filled by nongovernmental organizations, including the complex relationship that may develop with other actors, including firms, regulatory partners, and national and international authorities.

In chapter 3, John Kraemer and Mark Siedner map the Ebola epidemic's effect on health outcomes and systems in Guinea, Liberia, and Sierra Leone. Kraemer and Siedner provide a comprehensive review of existing literature—academic, news media, and other reports—to assess how Ebola caused short- and long-term harm to health that exceeded the direct consequences for those infected. Those harms include not only the loss of healthcare workers and facilities but also fear and deterrence that caused people in afflicted areas to stop even seeking health services. They identify opportunities for building stronger and more resilient health systems, focusing on measures that would improve outcomes during both routine and emergency situations. They specifically address efforts to invest in rural community health centers, train healthcare workers, and preventative measures that are both consistent with the IHR and far more cost-effective than ex post curative care and containment like that undertaken by wealthy countries and international organizations after the outbreak had crossed international borders.

In chapter 4, Sugy Choi, Jong-koo Lee, and Daniel Lucey provide a contrasting analysis by examining an infectious disease threat in a high-resource setting: the outbreak of MERS-CoV in the Republic of Korea between May and July 2015, approximately the same window in which Ebola was spiraling out of control in

---

[37] On March 31, Ebola was confirmed in Liberia in Foya, near the border of Sierra Leone and Guinea. An MSF team set up isolation units and trained health staff in Foya and Monrovia, but cases soon dwindled. By mid-May there had been no cases for more than 21 days, the maximum incubation period of the virus. New cases would re-emerge in Liberia in June.

West Africa. The authors demonstrate that even in countries with advanced medical facilities and relatively strong compliance with IHR obligations, the failure to implement basic measures may have wide-reaching consequences. The patient who transported the virus to Korea was not informed about control measures regarding MERS-CoV after returning to Incheon Airport following a trip to the Middle East; he was asymptomatic when he returned, a full patient travel history was not taken until he had visited his fourth healthcare facility, and the virus infected 79% of its victims through "superspreading" healthcare workers and caregivers. One infected patient traveled to southern China. The authors provide a detailed analysis not only of how small gaps in preparedness may render significant negative effects but also of the practical aspects of effective outbreak containment processes, including (1) early and complete identification and investigation of all contacts; (2) robust quarantine/isolation and monitoring of all contacts and suspected cases; (3) full implementation of infection prevention and control measures, including active surveillance and follow-up; and (4) prevention of travel, especially internationally, of infected persons and contacts.

In chapter 5, Gail Hansen analyzes the threat posed by antimicrobial resistance—the set of traits and genetic elements, developed and then disseminated, by which bacteria survive treatment by antibiotics—not only to the infected person but also to the broader community, which collectively faces pathogenic bacteria that are more difficult to combat. Hansen demonstrates how misuse of antibiotics in human and animal medicine has magnified the natural tendency of microbes to adapt and favors the spread of antibiotic-resistant organisms. This misuse—"too short a time, or too small a dose, at inadequate strengths, or for the wrong disease"—allows resistant bacteria to survive and pass on resistant traits to other bacteria. The consequences of antibiotic-resistant bacteria include infections that would not have otherwise occurred, infections that are more difficult to treat, and increased severity of infections. Hansen details how and why the multiplication of resistant bacteria is far outpacing the development of new antibiotic therapies and also analyzes the measures recommended by the US National Action Plan for Combating Antibiotic-Resistant Bacteria and the WHO Global Action Plan on Antimicrobial Resistance.

Part II begins with Lawrence Gostin and Rebecca Katz's analysis in chapter 6 of the IHR, the governing framework for global health security for the past decade. The authors present criticisms leveled by major global commissions regarding the future effectiveness of the IHR and the leadership of WHO in the wake of the Ebola epidemic. Gostin and Katz review the historical origins of the IHR and its performance over the past 10 years and also analyze the ongoing panel efforts aimed at providing politically feasible recommendations for reform. They propose a series of recommendations that focus on the development and strengthening of IHR core capacities; independently assessed metrics; new financing mechanisms; harmonization with the Global Health Security Agenda, PVS Pathways, the Pandemic Influenza Preparedness Framework, and One Health initiatives; public health and clinical workforce development; Emergency Committee transparency and governance; tiered PHEIC processes; enhanced compliance mechanisms; and an enhanced role for civil society. Gostin and Katz conclude that empowering WHO and realizing the IHR's potential will shore up global health security—a vital investment in human and animal health—while reducing the vast economic consequences of the next global health emergency.

In chapter 7, David Fidler situates Gostin and Katz's analysis within the broader context of global health diplomacy. According to Fidler's account, the IHR, the Global Health Security Agenda, the UN Mission for Ebola Emergency Response, and other institutions reflect differing perspectives on whether "global health diplomacy" actually creates a conceptual break from the interests that diplomacy traditionally serves. When health is seen as a paramount objective, Fidler argues, the necessity of negotiating among states and nonstate actors to support and promote it becomes imbued with political purpose and ethical energy. By contrast, when health struggles to compete for priority with other political interests, negotiations involving health raise questions about the substance and sustainability of the commitments made. Fidler's chapter brings into particular focus the critical nexus between international regulatory authorities based at WHO, official and unofficial diplomats carrying out traditional, hard-nosed negotiation over national interests, and the ascendant role of global health as a normative force in international politics and law.

In chapter 8, Jennifer Kates and Adam Wexler step back from the broader debate on health diplomacy and the IHR and assess the flow of official development assistance data available through the Organization for Economic Cooperation and Development (OECD) Assistance Committee Database and Creditor Reporting System. Their review covers trends in overall official development assistance for health, as well as for infectious diseases specifically and as a share of health assistance. It also examines the roles played by each donor, with particular focus on the US government. In addition to OECD data, it uses data from the US Office of Management and Budget, Federal Agency Congressional Budget Justifications, congressional appropriations bills, and the US Foreign Assistance Dashboard for known funding provided through the US Department of State, US Agency for International Development, Centers for Disease Control and Prevention, National Institutes of Health, and the US Department of Defense. The chapter concludes with glimpses into future financing prospects and issues surrounding global funding for infectious diseases being used to influence the behavior of both foreign and domestic players.

In chapter 9, Kevin Klock examines three public-private partnership governance alternatives to state-based or international organization–based health preparedness paradigms. Focusing on the Global Fund to Fight AIDS, Tuberculosis, and Malaria, Gavi, the Vaccine Alliance, and the Global Alliance for Improved Nutrition, Klock sets the governance structures of those partnerships against the traditional state-centered and international organization models under which the majority of global infectious disease law and policy is now made. Klock provides a step-by-step analysis of how private sector governance norms may be substituted or applied proportionately to achieve positive outcomes for the prevention, detection, and management of infectious disease, especially for populations in low-resource countries.

In chapter 10, Seth Berkley assesses the effectiveness of Gavi—which he leads—in substantially reducing rates of diphtheria, pertussis, and tetanus; facilitating the development of an inexpensive vaccine for meningitis A; expanding access to human papillomavirus vaccine; facilitating the transition of recipient countries to donor countries; and providing an economic and decision-making model that brings together the entire field of vaccinology. Berkley's chapter broadens the scope through which the social impact of vaccines is viewed—a scope traditionally focused on infectious disease—to include the full range of public health threats that vaccines combat, the substantial contribution vaccines play in alleviating the most severe forms of poverty around the world, and the role of routine immunization programs as the foundation of national primary healthcare and public health systems. Berkley outlines specific development, delivery, and financing mechanisms that may facilitate the achievement of access to new and underused vaccines for children living in the world's poorest countries, as well as the synergies that access to those vaccines will play in the broader fight against infectious disease, antibiotic resistance, and global poverty.

In chapter 11, Veronica Miller provides an overview of the critical challenges facing the global pharmaceutical and biomedical technology development system, as well as the public-private partnerships that facilitate wider access to better medicines and vaccines and ensure the supply of essential, existing ones to fight infectious disease. Starting from the recognition that drug development costs have soared and regulatory requirements have increased, Miller explains how clinical trial practices may be adapted to facilitate development and approval processes for new drugs, link economic and regulatory policies to keep the drug supply safe, and coordinate stakeholders toward a common mission of access to medicines. Specifically, she examines the role that adaptive trial designs and new approaches to clinical endpoints may play in opening possibilities for facilitating drug development, drawing on lessons from HIV and hepatitis C treatments.

In chapter 12, Annick Antierens places Miller's analysis in the Ebola context by providing an extensive account of how medical therapies and candidate vaccines were developed for Ebola virus disease, the financial and governmental partnerships that led them to be managed by major pharmaceutical firms and government agencies, and the difficulties encountered in attempting to ensure respect for the rights of human research subjects in Guinea, Liberia, and Sierra Leone could also meet ethical and human rights obligations to those populations as *patients*. Because trials involved facilities run by nongovernmental organizations, ethics and research protocols were reviewed both by participating government agencies and by those organizations. Nongovernmental organizations, for example, refused to allow studies on efficacy in affected countries and especially in at-risk populations to use placebos or active control arms. Antierens's chapter highlights the logistical and ethical complexities that arise when therapies and vaccines are developed in the course of a public health emergency.

In chapter 13, Saad Omer and Sam Halabi examine the evidence, strategies, and challenges surrounding vaccine safety as novel technologies and expanding coverage introduce new factors to consider in maintaining the safety profile of current and new vaccines. While the fundamental principle behind vaccination remains the same—administration of agent-specific, but relatively harmless, antigenic components that in vaccinated individuals induce protective immunity against the corresponding infectious agent—the technologies behind antigenic components have evolved. The chapter provides concrete recommendations on how the regulatory process that assures vaccine safety and efficacy may be adapted to respond to these technologies. The authors also review postlicensure vaccine safety and adverse event reporting systems at both the national and the international level. They assess weaknesses in the global system for adverse event monitoring, especially in light of advances in immunization coverage programs in low-income countries, and propose potential solutions to address those weaknesses.

In chapter 14, Mary Marovich examines the set of problems developed by Antierens, Omer, and Halabi and studies them in the context of the only HIV vaccine candidate regimen at the phase III trial stage: RV144. Marovich examines the experience with RV144 not only for the lessons learned about biomedical research and innovation aimed at a difficult medical problem but also for the financing, logistical, and stakeholder aspects of the effort that illustrated the planning and foresight necessary to develop, finance, and then distribute a safe and efficacious HIV vaccine, as well as the engagement with all constituencies as to the limits, if any, of that vaccine's mechanism of action. Her chapter discusses how the results of the RV144 phase III trial encouraged the formation of the Pox-Protein Public-Private Partnership (P5), which now includes the Bill and Melinda Gates Foundation, the HIV Vaccine Trials Network, Novartis Vaccines and Diagnostics/GSK, Sanofi Pasteur, the South African Medical Research Council, the US Military HIV Research Program, as well as NIAID's Division of AIDS. The chapter concludes by examining how the P5 plans to build on the RV144 study and also what an effective Global Vaccine Access Plan must include if a successful HIV vaccine candidate is ever developed.

In chapter 15 Martin Cetron, analyzes two common but controversial public health interventions at issue in public health emergencies—isolation and quarantine—in their civil rights and human rights contexts. Outlining the national and international legal regimes that have been adopted to assure a balance between civil rights and public health security, Cetron details how the response to Ebola raised once again the matter of the appropriate balance between measures that address the outbreak and the policies necessary to protect population health. Although there were wide calls for isolation and quarantine, as well as majority support for suspension of air travel from "Ebola-stricken" countries, Cetron identifies and explains the consensus in the public health community that such an approach would magnify the problem. Shutting off the afflicted countries would create barriers for humanitarian and medical staff to treat patients and provide support; other, more hazardous travel routes would spring up; and the effect on the local economies would be severe. Using sensible screening measures, Cetron argues, it is possible to leave access to the countries open while allowing as many able healthcare workers as possible to assist in the response. Cetron concludes by re-emphasizing the understanding codified in state, federal, and international law that the balance between civil liberties and public health protection should, when possible, err on the side of protection of rights out of respect for both human rights principles and pragmatic disease response.

In the epilogue, Renée Fox—one of the earliest and most accomplished academic ethnographers of Ebola, the communities that faced it, and the medical professionals who responded to it—draws parallels not only between the first confrontations between the public health community and Ebola but also between her own experience as a survivor of polio in the United States and the social and medical norms that prevailed then. She provides a powerful account of the hubris that led the medical professional class to delude itself into believing in the 1960s and 1970s that the human fight against infectious disease was nearing its end and of the episodes that shook the public health community back into awareness that, as Anthony Fauci phrased it, "Winning does not mean stamping out every last disease, but rather getting out ahead of the next one."[38] Fox closes by offering glimpses into what the Zika virus means as the newest threat in the perpetual effort humanity must mount against infectious disease.

References

Centers for Disease Control and Prevention. Ebola Viral Disease Outbreak—West Africa, 2014. Accessed July 24, 2015, at http://www.cdc.gov/mmwr/preview/mmwrhtml/mm6325a4.htm.
———. Ebola Virus Disease (EVD) Information for Clinicians in U.S. Healthcare Settings. Available at http://www.cdc.gov/vhf/ebola/healthcare-us/preparing/clinicians.html.
———. CDC Concludes Zika Causes Microcephaly and Other Birth Defects, Apr. 13, 2016 available at http://www.cdc.gov/media/releases/2016/s0413-zika-microcephaly.html
Center for Strategic and International Studies. The road to recovery: rebuilding Liberia's health system. Available at http://csis.org/files/ publication/120822_Downie_RoadtoRecovery_web.pdf.

---

[38] David M. Morens and Anthony S. Fauci, *Emerging infectious diseases: threats to human health*, PLOS Pathogens (July 4, 2013), available at http://journals.plos.org/plospathogens/article?id=10.1371/journal.ppat.1003467.

Commission on a Global Health Risk Framework for the Future. *The Neglected Dimension of Global Security: A Framework to Counter Infectious Disease Crises*, National Academy of Medicine (2016). Available at www.nam.edu/GHRF.

Fauci, A. S. *Ebola—underscoring the global disparities in health care resources*. 37(12) New England Journal of Medicine (2014).

Fauci, A. S., and Morens, D. *Zika virus in the Americas—yet another arbovirus threat*. 374: New England Journal of Medicine 601–604 (Jan. 13, 2016).

Fidler, D. *The globalization of public health: the first 100 years of international health diplomacy*. 79 Bulletin of the World Health Organization 842, 843 (2001).

Gostin, L., and Friedman, E. *A retrospective and prospective analysis of the West African Ebola virus disease epidemic: robust national health systems at the foundation and an empowered WHO at the apex*. 385 Lancet 1902–1909 (2015).

Howard-Jones, N. The Scientific Background of the International Sanitary Conferences 1851–1938 (1975). Available at http://whqlibdoc.who.int/publications/1975/14549_eng.pdf.

Katz, R., and Fischer, J. *The Revised International Health Regulations: a framework for global pandemic response*. 3 Global Health Governance 1, 2 (2010).

Lozano, R., Mohsen Naghavi, Kyle Foreman, Stephen Lim, Kenji Shibuya et al. *Global and regional mortality from 235 causes of death for 20 age groups in 1990 and 2010: a systematic analysis for the Global Burden of Disease Study 2010*. 380(9859) Lancet 2095–2128 (2012).

Marcones, C. B., and Ximines, M. F. *Zika virus in Brazil and the danger of infestation by Aedes(Stegomyia) mosquitoes*. Revista da Sociedade Brasileira de Medicina (Journal of the Brazilian Society of Tropical Medicine) (Dec. 22, 2015).

Matanock A., Arwady M. A., Ayscue P., Forrester J. D., Gaddis B., Hunter J. C., et al. *Ebola virus disease cases among health care workers not working in Ebola treatment units—Liberia, June–August, 2014*. 63(46) MMWR Morb Mortal Wkly Rep 1077–1081 (Nov. 21, 2014).

Moon, Suerie, et al. *Will Ebola change the game? Ten essential reforms before the next pandemic. The report of the Harvard-LSHTM Independent Panel on the Global Response to Ebola*. 386(10009) Lancet 2204–2221 (Nov. 28, 2015).

Sack, Kevin, Sheri Fink, and Adam Nossiter. *Ebola's Deadly Escape*. New York Times (Dec. 29, 2014).

UN Secretary-General's High-Level Panel on Global Response to Health Crises (Jan. 2016). Available at http://www.un.org/News/dh/infocus/HLP/2016-02-05_Final_Report_Global_Response_to_Health_Crises.pdf.

World Health Organization. Ebola Virus Disease. (2015). Accessed July 24, 2015, at http://www.who.int/mediacentre/factsheets/fs103/en/.

———. Global Health Observatory data repository, absolute numbers, data by country. Available at http://apps.who.int/gho/data/node. main.A1443?lang=e.

———. Outbreaks Chronology: Ebola Virus Disease. Accessed July 24, 2015, at http://www.cdc.gov/vhf/ebola/outbreaks/history/chronology.html.

———. Report of the Ebola Interim Assessment Panel (July 2015). Available at http://who.int/csr/resources/publications/ebola/report-by-panel.pdf.

———. Report of the Review Committee on the Functioning of the International Health Regulations (2005) in relation to Pandemic (H1N1) 2009. Available at http://apps.who.int/gb/ebwha/pdf_files/WHA64/A64_10-en.pdf.

———. WHO Director-General Summarizes the Outcome of the Emergency Committee Regarding Clusters of Microcephaly and Guillain-Barre Syndrome (Feb., 1, 2016). Available at http://www.who.int/mediacentre/news/statements/2016/emergency-committee-zika-microcephaly/en/.

PART I

CURRENT AND EMERGING INFECTIOUS DISEASE CHALLENGES

1

The Ebola Epidemic of 2014–2015

A Perfect Storm

ANTHONY S. FAUCI

The 2014–2015 outbreak of Ebola virus infections in West Africa is by far the most severe ever recorded. The rapid spread of the disease can be attributed to a "perfect storm" of converging and compounding factors: poor countries with histories of conflict, political unrest, and resultant mistrust of government; densely populated cities; severely limited healthcare infrastructure; and long-standing cultural practices that enhance the potential for contact with infectious bodily fluids. This chapter provides an overview of Ebola viruses, their routes of transmission, and the clinical manifestations of Ebola virus disease (EVD). The chapter then assesses the factors facilitating the spread of Ebola from Guinea to Liberia and Sierra Leone, and then elsewhere during the 2014–2015 outbreak. It concludes by analyzing the lessons that this outbreak can teach about prevention, detection, and management of the inevitable future emergences of infectious diseases.

The Origin, Transmission, and Clinical Course of Ebola Virus Disease

Ebola viruses, along with Marburg viruses, are members of the filovirus family, a group whose members are characterized by their filamentous viral structure. Each filovirus encodes its genome in single-stranded negative-sense RNA. Five species of Ebola virus cause a wide spectrum of disease:

1. *Zaire ebolavirus* has a reported case fatality rate of 30% to 90%;
2. *Sudan ebolavirus* has a reported case fatality rate of about 50%;
3. *Bundibugyo ebolavirus* has a reported case fatality rate of approximately 30%;

4. *Taï Forest ebolavirus* has caused one known nonfatal human infection; and
5. *Reston ebolavirus* primarily affects nonhuman primates.[1]

Zaire ebolavirus is the species implicated in the 2014–2015 outbreak in West Africa.

The transmission cycle of Ebola viruses has two components: an enzootic and an epizootic cycle. With regard to the former, it is believed that Ebola viruses circulate in fruit bats, although relatively little is known about how the viruses are maintained or transmitted within these or other animal populations.[2] The epizootic cycle is somewhat better understood. Epizootic transmissions, likely from fruit bats to nonhuman primates (and possibly other species), appear to occur sporadically, causing high mortality among infected primates.[3] The specific means of transmission from animals to humans is under investigation, although contact with infected bodily fluids such as blood or feces has been hypothesized.[4] Because so little is known about how the virus first passes to humans, and thus triggers human-to-human transmission, the epidemic potential of any given outbreak is unpredictable.[5] Ebola viruses can be transmitted to humans in many ways, including through contact with bodily fluids of an infected patient or cadaver, via contaminated objects (fomites), or through contact with infected animals.[6]

The clinical course of EVD begins with an individual's exposure to the virus through one of the aforementioned sources. The incubation period for the virus lasts from 8 to 10 days on average, although at extremes it may range from 2 to 21 days.[7] The virus is detectable and transmissible when the individual becomes symptomatic. In the first 3 days of symptomatic disease, most patients experience weakness and fever. During days 4 to 7, some patients will begin to show progressive disease, manifesting as vomiting and diarrhea. From days 8 to 10, those who are severely ill can begin to show symptoms of confusion, possible minor bleeding, and shock, generally due to fluid loss from vomiting and diarrhea. Patients with severe disease who are treated in a low-resource setting have a high mortality rate, often exceeding 50%. In higher-resource settings, with advanced life-support measures offered in intensive care units, a high percentage of patients have survived, although the small number of patients treated in such settings precludes any definitive statement about the true survival rate there.

---

[1] Anthony S. Fauci, *Ebola—underscoring the global disparities in health care resources*, 37(12) New England Journal of Medicine, 1084–86 (2014); World Health Organization, Ebola Virus Disease, available at http://www.who.int/mediacentre/factsheets/fs103/en/.

[2] Fauci, *supra* note 1.

[3] Centers for Disease Control and Prevention (CDC),Virus Ecology Graphic. Ebolavirus Ecology (2014), accessed July 25, 2015, at http://www.cdc.gov/vhf/ebola/resources/virus-ecology.html.

[4] *Id.*

[5] Fauci, *supra* note 1.

[6] World Health Organization, *supra* note 1.

[7] CDC, Ebola Virus Disease (EVD) Information for Clinicians in U.S. Healthcare Settings, available at http://www.cdc.gov/vhf/ebola/healthcare-us/preparing/clinicians.html.

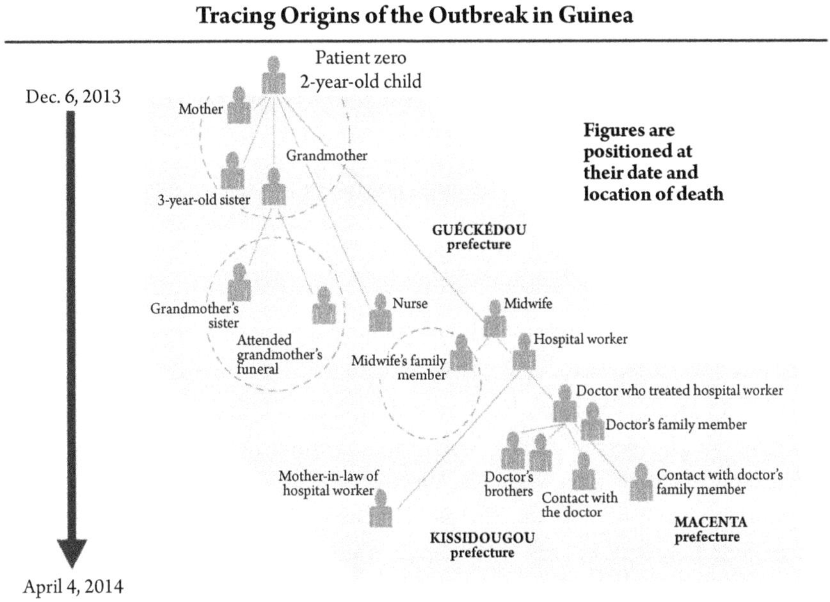

Tracing Origins of the Outbreak in Guinea

Figure 1.1 Tracing origins of the outbreak in Guinea.

The 2014–2015 Outbreak of Ebola Virus Disease
Origin and Spread

On March 21, 2014, the Guinea Ministry of Health reported an outbreak of an illness characterized by fever, severe diarrhea, vomiting, and a high case fatality rate (59%) among 49 persons.[8] Subsequent data suggested that the outbreak likely began in December 2013, when a 2-year-old boy contracted Ebola virus in Guéckédou prefecture. The boy reportedly was infected after contact with bats. He soon fell ill and died, and a funeral followed. This funeral and its associated rituals resulted in the further spread of the Ebola virus among family members and friends within the community. Immediate family members then came into contact with more distant relatives, who also became ill and died, as did healthcare workers. Funeral practices and contact between health workers and other patients resulted in the rapid spread of the virus. Porous borders in this forested region of Guinea led to spillover of the virus to Liberia and Sierra Leone. Mobile populations soon brought the virus to capital cities, further facilitating spread of the outbreak. This process is depicted in Figure 1.1.

Between June and December 2014, weekly reports of new cases of EVD reached as high as 500 to 700 in Sierra Leone and Liberia (Figure 1.2).

---

[8] CDC, Ebola Viral Disease Outbreak—West Africa (2014), available at http://www.cdc.gov/mmwr/preview/mmwrhtml/mm6325a4.htm.

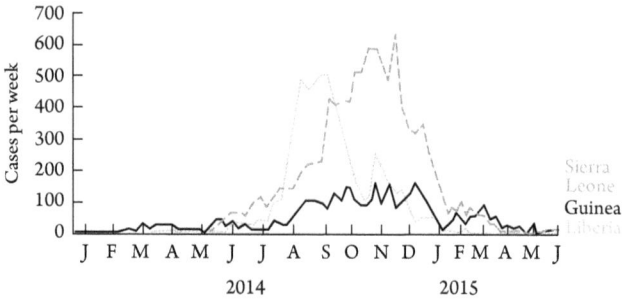

Figure 1.2 New confirmed and probable cases of Ebola infection per week.

The World Health Organization declared a public health emergency of international concern on August 8, 2014. It was this announcement and reports of infections among health worker volunteers from the United States and Europe that galvanized attention worldwide. The global community brought its public health and disaster relief resources to bear to combat the outbreak, partnering closely with affected-country governments and nongovernmental organizations. The United States sent epidemiologists and others from the Centers for Disease Control and Prevention (CDC), scientists from the National Institutes of Health (NIH), military support (to construct Ebola treatment units), and broader economic support to mitigate the deleterious effects of the outbreak on food and housing security. Other nations, international organizations and charities, and foundations, along with the World Health Organization and other United Nations agencies, contributed extensively to the response as well.

While specific elements of the response varied across the region, the essential components were the same. These included (1) public education, (2) case identification, (3) prompt isolation, (4) contact tracing, (5) hygienic treatment practices, (6) personal protective equipment (PPE) for healthcare workers and caregivers, (7) aggressive supportive care, and (8) safe burial practices.

With the mobilization of the global public health community and the efforts of affected countries, by March 2015, a marked diminution of transmission in Guinea, Liberia, and Sierra Leone had occurred. Liberia was officially declared Ebola free as of May 9, 2015. By June 2015, the number of new cases each week in the other two countries was low, but not zero—there remained small pockets of active cases with about 3 to 15 cases reported each week. Unfortunately, even a small number of Ebola cases could spark a wide-scale outbreak, and so a consensus emerged that the goal of no new infections must be reached in all affected countries.

Factors Influencing the Rapid Spread of Ebola

The 2014–2015 outbreak of EVD is unprecedented in magnitude but was preceded by numerous prior outbreaks, the first of which was recognized as Ebola in 1976.[9] Subsequently, 24 outbreaks occurred, resulting in a cumulative total of 2,500 cases and 1,500 deaths (prior to the 2014–2015 outbreak).[10] By July 2015, the West African Ebola outbreak was nearly eight times larger than all other outbreaks combined. Several factors contributed to the magnitude in 2014–2015. Those factors reveal key deficiencies both in the global distribution of public health resources and in the mechanisms the World Health Organization has available to address public health emergencies of international concern.

The Ebola outbreak of 2014–2015 originated in severely under-resourced countries with limited public health infrastructure and no prior experience controlling Ebola.[11] Liberia, for example, has approximately one physician for every 77,000 people. Not only are there few health professionals, but those professionals and the hospitals and clinics where they work face multiple health threats, including malaria, tuberculosis, diarrheal diseases, and many other endemic diseases, with limited infrastructure and a frequent dearth of basic supplies. Moreover, many diseases endemic to the region have clinical manifestations that can easily be confused with mild EVD.[12] Add to these challenges the first introduction of Ebola virus to major urban centers, and one can begin to understand the scope of the challenge presented by this outbreak.

The geopolitical context in which the outbreak occurred also contributed to the difficulties in initiating and coordinating the public health response. Travel across borders between the three countries occurs frequently; however, coordination of public health activities such as contact tracing was limited when the outbreak began. Moreover, a recent history of conflict left many people distrustful of authority, including health officials.[13] In addition, traditional burial practices, such as the bathing and embracing of corpses, are culturally important across this region and facilitated transmission of the disease.[14]

The Spread of Ebola to the United States

While this "perfect storm" of factors explains the rapid spread and heavy toll Ebola exacted in the three most affected countries, the care of Ebola patients transported to the United States for treatment and the inadvertent introduction of the virus into the country by an infected patient provide additional important lessons. In this regard, disease management was challenging even in high-resource settings where

---

[9] World Health Organization, Ebola Virus Disease, available at http://www.who.int/mediacentre/factsheets/fs103/en/; CDC, Outbreaks Chronology: Ebola Virus Disease, available at http://www.cdc.gov/vhf/ebola/outbreaks/history/chronology.html.

[10] Id.

[11] Fauci, *supra* note 1.

[12] Id.

[13] Id.

[14] Id.

healthcare workers had access to information, equipment, and facilities necessary for the safe care of Ebola patients.

The first such case followed the air evacuation on August 2, 2014, from Liberia to an Atlanta hospital of a US physician who became infected with the Ebola virus while caring for patients. This evacuation process was done in a controlled manner under strict safety protocols. The case of a Partners in Health (PIH) healthcare worker evacuated from Sierra Leone to the NIH on March 13, 2015, also showed the importance of assessing all risks with respect to Ebola exposure and treatment. This patient was completely contained during transport and care. All NIH staff caring for the patient worked in teams, donning and doffing full PPE under careful supervision. The medical staff carefully monitored the clinical status of the patient, paying particular attention to fluid and electrolyte balance. It had been hypothesized that as long as fluid levels were monitored and the patient remained euvolemic, the patient would be fine. Although it is difficult to arrive at precise numbers, this is likely true in approximately 80% or more of cases. However, in approximately 20% of cases, including this particular patient, the virus continues to attack organs, leading to respiratory and heart failure, encephalitis, and other complications. Advanced life support was initiated, and fortunately, the patient survived.

A different scenario occurred following the inadvertent importation of Ebola virus to the United States by Thomas Eric Duncan.[15] He departed Monrovia, Liberia, on September 19, 2014, and remained asymptomatic as he traveled through Brussels, Belgium, arriving in Dallas, Texas, on September 20. On September 24, Mr. Duncan began experiencing symptoms, and two days later he visited the emergency room at Texas Health Presbyterian Hospital. The hospital discharged him that day, not suspecting Ebola. On September 28, Mr. Duncan became very ill and returned to the emergency room by ambulance.[16] He died on October 8, 2014. Two intensive care unit nurses at the hospital contracted Ebola while caring for Mr. Duncan. Those nurses had not received sufficient training and therefore were not wearing completely adequate PPE for an intensive care setting. For example, areas of the nurses' skin and hair on the head were exposed.[17]

In total, 11 individuals infected with Ebola received care in the United States. Several healthcare institutions had designated facilities qualified to provide intensive care treatment to Ebola patients in an isolation setting. In this regard, the Biocontainment Patient Care Unit at the Nebraska Medical Center, the Emory University Hospital Isolation Unit in Atlanta, and the Special Clinical Studies Unit at the NIH Clinical Center each played a key role in caring for individuals in the United States.

---

[15] Betsy McKay and Ana Campoy, *First case of Ebola in U.S. is confirmed*, Wall Street Journal (Oct. 1, 2014), available at http://www.wsj.com/articles/ebola-virus-first-us-case-confirmed-1412111463.

[16] *Id.*

[17] Manny Fernandez, *2nd Ebola case in U.S. stokes fears of health care workers*, New York Times (Oct. 12, 2014), available at http://www.nytimes.com/2014/10/13/us/texas-health-worker-tests-positive-for-ebola.html?_r=0.

Even though a handful of well-equipped US facilities were able to respond to the challenges of caring for patients with Ebola, there were highly vocal governmental and public calls for additional safeguards, including suspension of travel from Africa and the quarantine of healthcare workers potentially exposed to Ebola. While understandable as a measure to reduce the risk of inadvertent importation, travel bans isolate the disease-stricken countries, hobbling efforts to contain the disease's spread. This could allow an outbreak to continue unabated and eventually lead to more inadvertent exportations of disease. By contrast, exit screening—examination for symptoms, fever, or other signs of illness—at the point of departure appears to be a more useful public health response. If a traveler had been in contact with an Ebola patient and showed symptoms, that traveler could be isolated and treated. In the United States, travelers returning from affected countries were directed to five airports, at which entry screening was conducted. Specifically, travelers were screened for fever, presence of symptoms, and history of contact with an Ebola patient. If warranted, they could be isolated and further evaluated by qualified health professionals.

Some state governments advocated quarantine requirements for healthcare volunteers returning from affected countries. The states of New York and New Jersey imposed mandatory quarantines for all people entering the country through Newark Liberty Airport or John F. Kennedy International Airport if they had had direct contact with Ebola patients in Guinea, Liberia, or Sierra Leone.[18] As with entry and exit screening as alternatives to travel bans, it is possible to monitor healthcare workers traveling to and from affected areas without imposing complete isolation. While the New York and New Jersey policies were ultimately reversed, they demonstrated the pressures applied to governments seeking to protect their populations from public health threats. Public health measures must be guided by both scientific evidence and civil rights considerations in order to balance the rights of healthcare workers and the consequences for outbreak control against the risks to the US population.

Building Capacity After the 2014–2015 Outbreak of Ebola Virus Disease: Biomedical Innovation and Healthcare Infrastructure Support

Medical Countermeasures: Diagnostics, Vaccines, Therapeutics

The response to the 2014–2015 outbreak of EVD created valuable opportunities to understand more about the disease and to develop both medical and nonmedical interventions. From a diagnostic standpoint, it is important to rapidly diagnose EVD to exclude the possibility of other treatable febrile diseases that are much more

---

[18] Marc Santora, *First patient quarantined under strict new policy tests negative for Ebola*, New York Times (Oct. 25, 2014), available at http://www.nytimes.com/2014/10/25/nyregion/new-york-ebola-case-craig-spencer.html.

prevalent than Ebola in Africa. For example, it would be unwise to place a febrile malaria patient in a holding room with Ebola patients. One outcome of the response to the 2014–2015 outbreak was the development of several rapid diagnostic tests for Ebola that reduce the time from the presentation of the patient to diagnosis and treatment.[19]

The outbreak also accelerated the development of Ebola vaccine candidates that had been in various stages of research for at least 15 years. As of July 2015, two vaccine candidates, NIAID/GSK cAd3 and NewLink/Merck rVSV-EBOV, were in various stages of clinical trials in the three most affected countries. A phase I trial of the NIAID/GSK Ebola vaccine candidate was launched in 2014 at the NIH with 20 healthy US volunteers. The NIAID/GSK vaccine candidate uses as a vector chimpanzee adenovirus type 3 (cAd3)—similar to human viruses that can cause the common cold—into which is introduced the Ebola glycoprotein gene; the gene expresses the viral glycoprotein, which stimulates an immunological response in the vaccine recipient.[20] A preliminary report of the phase I trial showed the vaccine candidate was well tolerated: only 2wo of 20 healthy participants had fevers, which resolved within 24 hours.[21] The report further showed antibody and CD8+ T cell responses that were consistent with those that protected nonhuman primates. A phase II trial in Liberia designed with this vaccine candidate, the NewLink/Merck candidate, and a placebo is continuing follow-up after enrolling 1,500 participants. The trial is being conducted by the Partnership for Research on Ebola Virus in Liberia (PREVAIL), a clinical research partnership between the NIH and the government of Liberia.

The NewLink/Merck rVSV-EBOV vaccine candidate uses a recombinant vesicular stomatitis virus (rVSV) as a vector, which delivers the Ebola glycoprotein gene. Two phase I clinical trials took place involving 52 healthy adult volunteers.[22] The preliminary report showed the vaccine candidate was also generally well tolerated. Follow-up in the Phase II PREVAIL trial is ongoing in Liberia, and a stepped-wedge phase II trial of the vaccine in Sierra Leone and a ring vaccination trial in Guinea are currently underway.

Janssen, a division of Johnson & Johnson, in association with Bavarian Nordic, also developed a prime-boost vaccine regimen, AdVac EBOV + MVA. This regimen combines a priming dose of AdVac EBOV, which uses an adenovirus vector

---

[19] Alexandra Sifferlin, *A rapid Ebola test can diagnose the disease in just minutes*, Time (June 25, 2015), available at http://time.com/3936502/rapid-ebola-test/.

[20] Julie Ledgerwood et al., *Chimpanzee adenovirus vector Ebola vaccine—preliminary report*, New England Journal of Medicine (Nov. 26, 2014), available at http://www.nejm.org/doi/full/10.1056/NEJMoa1410863.

[21] *Id.*

[22] J. A. Regules et al., *A recombinant vesicular stomatitis virus Ebola vaccine—preliminary report*, New England Journal of Medicine (Apr. 1, 2015), available at http://www.nejm.org/doi/pdf/10.1056/NEJMoa1414216.

to deliver the Ebola glycoprotein gene, followed by a boost with modified vaccinia Ankara. Phase I trials are fully enrolled. Because infection rates of the Ebola virus decreased rapidly, it was impossible to prove efficacy of the various vaccine candidates in Liberia and Sierra Leone, although the trials are nevertheless generating important data regarding safety and immunogenicity. However, the ring vaccine trial in Guinea with the rVSV candidate appeared to confer protection before the number of cases decreased dramatically as a result of public health measures.[23]

NIAID, in partnership with the Liberian government, also launched a clinical trial designed to obtain safety and efficacy data on the investigational therapeutic ZMapp as a treatment for Ebola.[24] ZMapp is a cocktail of three monoclonal antibodies targeting the surface glycoprotein of the Ebola virus, preventing it from entering a cell. ZMapp is currently being studied in adults and children testing positive for Ebola virus disease.[25] One group is treated using optimized standard of care, including careful electrolyte and fluid management, plus antibiotics as needed. The other group is treated using this same optimized standard of care and also receives ZMapp.

Supporting the Development of Healthcare Infrastructure

While Ebola vaccines, diagnostics, and therapeutics advanced as a result of the epidemic, management of future outbreaks will depend on public health preparedness strategies that emphasize enhanced disease surveillance and bolstering of healthcare infrastructure. The Global Health Security Agenda (GHSA), for example, was created to accelerate the development of capacity needed to prevent, detect, and rapidly respond to outbreaks before they become epidemics.[26] Implementing the GHSA will also help move toward eliminating, to the greatest extent possible, disparities between the healthcare infrastructure in the developed and developing worlds. The global public health response to EVD in West Africa has helped lay some foundations in that direction.

For example, clinical laboratory capacity was improved at Redemption Hospital in Monrovia, Liberia, by providing laboratory equipment and training health workers on equipment use, infection prevention, and control measures.[27] The Center of

---

[23] Ana Maria Henao-Restrepo et al., *Efficacy and effectiveness of an rVSV-vectored vaccine expressing Ebola surface glycoprotein: interim results from the Guinea ring vaccination cluster-randomised trial*, 386(9996) Lancet, 857–866 (Aug. 29, 2015), available at http://www.thelancet.com/pdfs/journals/lancet/PIIS0140-6736(15)61117-5.pdf.

[24] National Institutes of Health, *Liberia-U.S. Clinical Research Partnership Opens Trial to Test Ebola Treatments*, available at http://www.nih.gov/news/health/feb2015/niaid-27.htm.

[25] *Id.*

[26] US Department of State, The U.S. Government Response to the Ebola Outbreak (Nov. 12, 2014), available at http://www.state.gov/s/dmr/remarks/2014/233996.htm.

[27] Melanie Mayhew, Health Workers on Ebola Frontlines Serve Countries, Risk Own Lives (Apr. 7, 2015), available at http://www.worldbank.org/en/news/feature/2015/04/06/healt-workers-on-ebola-frontlines-serve-countries-risk-own-lives.

Excellence for Infectious Disease Control, a healthcare capacity-building program, was established at the John F. Kennedy (JFK) Medical Center in Monrovia to prevent, treat, and control infectious diseases as part of the post-Ebola recovery. The JFK Medical Center lost many of its medical personnel to EVD, reducing the hospital's already overworked staff. The CDC, NIH, and US Army Medical Research Institute for Infectious Diseases worked with the Liberian Institute for Biomedical Research (LIBR) to establish laboratories and train staff in order to expand capacity to conduct testing for Ebola and other diseases.[28] Likewise, PREVAIL was initiated to conduct clinical research to develop vaccines and treatments for the Ebola virus.[29] This Liberian-US research partnership has since been extended to a regional research network in Sierra Leone, Guinea, and Mali.[30] It is worth emphasizing that these kinds of collaborations are crucial to building sustainable healthcare systems for the future. The healthcare systems of developing countries cannot be sustained solely by donations of richer nations and philanthropies. Stakeholder governments must play a larger role, including investments in health infrastructure and training of health professionals.

In addition to investments in biomedical innovation and healthcare infrastructure, medical researchers must follow, in a systematic way, those who survived the disease. While the current debate has largely focused on the high case fatality rate associated with Ebola, those who survive may face a range of chronic sequelae that are as yet poorly understood. In order to respond to the long-term public health burden imposed by Ebola, it is essential to fill this knowledge gap. In this regard, PREVAIL has an ongoing study in Liberia that aims to enroll as many as 7,500 survivors and their close contacts, monitoring for arthritis, cognitive impairments, visual defects, and other signs and symptoms anecdotally reported by Ebola survivors.[31]

Conclusion

Emerging infectious diseases are a continuing and perpetual challenge. History tells us such outbreaks will continue. In order to address them, it is essential to erase the health disparities between rich and poor nations.

---

[28] Embassy of the United States, The United States Increases Its Assistance for Anti-Ebola Efforts in West Africa (Aug. 19, 2014), available at http://monrovia.usembassy.gov/event_dart_91914.html.

[29] Ebola Communication Network, The Liberia-US Joint Clinical Research Partnership (Feb. 2015), available at http://ebolacommunicationnetwork.org/wp-content/uploads/2015/02/Research-on-Ebola-Vaccines.pdf.

[30] Id.

[31] National Institutes of Health, Study of Ebola Survivors Opens in Liberia (June 2015), available at http://www.nih.gov/news/health/jun2015/niaid-17.htm.

References

Baize, S., Pannetier D., Oestereich, L., Rieger, T., Koivogui, L., Magassouba, N., Soropogui, B., Sow, M. S., Keïta, S., De Clerck, H., Tiffany, A., Dominguez, G., Loua, M., Traoré, A., Kolié, M., Malano, E. R., Heleze, E., Bocquin, A., Mély, S., Raoul, H., Caro, V., Cadar, D., Gabriel, M., Pahlmann, M., Tappe, D., Schmidt-Chanasit, J., Impouma, B., Diallo, A. K., Formenty, P., Van Herp, M., and Günther, S. *Emergence of Zaire Ebola virus disease in Guinea*. 371(15) New England Journal of Medicine 1418–25 (2014).

Centers for Disease Control and Prevention. Ebola Viral Disease Outbreak—West Africa, available at http://www.cdc.gov/mmwr/preview/mmwrhtml/mm6325a4.htm.

———. Ebola Virus Disease (EVD) Information for Clinicians in U.S. Healthcare Settings. Available at http://www.cdc.gov/vhf/ebola/healthcare-us/preparing/clinicians.html.

———. Virus Ecology Graphic. Ebolavirus Ecology. Available at http://www.cdc.gov/vhf/ebola/resources/virus-ecology.html.

Ebola Communication Network. The Liberia-US Joint Clinical Research Partnership (2015). Accessed July 25, 2015, at http://ebolacommunicationnetwork.org/wp-content/uploads/2015/02/Research-on-Ebola-Vaccines.pdf.

Embassy of the United States. The United States Increases Its Assistance for Anti-Ebola Efforts in West Africa (2014). Accessed July 25, 2015, at http://monrovia.usembassy.gov/event_dart_91914.html.

Fauci, A. S. *Ebola—Underscoring the Global Disparities in Health Care Resources*. 37(12) New England Journal of Medicine (2014).

Fernandez, M. 2nd Ebola Case in U.S. Stokes Fears of Health Care Workers (2014). Accessed July 24, 2015, at http://www.nytimes.com/2014/10/13/us/texas-health-worker-tests-positive-for-ebola.html?_r=0.

Flynn, A. G. Partners in Health Ebola-Infected Clinician Discharged Virus Free From NIH Facility (2015). Available at http://www.masslive.com/news/index.ssf/2015/04/partners_in_health_ebola-infected_clinician_discharged_virus-free_from_nih_facility.html.

Henao-Restrepo, A. M., Longini, I. M., Egger, M., Dean, N. E., Edmunds, J., Camacho, A., Carroll, M. W., Doumbia, M., Draguez, B., Duraffour, S., Enwere, G., Grais, R., Gunther, S., Hossmann, S., Kondé, M. K., Kone, S., Kuisma, E., Levine, M. M., Mandal, S., Norheim, G., Riveros, S., Soumah, A., Trelle, S., Vicari, A. S., Watson C. H., Kéïta, S., Kieny, M. P., and Røttingen, J. A. *Efficacy and Effectiveness of an rVSV-Vectored Vaccine Expressing Ebola Surface Glycoprotein: Interim Results From the Guinea Ring Vaccination Cluster-Randomised trial*. 386(9996) Lancet 857–866 (Aug. 29, 2015).

Holley, P. *In Liberia Ebola outbreak is declared officially over*, Washington Post (May 9, 2015).

Kaeser, C., McKay, B., Umlauf, T., and McEnaney, C. *How the 2014 Ebola crisis unfolded*. Wall Street Journal (Sept. 8, 2014).

Kim, J. Y. *The path to zero Ebola cases*, New York Times (Dec. 11, 2014).

Ledgerwood, J. E., DeZure, A. D., Stanley, D. A., Laura Novik, L., Enama, M. E., Berkowitz, N. M., Hu, Z., Joshi, G., Ploquin, A., Sitar, S., Gordon, I. J., Plummer, S. A., Holman, L. A., Hendel, C. S., Yamshchikov, G, Roman, F., Nicosia, A., Colloca, S., Cortese, R., Bailer, R. T., Schwartz, R. M., Roederer, M., Mascola, J. R., Koup, R. A., Sullivan, N. J., Graham, B. S., and the VRC 207 Study Team. *Chimpanzee adenovirus vector Ebola vaccine—preliminary report*. New England Journal of Medicine (2014).

Mayhew, M. Health Workers on Ebola Frontlines Serve Countries, Risk Own Lives (Apr. 7, 2015). Available at http://www.worldbank.org/en/news/feature/2015/04/06/healt-workers-on-ebola-frontlines-serve-countries-risk-own-lives.

McKay, B., and Campoy, A. *First case of Ebola in U.S. is confirmed*. Wall Street Journal (Oct. 1, 2014).

Morse, D. *Nina Pham, nurse who contracted Ebola, is now free of virus and leaves NIH*. Washington Post (Oct. 24, 2014).

National Institutes of Health. Liberia-U.S. Clinical Research Partnership Opens Trial to Test Ebola Treatments (2015). Available at http://www.nih.gov/news/health/feb2015/niaid-27.htm.

———. Study of Ebola Survivors Opens in Liberia (2015). Available at http://www.nih.gov/news/health/jun2015/niaid-17.htm.

Regules, J. A., Beigel, J. H., Paolino, K. M., Voell, J., Castellano, A. R., Muñoz, P., Moon, J. E., Ruck, R. C., Bennett, J. W., Twomey, P. S., Gutiérrez, R. L., Remich, S. A., Hack, H. R., Wisniewski, M. L., Josleyn, M.D., Kwilas, S. A., Van Deusen, N., Mbaya, O. T., Zhou, Y., Stanley, D. A., Bliss, R. L., Cebrik, D., Smith, K. S., Shi, M., Ledgerwood, J.E., Graham, B. S., Sullivan, N. J., Jagodzinski, L. L., Peel, S. A., Alimonti, J. B., Hooper, J. W., Silvera, P. M., Martin, B. K., Monath, T. P., Ramsey, W. J., Link, C. J., Lane, H. C., Michael, N. L., Davey, Jr., R. T. , and Thomas, S. J. for the rVSV∆G-ZEBOV-GP Study Group. A Recombinant Vesicular Stomatitis Virus Ebola Vaccine—Preliminary Report. New England Journal of Medicine (Apr. 1, 2015).

Samadi, D. B. How to stop Ebola in America: ban air travel from West Africa. Fox News (Oct. 15, 2014). Available at http://www.foxnews.com/health/2014/10/15/how-to-stop-ebola-in-america-ban-air-travel-from-west-africa/.

Santora, M. *First patient quarantined under strict new policy tests negative for Ebola*. New York Times (Oct. 25, 2014).

US Department of State. The U.S. Government Response to the Ebola Outbreak (2014). Available at http://www.state.gov/s/dmr/remarks/2014/233996.htm.

World Health Organization. Ebola Virus Disease (2015). Available at http://www.who.int/mediacentre/factsheets/fs103/en/.

———. Outbreaks Chronology: Ebola Virus Disease (2015). Available at http://www.cdc.gov/vhf/ebola/outbreaks/history/chronology.html.

2

Treating, Containing, Mobilizing

The Role of Médecins Sans Frontières in the West African Ebola Epidemic Response

HEATHER PAGANO AND MARC PONCIN

The 2014–2016 Ebola epidemic in West Africa, 67 times the size of the largest previously recorded Ebola outbreak, with 28,639 cases and 11,316 deaths,[1] stunned the world, revealing the global health community's collective shortcomings in the face of a virulent and deadly disease. The epidemic also changed Médecins Sans Frontières (MSF), one of the key responders to the crisis, driving the medical humanitarian organization beyond its standard emergency operational role. Responding to the Ebola crisis in Guinea, Liberia, and Sierra Leone, as well as the spillover into Nigeria, Mali, and Senegal, was one of the largest emergency operations in MSF's 44-year history.[2] The cost was high: 28 MSF staff were infected in the outbreak, and 14 died.

The demands of this emergency drove MSF beyond its usual operational scope to training other organizations; assuming a leading role in strategic decisions at national levels; participating in clinical trials of experimental drugs, vaccines, and diagnostic tests with scientific partners; and taking part in lessons-learned workshops and conferences with governments, multilateral institutions, and academic groups. This was an evolution based on pragmatism, linked to four main factors: the deterioration of the epidemiological situation that overwhelmed capacity on the ground; few expert actors with limited capacity; technical and political failures at

---

[1] Jonathan Corum, *A history of Ebola in 24 outbreaks*, New York Times (Dec. 29, 2014) (noting 425 cases in Uganda in 2000); World Health Organization, West Africa epidemic numbers, Ebola situation report (Feb. 3, 2016).

[2] MSF responded to the Ebola epidemic in the three most affected countries—Guinea, Sierra Leone, and Liberia—and also responded to the spread of cases to Nigeria, Senegal, and Mali, as well as a separate epidemic in Democratic Republic of Congo in 2014. In total, the organization spent more than 96 million euros on tackling the epidemic.

local and international levels; and the moral and professional necessity to conduct trials of new therapies to find more efficient medical treatment beyond the supportive care provided in past outbreaks.

MSF's independent and flexible funding, preparedness to mitigate risks, and logistics capacity, combined with previous experience with filovirus outbreaks, positioned the organization as one of the first responders. However, due to the unprecedented scale of the outbreak and limited resources, MSF was faced with new, complex, and difficult strategic decisions. The typical six-pillar approach[3] to managing an Ebola outbreak was under strain from the onset, due the size and geographical spread of the epidemic. Pragmatic changes and alternative, often suboptimal, solutions had to be found each time a conventional strategy failed. In previous outbreaks, MSF had only ever needed to operate one, or exceptionally two, Ebola management centers (EMCs) at a time. During this epidemic, the organization set up and managed 15 EMCs and transit centers in the three most-affected countries, operating up to 8 simultaneously.

In this chapter, we examine the evolving role of MSF as the epidemic spread. Ultimately, the Ebola epidemic created vast shifts in the global health landscape, revealing strengths and, more commonly, weaknesses in various sectors of the global health community. MSF was not unaltered by this crisis and as a result underwent change as an organization.

From Misdiagnosis to Mistrust

Had the virus not gone undetected in the first phase of the epidemic, the outbreak may not have spiraled out of control. A lack of detection is consistent with past experience with Ebola outbreaks. It often takes considerable time for the first cases to be confirmed. The past eight large outbreaks took on average 2 months to be recognized and investigated.[4] Symptoms are easily mistaken for those of other diseases such as cholera and malaria, and experts able to correctly diagnose Ebola and other hemorrhagic fevers were few, even among organizations experienced in Ebola outbreaks, such as MSF, the World Health Organization (WHO), and the US Centers for Disease Control and Prevention (CDC).

---

[3] In the past, partners in Ebola collaborated in tandem to control Ebola outbreaks with a formula that evolved into six core pillars: (1) isolate and care for patients, (2) make burials safe, (3) engage communities, (4) conduct disease surveillance, (5) trace contracts, and (6) re-establish healthcare systems. Engaging in one without another will fail to bring Ebola under control, particularly neglecting to gain the trust of the affected communities. Figure 2.1 illustrates the extensive presence of MSF perssonel and facilities in the three most affected countries:

[4] Corum, *supra* note 1.

Map of the region

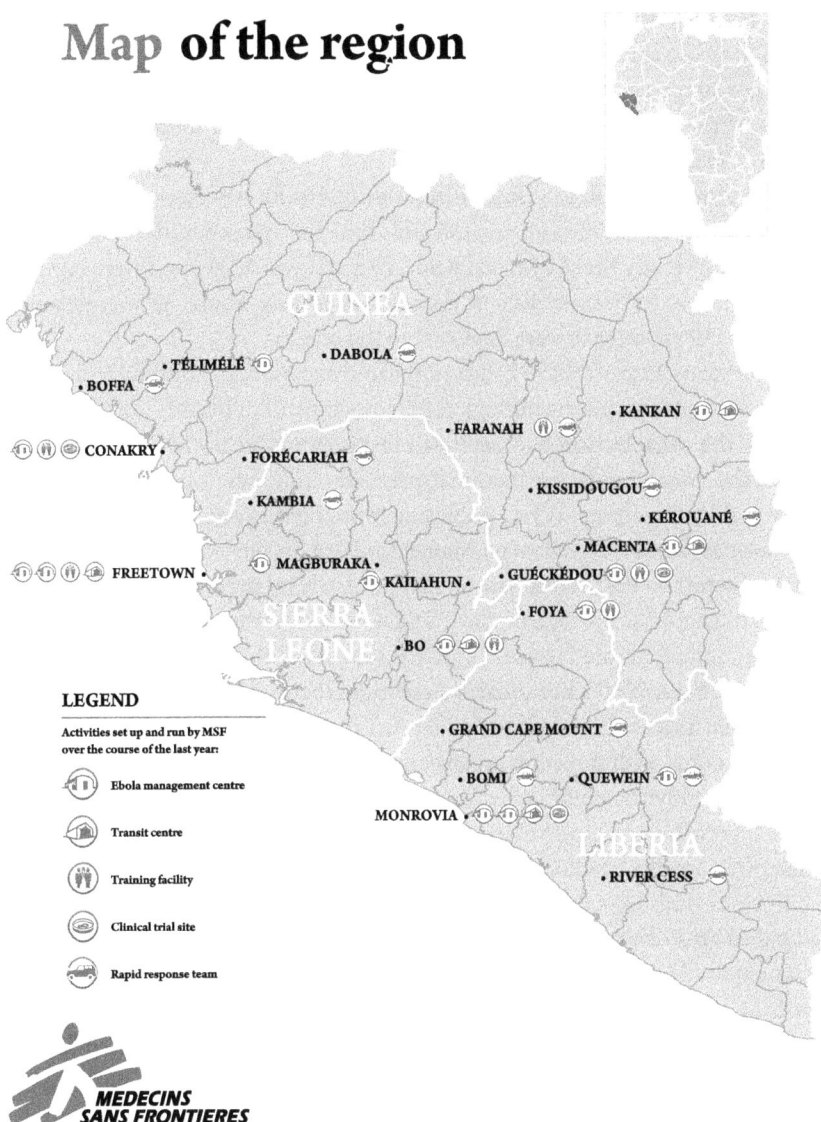

Figure 2.1 West African Ebola Outbreak: MSF Activities in Liberia, Sierra Leone & Guinea.

This outbreak reportedly began with a child in Guinea's forest region who died on December 28, 2013.[5] At the end of January, a joint MSF and Guinea Ministry

---

[5] Almudena Mari Saez et al., *Investigating the zoonotic origin of the West African Ebola epidemic* 7(1) EMBO Molecular Medicine, 17–23 (2014), available at http://embomolmed.embopress.org/content/early/2014/12/29/emmm.201404792.

of Health team investigated five cases of severe diarrhea in the young child's village of Meliandou. The clinical and epidemiological evidence presented from these five cases did not suggest the Ebola virus, which was also unknown in the region. It was concluded it was not cholera and that further cases would be followed up by the Ministry of Health.

However, on March 14, the Guinea Ministry of Health reported an outbreak of a "mysterious disease" in the same region. This time the symptoms described in the report matched closely those of a viral hemorrhagic fever (VHF) and were brought to the attention of MSF specialists in Europe. Suspecting Ebola, MSF emergency teams with VHF experience were deployed to the region.

In the previous 20 years, MSF had accumulated experience in dealing with Ebola outbreaks, since its first intervention in the Democratic Republic of Congo in 1995. Since then, the organization had deployed in Ebola outbreaks in nine countries, alongside the usual Ebola international partners. This new outbreak, however, would be unlike the others. WHO published formal notification of an outbreak of the Ebola virus disease in Guinea on March 23, 2014. In the following months, the operational setup on the ground was guided primarily by the classical approach. In support of the national authorities, the US CDC sent in a team of Ebola experts, the Red Cross conducted safe burials, UNICEF supported the Ministry of Health in social mobilization, WHO headquarters provided logistical and technical support to the regional and country offices that led the response, and MSF teams opened EMCs and worked with the other organizations.

In the past, filovirus outbreaks primarily took place in remote areas where the six-pillar approach was simpler to implement. A key challenge of this outbreak from the onset was not the absolute number of cases, which until June remained similar to previous outbreaks, but the dispersal of small numbers of cases over a wide geographical area. This multiplied the human resources, logistics, and laboratory capacity required in each individual location to bring the epidemic under control.

For MSF teams, the unusual epidemiological profile was a red flag from the end of March: unconnected chains of transmission in multiple locations, epidemiological spread to a major urban center—Guinea's capital, Conakry—and alerts in neighboring Liberia.[6] On March 31, 2014, MSF declared the outbreak unprecedented due to "an epidemic of a magnitude never before seen in terms of the distribution of cases."[7] With their warning having little effect, MSF felt alone in voicing concern

---

[6] On March 31, Ebola was confirmed in Liberia in Foya, near the border of Sierra Leone and Guinea. An MSF team set up isolation units and trained health staff in Foya and Monrovia, but cases soon dwindled. By mid-May there had been no cases for more than 21 days, the maximum incubation period of the virus. New cases would re-emerge in Liberia in June.

[7] MSF, Guinea: Mobilisation against an Unprecedented Ebola Epidemic (Mar. 31, 2014), available at http://www.msf.org/article/guinea-mobilisation-against-unprecedented-ebola-epidemic.

publicly and calling for greater action. Indeed, this warning of March 31 would initially draw criticism from other health actors.[8]

Ebola had been silently spreading in the region for 3 months; in time, it would be fueled by population mobility, mistrust of authorities, fear of the unknown disease, unsafe burial practices, poor surveillance systems, weak national health systems, and a lack of commitment at the higher levels of the affected governments that left the ministries of health stranded. The biogeography of the epidemic exacerbated this already precarious situation, with the virus surfacing at the junction of three countries where borders are porous. The region is characterized by high population mobility, in part due to poverty where people regularly move in search of work, as well as frequent visits to extended family members dispersed across national borders.[9]

Previous Ebola outbreaks demonstrated the importance of earning the acceptance of the community because, without it, the risk rises that the sick are hidden or that mistrustful communities assail or threaten health workers. In the West African outbreak, social mobilization was a shared responsibility among various health actors under the coordination of the ministries of health and UNICEF. From March to July 2014, gaining trust from the communities proved to be the most crucial, yet the weakest, link. To stop the spread of the virus, substantial empowerment and investment in the affected communities, based on clear understanding of their culture and traditions, is required. Conducting safe burials, for example, must be based on an understanding of the community's practices and beliefs around death. Recent violent conflicts and poor health infrastructure made trust-building even more difficult than before.

Prior to the Ebola outbreak, the dysfunctional health services in all three fragile states, as well as inadequate infrastructure, "contributed to a profound distrust of the authorities who were unable to provide basic services, of which health was only one."[10] The reasons for the deficiencies range from recent protracted civil wars in Sierra Leone and Liberia to corruption, including in the health sector, a lack of investment in healthcare, and poor health services with critical shortages of qualified medical staff and fragile drug supply systems. It is, then, unsurprising that there was little trust in the healthcare system when Ebola struck.

---

[8] Saliou Samb, *WHO says Guinea Ebola outbreak small as MSF slams international response*, Reuters (Apr. 1, 2014), available at http://www.reuters.com/article/us-guinea-ebola-idUSBREA301X120140401.

[9] World Health Organization, Factors that contributed to undetected spread of the Ebola virus and impeded rapid containment (Jan. 2015), available at http://www.who.int/csr/disease/ebola/one-year-report/factors/en/.

[10] ICG, The politics behind the Ebola crisis, Africa Report N°232 (Oct. 28, 2015), available at http://www.crisisgroup.org/en/regions/africa/west-africa/232-the-politics-behind-the-ebola-crisis.aspx.

Once the virus was confirmed, many affected communities rejected proposed control measures out of fear and disbelief.[11] Unable to comfort their sick, accompany them to the hospital, or mourn or bury their family members, those in the affected communities instead witnessed foreigners in spacesuits who appeared in their villages and took away their loved ones, only half of whom returned. At the peak of the epidemic, people were often neither informed when their relatives died nor given the chance to bury them.

Public health messages at the onset of the outbreak proved disastrous. Poorly crafted messages such as "Ebola kills up to 9 out of 10 people" and "there is no treatment or vaccine" discouraged communities from seeking care in Ebola treatment centers and led to intentional hiding of cases. Top-down communications from the aid community, including MSF, and insufficiently engaging or relying on the local community to put in place control measures were critical mistakes.[12]

In Guinea, the distrust was compounded by past political manipulations linked to ethnicities, which magnified the resistance against control measures and led to direct violence against aid actors, including MSF, with rocks thrown at ambulances and forced temporary closures of EMCs. In the forest region, communities are still divided after secular conflicts that generated distrust in the national authorities.[13] Control measures recalled previous episodes of authoritarianism by a central state disrespectful of local cultures and were met with resistance.[14] In Sierra Leone and Liberia, as well as Guinea, several communities refused to believe that the Ebola outbreak was real, "judging it to be part of a government conspiracy to secure new funding from Western donors."[15]

---

[11] Historically communities affected by filovirus outbreaks have reacted out of fear, disbelief, and hostility. This was the case for MSF in Kikwit, Democratic Republic of Congo, in 1995; at the border of Gabon and Congo in 2001–2002; in Congo again in 2003; and in Angola in 2005. Phillipe Calain and Marc Poncin, *Reaching out to Ebola victims: coercion, persuasion or an appeal for self-sacrifice?*, 147 Soc. Sci. Med. 126–133 (2015), available at http://www.sciencedirect.com/science/article/pii/S0277953615302021.

[12] ICG, *supra* note 10; World Health Organization, Report of the Ebola interim assessment panel—July 2015 (2015), available at http://www.who.int/entity/csr/resources/publications/ebola/report-by-panel.pdf?ua=1.

[13] Julienne Anoko, Communication with rebellious communities during an outbreak of Ebola virus disease in Guinea: an anthropological approach, Ebola Response Anthropology Platform (2015), available at http://www.ebola-anthropology.net/case_studies/communication-with-rebellious-communities-during-an-outbreak-of-ebola-virus-disease-in-guinea-an-anthropological-approach/.

[14] Mathieu Fribault, *Ebola in Guinea: historic violence and regimes of doubt*, 11 Anthropologie & Santé: Revue Internationale Francophone d'Anthropologie de la Santé (2015). French available at http://anthropologiesante.revues.org/1761.

[15] Adam Kamradt-Scott et al., *Civil-military cooperation in Ebola and beyond*, 387(10014) Lancet 104–105 (2016), available at http://www.thelancet.com/journals/lancet/article/PIIS0140-6736%2815%2901128-9/abstract.

Conflicting Messages

Though the surveillance data were poor from the outset, the worrying geographical spread of cases should have been sufficient to raise serious concern. Yet the national authorities in Guinea and Sierra Leone, as well as WHO, minimized the severity of the crisis, in part for political reasons.[16] Guinea's president predicted "rapid and final success" against the epidemic in late March 2014 and stated that the situation was "well under control" a month later.[17] Health officials in Guinea, and later also in Sierra Leone, were instructed to report only confirmed Ebola cases, leaving out suspected and probable cases, in an effort to artificially limit the numbers and the magnitude of the epidemic.[18] Fear of driving away investors and economic concerns compelled the government to downsize the perception of the outbreak's severity. These concerns were understandable: neighboring countries either closed their borders or restricted travel, while foreign workers from private companies left.[19]

National authorities in Guinea resisted, with some annoyance, MSF's March 31 declaration on the unprecedented nature of the outbreak. In May 2014, the president publicly accused the organization of spreading panic as a fundraising ploy.[20] The MSF representative was summoned to the president's office and informed that only WHO had the authority to communicate public messages on the outbreak, and that MSF was to fall in line with its assessments.[21] When it became clear that the outbreak was out of control, the national governments reversed course. They

---

[16] Maria Cheng and Raphael Satter, *Emails: UN health agency resisted declaring Ebola emergency*, AP (Mar. 20, 2015), available at http://bigstory.ap.org/article/2489c78bff86463589b41f3faaea5ab2/emails-un-health-agency-resisted-declaring-ebola-emergency. *A note on IHR*: Today's global health system, and the International Health Regulations in particular, rely on the state acting in good faith in epidemics. However, MSF's field experience in numerous infectious disease outbreaks demonstrates that states have little incentive to declare disease outbreaks, react to them with full force, or call for assistance in case their capacity is overstretched. An important lesson Ebola demonstrated on a much wider scale is that countries experiencing an outbreak must find incentives in the system, not economic or political punishment.

[17] Adam Nossiter, *Ebola now preoccupies once-skeptical leader in Guinea*, New York Times (Nov. 30 2014), available at http://www.nytimes.com/2014/12/01/world/africa/ebola-now-preoccupies-once-skeptical-leader-in-guinea.html?_r=2.

[18] Paul Schemm, *WHO reduces Ebola death toll in Sierra Leone*, Yahoo.com (June 25, 2014), available at http://news.yahoo.com/reduces-ebola-death-toll-sierra-leone-160340050.html.

[19] Suerie Moon et al., *Will Ebola change the game? Ten essential reforms before the next pandemic. The report of the Harvard-LSHTM Independent Panel on the Global Response to Ebola*, 386(10009), Lancet 2204–2221 (Nov. 28, 2015).

[20] Boubacar Diallo, Ebola en Guinée: Quand Alpha Conde s'en prend à MSF, l'ONG de son "ami-jumeau" Bernard Kouchner, Africaguinee.com (May 12, 2014), French available at http://www.africaguinee.com/articles/2014/05/12/ebola-en-guinee-quand-alpha-conde-s-enprend-msf-l-ong-de-son-ami-jumeau-bernard.

[21] Personal experience of author M. Poncin, then emergency coordinator in Guinea.

then sought MSF's assessments of the outbreak and response, particularly after an August 2014 visit by MSF international president Dr. Joanne Liu to the 3 countries and meetings with those countries' presidents.

It was not until the end of May 2014 that the outbreak in Sierra Leone was confirmed, though it had been silently spreading for months and then went on to reignite the epidemic in Liberia.[22] Prior to this date, not all suspicions of cases were followed up, including alerts MSF had sent to the Sierra Leone authorities in March, and weak surveillance missed the presence of the virus long before its official confirmation. As in Guinea, Sierra Leone's minister of health and sanitation in Freetown was upset by MSF's alarms and instructed MSF to stop its dismaying communication.[23]

The first Ebola cases in Sierra Leone from the end of May were referred to Kenema Government Hospital, a Ministry of Health–run facility experienced in treating Lassa, another viral hemorrhagic fever. Over the following weeks, the rapid increase in cases strained the hospital's capacity. The subsequent chaotic situation in Kenema during the summer of 2014 was illustrative of the dramatic evolution of the outbreak and the dangers of managing an Ebola center without adequate infection control. More than 40 health workers succumbed to the virus in Kenema, while "shoddy supplies, little support and infighting exacerbated the chaotic situation," according to an Associated Press investigation.[24]

In late June 2014, MSF opened a 32-bed EMC in Sierra Leone's Kailahun district, near the Guinean border; the center was quickly overwhelmed with patients and had to be expanded to 65 beds. MSF received little clear information about or overview of the epidemiology of the outbreak, due in part to a lack of effective collaboration with other actors on the ground.[25] The delayed recognition of the outbreak meant the intervention came too late, while the high numbers of patients meant that the MSF team had to prioritize patient care and reduce critical outreach activities. Controlling the epidemic by preventing the spread of the virus and breaking disparate transmission chains through contact tracing, surveillance, or community mobilization proved nearly impossible.

In contrast to Guinea and Sierra Leone, authorities in Liberia recognized the seriousness of the epidemic immediately, but by then available support was dwindling. MSF received nearly daily phone calls from the Liberian Ministry of Health

---

[22] Kevin Sack, Sheri Fink, and Adam Nossiter, *Ebola's Deadly Escape*, New York Times, (Dec. 29, 2014).

[23] Internal MSF email dated April 4, 2014, from MSF head of mission in Sierra Leone to MSF headquarters, following an Ebola National Task Force meeting in Freetown.

[24] Maria Cheng, Raphael Satter, and Krista Larson, *AP investigation: bungling by UN agency hurt Ebola response*, AP (Sept. 20, 2015), available at http://bigstory.ap.org/article/3ba4599fdd754cd-28b93a31b7345ca8b/ap-investigation-bungling-un-agency-hurt-ebola-response.

[25] MSF, Pushed to the Limit and Beyond, Geneva, Médecins Sans Frontières (2015), available at http://www.msf.org.uk/article/ebola-pushed-to-the-limit-and-beyond-msf-report.

requesting support in June, but, already overstretched in Guinea and Sierra Leone, the organization did not have sufficient Ebola-experienced personnel to respond to the extent required.

The lack of national leadership in the early phase was coupled with that of the world's public health guardian, the World Health Organization. After initially disputing MSF's March 31 declaration, WHO on April 8 held a press conference acknowledging that the epidemic was "one of the most challenging outbreaks ever faced." However, translating this recognition into robust action did not follow on the scale required.

WHO ultimately failed in its leadership role in guiding, supporting, and facilitating international, regional, and national epidemic management for a variety of reasons, many inherent to the structure of the organization itself.[26] National guidance for the authorities was deficient, while practicalities were not ensured, such as regular payment of surveillance teams and provision of necessary logistical means (e.g., transport and training) to carry out their duties. Considering the regional dimension of the outbreak and the population mobility, a strong surveillance system across borders was needed, but collaboration and communication between the countries was poor or nonexistent, and imported cases in new areas were not investigated thoroughly.

WHO inaction was also a product of political and economic pressures. Internal documents from early June 2014 show that the organization's leadership feared a declaration of public health emergency could be seen as a "hostile act" and "could anger the African countries involved, hurt their economies or interfere with the Muslim pilgrimage to Mecca."[27] In early July, the WHO assistant director-general, Dr. Keiji Fukuda, stated at a press conference that the outbreak was serious, but that all actions to deal with an Ebola epidemic were being implemented, and the epidemic was "not out of control."[28] This statement directly contradicted another warning MSF issued days earlier. Following its teams' estimation of active transmission of the virus in more than 60 locations, MSF publicly declared that the outbreak was "out of control," the organization was at its maximum capacity, and a

---

[26] Moon et al, *supra* note 19; WHO, Report of the Ebola interim assessment panel—July 2015, available at http://www.who.int/entity/csr/resources/publications/ebola/report-by-panel.pdf?ua=1; Laurie Garrett, *Ebola's lessons: how the WHO mishandled the crisis*, Foreign Affairs (Aug. 18, 2015), available at https://www.foreignaffairs.com/articles/west-africa/2015-08-18/ebolas-lessons?campaign=Garrett; National Academy of Medicine, The Neglected Dimension of Global Security: A Framework to Counter Infectious Disease Crises, Commission on a Global Health Risk Framework for the Future (2016), available at http://www.nap.edu/catalog/21891/the-neglected-dimension-of-global-security-a-framework-to-counter.

[27] Cheng and Satter, *supra* note 16.

[28] Boubacar Diallo, Ebola en Afrique de l'Ouest: "l'épidémie n'est pas hors de contrôle," selon l'OMS, Africaguinee.com (July 10, 2014), available at http://www.africaguinee.com/articles/2014/07/10/ebola-en-afrique-de-l-ouest-l-epidemie-n-est-pas-hors-de-controle-selon-l-oms.

massive deployment of resources was needed on the ground.[29] With such conflicting messages, it is little wonder that the initial international response was slow and confused. National governments typically take greater heed of the assessments of the UN than of nongovernmental organizations (NGOs); this explains in part why MSF's warnings went unheard.

MSF's "out of control" declaration followed a stark message sent by the field team in Guinea to MSF headquarters in June. It warned that at the moment when cases were on the rise across the country, the MSF teams were exhausted, gaps in human resources were increasing, and operational standards were being undermined with increased risk-taking, causing fear of potential staff contamination.[30]

It was not until July 2014 that WHO set up a meeting between the three national heads of government and established a regional coordination body in Conakry. While this commenced global reporting of cases, it resulted in little improvement for provision of care for patients or epidemic containment. The coordination between international and national partners remained weak and inefficient, at both national and regional levels. According to MSF: "decisions on setting priorities, attributing roles and responsibilities, ensuring accountability for the quality of activities, and mobilizing the resources necessary were not taken on the necessary scale."[31] By late July, more than 1,400 people had been infected and 800 deaths had been recorded, yet MSF remained one of the very few international aid organizations caring for infected people for most of this period, running four EMCs, as well as smaller transit units.

From Global Fear to Political Action

By early August 2014, Liberia, Sierra Leone, and Guinea had all declared a state of national emergency in recognition of the severity of the crisis. The health authorities and governments were struggling under the weight of the epidemic, and coordination remained weak.

In epidemics or emergency response, MSF does not generally intervene actively at the national level in developing strategies or coordinating other actors because this is the role of national authorities with the support of the United Nations. The ministries of health are MSF's usual counterpart in the field, although they are often one of the less influential ministries in government.

---

[29] MSF, Ebola in West Africa: epidemic requires massive deployment of resources (June 21, 2014), available at http://www.msf.org/article/ebola-west-africa-epidemic-requires-massive-deployment-resources.

[30] Internal MSF email of author M. Poncin, then emergency coordinator in Guinea, to MSF headquarters, dated June 11, 2014.

[31] MSF, *supra* note 25.

As the outbreak burgeoned, national governments asked MSF for further support, and by midsummer the organization began occupying the unusual role of technical adviser, particularly in Guinea and Liberia, on control strategies and coordination with other actors. For example, the MSF team in Guinea shared its concerns with the minister of health and the president in August on the poor functioning of national and international coordination, and suggested possible actions for managing the crisis and establishing prompt and appropriate response measures.[32] The recommendations contributed to the establishment in September of a new and more efficient national coordination cell, an illustration of what has been described as "MSF's role of the ship's bow, guiding the international efforts."[33]

Such input and liaison with higher levels of government were atypical for MSF, and its involvement was far from ideal; the organization lacked experience in external coordination, and its standard periodic rotations of coordination staff often meant that advising individuals held their positions too briefly to build proper relationships with their national counterparts. This evolution during the epidemic was ultimately linked to three main factors: the organization's past experience with the virus, WHO technical and political missteps that failed to give direction or coordinate with other actors, and the fact that the epidemic was labeled a health rather than a humanitarian crisis, meaning "that the surge capacity, emergency funding, and coordination structures typical of a large-scale disaster response were not triggered, and the formal cluster system was not activated across the board."[34]

The outbreak spiraled further out of control in August, with case numbers increasing dramatically in Liberia and Sierra Leone. Although conditions for such a declaration had been met at least 2 months earlier,[35] it was not until August 8, 2014, that WHO declared the outbreak to be a "public health emergency of international

---

[32] Formal MSF letter sent by email to the minister of health, August 25, 2014.

[33] François Grünewald, *Ebola: comment le virus est sorti de la clairière*, 40 Humanitaire 32–43 (2015), available at http://humanitaire.revues.org/3135.

[34] DuBois et al, The Ebola response in West Africa: exposing the politics and culture of international aid, Working and Discussion Paper, ODI (Oct. 2015), available at http://www.odi.org/publications/9956-ebola-response-west-africa-exposing-politics-culture-international-aid.

[35] The epidemic more than met the following criteria examples for a PHEIC: high case fatality; significant public health risk; cases reported among health staff; event in an area of high population density; inadequate human, financial, material, and technical resources; insufficient laboratory and epidemiological capacity; lack of drugs or vaccines; existing surveillance system inadequate to detect new cases in a timely manner; occurrence of the event itself unusual for the area; international travel (in the subregion); highly mobile population; and the event causing requests for more information by foreign officials and international media. From the annex of "Examples for the application of the decision instrument for the assessment and notification of events that may constitute a public health emergency of international concern" (*International Health Regulations*, 2nd ed. Geneva: World Health Organization 44–46 (2005).).

concern" under the International Health Regulations, at which point more than 1,000 people had died.

The world began to take the crisis seriously. Multiple reasons have been theorized as to why the international awakening was slow in the many expert panels and academic articles dedicated to the subject, but two seemed clear from MSF's perspective. On July 25, the virus had reached Nigeria via an air passenger from Liberia, sparking fears that Ebola would spread in Africa's most populous nation.[36]

The second reason, and undoubtedly the most convincing one for wealthy countries, was the realization that Ebola could travel and become an international security threat. At the end of July, two US nationals from the US aid group Samaritan's Purse became infected in Monrovia, and the organization suspended all operations in Liberia. The subsequent evacuation of these individuals to the United States for treatment raised global awareness of the threat Ebola posed. The suspension of Samaritan's Purse EMCs, the only two available in Liberia, was also a wake-up call for MSF. In the absence of any others to take them over, MSF "decided to push beyond its threshold of risk, and took over the two centers, sending coordinators without Ebola-experience and staff with only two days of Ebola training.[37] Given the explosion of cases in the region, it was clear that deploying further MSF teams would not be sufficient and that further support from other organizations was necessary.

Ebola-specific expertise was scarce when the outbreak began, including in MSF, with only approximately 10 viral hemorrhagic fever specialists and 30 staff with previous Ebola experience. The virus itself was also the cause of much of the initial inertia. The deadly and contagious disease with distressing symptoms and no proven treatment provoked an "atmosphere of fear unparalleled in a sector well-used to danger."[38] Fear spread more quickly than the infections and was a major impediment for international aid agencies. MSF was also not immune; organizational reluctance to deploy inexperienced staff delayed mobilization of the organization's full capacity.

In recognition of the growing shortage of qualified staff in all sectors, and its critical need for confrères in the fight against the epidemic, MSF opened its Ebola training centers for external organizations focusing on medical management and infection and prevention control measures for safely running EMCs. More than 1,000 MSF staff and personnel from external organizations were trained at the MSF centers in Europe, with thousands more trained on-site in the affected countries. This had a knock-on effect with other organizations, which scaled up their activities and went on to train others in turn.

In addition to facing the tangible threat of danger in the field, MSF international staff encountered extreme reactions on their return home. They were often shunned

---

[36] The Nigerian government utilized a dedicated public health emergency operations center previously set up for polio, while extensive contact tracing efforts helped avoid a widespread epidemic.

[37] MSF, *supra* note 25.

[38] DuBois et al., *supra* note 34.

by their family and friends, uninvited to gatherings, or banished from staying at or visiting the family home. The communities in the affected countries ostracized locally hired staff, resulting in other difficulties in addition to the mental health effects of the grueling tasks required to manage the crisis.[39]

Fear also compelled many countries to impose trade and travel measures that "lacked scientific and public health justifications and few bothered to explain their actions," in contravention of the International Health Regulations.[40] Some governments restricted the movements of healthy returning aid workers, justifying strict quarantine measures to mitigate public anxiety rather than applying measures based on science and evidence.[41] Airlines refused to fly to the region, with few notable exceptions. MSF conducted information-sharing sessions with SN Brussels Airlines staff to help assuage fears in an effort to keep the flights; to the organization's relief, this effort was successful.

Medical evacuations of infected staff were another deep concern, with fears that MSF would not be able to recruit international staff if there was no option to evacuate them if they fell ill. MSF spent precious time lobbying for the European Union to pool resources and put planes on standby in West Africa or Europe, but "the proposals ran into arguments over who would provide the aircraft, who would foot the bill, and most contentious, who would take overall control."[42]

With the WHO declaration and Ebola's new threat to wealthy nations, the outbreak became worldwide daily news. MSF participated in hundreds of media interviews per day, regularly calling for more assistance. Still, mass international support was not deployed in August or September 2014.

The number of new Ebola cases in Liberia skyrocketed by August, rising from fewer than 10 in June to more than 1,000 in the space of 2 months. The six-pillar approach crumbled due to the spread and volume of cases; MSF staff in the field and in headquarters scrambled to adjust their treatment and control options to the exploding epidemic. In Monrovia, MSF had to construct the largest EMC in history, with a capacity of 250 beds.[43] Despite this scale-up, the center was almost

---

[39] Helene Cooper, *They helped erase Ebola in Liberia. Now Liberia is erasing them*, New York Times (Dec. 9, 2015), available at http://www.nytimes.com/2015/12/10/world/africa/they-helped-erase-ebola-in-liberia-now-liberia-is-erasing-them.html.

[40] David Heymann et al., *Global health security: the wider lessons from the West African Ebola virus disease epidemic*, 385(9980) Lancet 1884–1901 (May 9, 2015).

[41] Kaci Hickox, *Caught between civil liberties and public safety fears: personal reflections from a healthcare provider treating Ebola*, 11 J. Health & Biomedical Law 9–23 (2015).

[42] Sheri Fink, *Ebola crisis passes, but questions on quarantine persist*, New York Times (Dec. 2, 2015), available at http://www.nytimes.com/2015/12/03/health/ebola-crisis-passes-but-questions-on-quarantines-persist.html?_r=0.

[43] Prior to the West Africa epidemic, a 40-bed center was the largest the organization had built to respond to an Ebola outbreak.

immediately overwhelmed, and it could be opened for only 30 minutes each morning to fill the beds vacated by those who had died the night before.

The vastly insufficient bed numbers across Monrovia led MSF to distribute tens of thousands of family and home disinfection kits to provide some protection for household contacts of Ebola patients. The organization also dispensed antimalarial tablets to more than 650,000 people in Monrovia, with the dual aim of preventing malaria and reducing the pressure on EMCs from people incorrectly assuming they had Ebola. These were imperfect solutions as the organization attempted to adapt its operational strategy to respond to the reality on the ground.

The Option of Last Resort

On September 2, 2014, Dr. Joanne Liu, MSF international president, briefed the UN member states in New York on the status of the outbreak, stating that "the world had been losing the battle against Ebola for the past six months," emphasizing that the medical teams on the front line were exhausted, and calling for the deployment of civilian and military units with biological warfare expertise.[44]

This call was uncharacteristic for MSF, and the decision was made with reservations because, to guard its independence and ensure humanitarian access to patients, the organization maintains a deliberate distance from armed forces. In the case of the Ebola epidemic, the call was exceptional and based on the belief that the military would have the means and the know-how to intervene on the scale required and could stem the tide of the epidemic while aid agencies trained to deploy. The organization was cautious to clarify it was not making a request for armed stabilization, and that military assets and personnel should not be used for law enforcement, quarantine, containment, or crowd control measures—which could further destabilize the region and force more infected people underground. Fortunately, these concerns did not materialize in the subsequent military response.[45]

The statement of Dr. Liu to the UN was followed by another on September 18, 2014. Via videoconference from Monrovia, MSF's Liberian team leader, Jackson K. P. Naimah, addressed the emergency session of the UN Security Council, illustrating the severity of what was faced on the ground, stressing that the visibly ill

---

[44] Specifically, MSF called for field hospitals with isolation wards to be scaled up, trained personnel to be sent out and care for patients, mobile laboratories to be deployed, and air bridges to be established to move personnel and materials to and within West Africa. MSF, United Nations Special Briefing on Ebola (Sept. 2, 2014), available at http://www.doctorswithoutborders.org/news-stories/speechopen-letter/united-nations-special-briefing-ebola.

[45] Andre Heller Perache, "*To put out this fire, we must run into the burning building*": *a review of MSF's call for biological containment Teams in West Africa*, 64 Humanitarian Exchange (June 2015), available at http://odihpn.org/magazine/to-put-out-this-fire-we-must-run-into-the-burning-building%C2%92-a-review-of-msf%C2%92s-call-for-biological-containment-teams-in-west-africa/.

were being turned away from MSF's center for lack of space, and requesting urgent help.[46]

The UN Security Council, having determined that the epidemic constituted a threat to international peace and security, passed Resolution 2177 urging member states to provide more resources to combat the outbreak. The global community mobilized, with commitments of resources by the United States, the United Kingdom, France, the African Union, Cuba, China, the European Union, Russia, the World Bank, the International Monetary Fund, and others.

The UN Mission for Ebola Emergency Response (UNMEER) was created to coordinate the UN agencies' response, bypassing both WHO and the traditional UN body for emergency coordination, the Office for the Coordination of Humanitarian Affairs (OCHA). Despite acknowledgment that UNMEER provided better UN internal coordination and a cross-border view of the crisis, critical views have emerged about its expense, its slowness to deploy, its distance from the affected countries with its coordination based in Ghana, and how it bypassed the existing coordination mechanisms and deprioritized non-Ebola assistance and protection activities.[47] Indeed, as the WHO Ebola Interim Panel Assessment asserts, UNMEER was not the appropriate model for managing the large-scale emergency, and the establishment of a UN mission would not be recommended for future emergencies with health consequences.[48]

Although WHO was not charged with coordinating the UN response, positive changes on the ground developed, notably with the replacement of the country representatives, the deployment of more experienced staff to manage their Ebola activities, and direct operational support in surveillance and contact tracing in the affected countries.

Globally, political attention was raised and resources pledged in September 2014, but it was not until October that widespread international aid slowly began to be deployed in the affected countries, "taking months for funding, personnel, and other resources to reach the region."[49] By this stage, there had been around 9,000 cases, half of which had been treated by MSF. The slow response resulted in needless suffering and cost many lives. A report by the UK government quotes research indicating that as many as 12,500 cases of Ebola could have been prevented if interventions had been delivered 1 month earlier.[50]

---

[46] MSF addresses UN Security Council emergency session on Ebola, (Sept. 18, 2014), available at http://www.msf.org/article/msf-addresses-un-security-council-emergency-session-ebola.

[47] DuBois et al., *supra* note 34.

[48] World Health Organization, *supra* note 12.

[49] Moon et al., *supra* note 19.

[50] *Ebola's legacy: UK deficits and their global lessons*, 387(10017) Lancet 403 (Jan. 30, 2016), available at http://www.thelancet.com/journals/lancet/article/PIIS0140-6736%2816%2900209-9/fulltext?rss=yes.

More than 5,000 military personnel were deployed by the United States, the United Kingdom, France, China, Canada, and Germany, the majority of whose efforts were limited to support, coordination, and logistics for the work of NGOs and the local authorities instead of hands-on clinical care for Ebola patients. However, their deployment was "key to convincing several non-governmental organizations to maintain or establish operations in the affected countries."[51] In particular, the establishment of three medical facilities in each of the capital cities to treat local and foreign healthcare workers was reassuring for NGOs to deploy their staff and bolstered local healthcare workers and authorities.

The level and approach of international support differed across the three countries. In Guinea, MSF remained the only aid organization running EMCs until November 2014. MSF lobbied the French government in Conakry and Paris to step up its efforts and ultimately signed an agreement with the French Red Cross to assist it in setting up an Ebola center in Macenta, the epicenter of the epidemic at that time.[52] MSF constructed the center, trained the French Red Cross international and national staff, and provided support by ordering supplies through the MSF Supply Center. Supporting other NGOs in this way was yet another first for the organization.

The Long Road to Zero

The epidemic finally turned a corner toward the end of 2014, and case numbers began declining in the region. Strong community mobilization, particularly in Liberia, has been found to have been a major contributing factor to this decrease.[53] However, the outbreak persisted, with several challenges, particularly related to operational coordination among the multitude of actors, regional cooperation across borders, and contact tracing and surveillance, with new cases emerging without known links to existing cases.

Ongoing misconceptions about the virus and intense stigma continued, with some people suspected to have Ebola still avoiding treatment or reporting cases. Throughout the outbreak, health workers not only faced the risk of contamination but also were recurrently rejected by the communities they aimed to assist, sometimes experiencing direct violence. Assaults persisted into 2015 in Guinea and even

---

[51] Kamradt-Scott et al., *supra* note 15.

[52] Radio France International, *Ebola: à Macenta, un centre "quatre étoiles" contre l'épidémie* (Nov. 15, 2014), French available at http://www.rfi.fr/afrique/20141115-ebola-macenta-guinee-msf-croix-rouge-girardin.

[53] Sharon Alane Abramowitz et al., *Community-centered responses to Ebola in urban Liberia: the view from below*, 9(4) PLoS Negl Trop Dis. (2015), available at http://www.ncbi.nlm.nih.gov/pmc/articles/PMC4391876/.

extended into 2016 during the resurgence of cases in Sierra Leone.[54] Yet national health workers on the ground continued to "show immense courage and professionalism in dealing with such challenges despite minimal levels of support."[55]

Difficulties in adapting to the rapid changes and new hot spots of the outbreak were observed, with international resources continuing to be allocated where they were no longer the priority. In Monrovia, for example, more EMCs were being built in December despite an already adequate isolation capacity and a drop in cases in the capital. Yet new cases were appearing elsewhere in the country, and in some locations patients still had to travel up to 12 hours by road to reach an Ebola center and a functioning laboratory.[56] The bulk of the direct care of patients and work with the communities was carried out by local people, government authorities, and NGOs.

From December 2014 onward, MSF focused on improving its quality of care and activities across the three countries. Innovations were piloted such as improvements to the design of EMCs, the use of electronic, tablet-based patient data management in the high-risk zone, and further development of protocols for pregnant women. It was also in this period that the first Ebola experimental treatment trial in West Africa began, at MSF's center in Guéckédou, Guinea, on December 17.

Four months earlier, in August, an advisory panel convened by the director-general of WHO confirmed that using Ebola products not yet tested on humans was ethical given the nature of the epidemic. Research and development efforts were swiftly put into motion under WHO coordination. MSF contributed to the design of clinical protocols and, for the first time in the midst of an emergency, partnered with research institutions, WHO, ministries of health, and pharmaceutical companies to trial experimental treatments and vaccines.

In 2015, trials for the experimental treatments favipiravir and convalescent plasma took place in MSF's centers in Guinea, as did trials for the drug brincidofovir in Liberia. The trial of the rVSV-EBOV vaccine started in Guinea in March 2015, led by WHO, MSF, the Norwegian Institute of Public Health, and the Guinean health authorities. In July 2015, promising results of the vaccine trial were published in the *Lancet*, with the interim review stating 100% efficacy.[57] More research and analysis are needed, but the vaccine proffered long-awaited good news for those who might be exposed to the disease (i.e., contacts of infected patients and front-line workers).

---

[54] BBC, *Ebola outbreak: Sierra Leone clashes over market closure* (Jan. 26, 2016), available at http://www.bbc.com/news/world-africa-35409690.

[55] Marc Poncin, *Ebola healthcare workers: a hazardous and isolating job*, HPN (June 8, 2015), available at http://odihpn.org/blog/ebola-healthcare-workers-a-hazardous-and-isolating-job/.

[56] MSF, Ebola response: where are we now? (Dec. 2014), https://www.doctorswithoutborders.org/sites/usa/files/ebola_briefing_paper_12.14.pdf.

[57] Ana Maria Henao-Restrepo et al., *Efficacy and effectiveness of an rVSV-vectored vaccine expressing Ebola surface glycoprotein: interim results from the Guinea ring vaccination cluster-randomised trial*, 386 (9996) Lancet, 857–866 (Aug. 29, 2015), available at http://www.thelancet.com/pdfs/journals/lancet/PIIS0140-6736(15)61117-5.pdf.

Most MSF efforts in 2015 focused on keeping up the momentum required to reach zero cases in the region, with constant vigilance. A newfound challenge was discovered among the more than 17,000 survivors of the virus: Ebola may lie dormant and hide in parts of the body such as the eyes and testicles, long after leaving the bloodstream. Though the risk of re-emergence or transmission to others has been rare, many continue to experience health problems after they survived the disease. Memory loss, joint pain, eye inflammation, and mental health problems including depression and post-traumatic stress disorder have all been diagnosed in the MSF-run survivor clinics in Liberia, Guinea, and Sierra Leone, where medication is prescribed, mental health support is provided, and patients are referred to specialists for severe problems such as loss of vision. This unprecedented outbreak has revealed that perhaps the six-pillar approach might be updated with a seventh—care and follow-up of survivors as an integral component of Ebola outbreak management.

Conclusion

The 2014–2016 Ebola epidemic was among the largest responses in MSF's history, with more than 4,000 national staff and 1,300 international staff deployed to care for patients and help contain the outbreak. More than 10,300 patients were admitted to the MSF EMCs, of which 5,226 were confirmed Ebola cases, representing one-third of all WHO-confirmed cases.[58] The organization was compelled to take on responsibilities beyond its usual first responder mandate, with both successes and failures.

MSF's patient-driven medical and emergency focus in the Ebola outbreak saw the organization choose to prioritize patient care over other critical containment activities when the outbreak was spiraling out of control. But when reaching out to provide urgent care for patients in the initial months, MSF did not sufficiently consider the role the local communities should have taken to halt the epidemic.

Indeed, the isolated expertise of the organization meant that its medical-clinical approach dominated much of the early response. Because those involved with MSF are seen as "treatment specialists first and foremost seeing a world of patients requiring treatment," its calls for increased bed capacity had an influence on the subsequent priorities set by donors who advanced the construction of EMCs and deprioritized community engagement and other non-Ebola activities needed in the overall humanitarian response.[59] Instead of perceiving the local population simply

---

[58] As of February 1, 2016, a total of 28,592 suspect, probable, and confirmed Ebola cases were registered in Guinea, Liberia, and Sierra Leone; of these, 15,206 were confirmed Ebola cases. WHO, *supra* note 1.

[59] DuBois et al., *supra* note 34.

as patients or as a population that needed to understand and abide by the containment measures, the global health community should have considered the communities as direct stakeholders much earlier on as a critical means to end the outbreak.

In the international response mobilization, political leaders of the Global North also overlooked the affected communities and were quick to take action to protect their own citizens and interests but had been late to intervene in favor of those suffering in West Africa in the months before. The Ebola epidemic has been cited as a striking example of how national security matters currently prevail over public health achievement.[60] Securitizing health, with the protection of wealthy states as its key motivator, is gaining influence in the quotidian debates around global health security. Concerns grow that international responses in the future will be triggered only when an epidemic is perceived as an international health threat, rather than based on the health needs of those caught in an epidemic.

Though the patient-centered focus has drawbacks in its rather narrow view of a humanitarian response, MSF takes the solidarity approach over the security approach. The organization sees health security as the commitment to secure and improve the health of all without discrimination (i.e., that "the value of health cannot be dependent on its utility to the security of the wealthy").[61] As was done during the Ebola epidemic, MSF will continue to use its voice and credibility to encourage that patients remain at the center of any epidemic response.

From MSF's point of view, if the global management of infectious diseases is to succeed in the future, then the global health security framework must strike a better balance between guaranteeing national security, on one side, and the provision of care to those suffering the disease, on the other.

References

Abramowitz S, McLean K, McKune S, Bardosh K, Fallah M, Monger J, et al. *Community-centered responses to Ebola in urban Liberia: the view from below.* 9(4) PLoS Negl Trop Dis. (2015): e0003706.

Anoko, Julienne. *Communication with rebellious communities during an outbreak of Ebola virus disease in Guinea: an anthropological approach.* Ebola Response Anthropology Platform (2015). Available at http://www.ebola-anthropology.net/case_studies/communication-with-rebellious-communities-during-an-outbreak-of-ebola-virus-disease-in-guinea-an-anthropological-approach/.

BBC. *Ebola outbreak: Sierra Leone clashes over market closure* (Jan. 26, 2016).

Calain P, Poncin M. *Reaching out to Ebola victims: coercion, persuasion or an appeal for self-sacrifice?* 147 Soc. Sci. Med. 126–133 (2015).

---

[60] Philippe Calain and C. Abu-Sa'Da, *Coincident polio and Ebola crises expose similar fault lines in the current global health regime*, 9(29) Confl Health (2015), http://www.ncbi.nlm.nih.gov/pmc/articles/PMC4572646/.

[61] DuBois et al., *supra* note 34.

Calain P, Abu-Sa'Da C. *Coincident polio and Ebola crises expose similar fault lines in the current global health regime.* 9(29) Confl Health (2015).

Cheng M, Satter F. *Emails: UN health agency resisted declaring Ebola emergency.* AP (Mar. 20, 2015).

Cheng M, Satter R, Larson K. *AP investigation: Bungling by UN agency hurt Ebola response.* AP (Sept. 20, 2015).

Cooper H. *They helped erase Ebola in Liberia. Now Liberia is erasing them.* New York Times (Dec. 9, 2015).

Corum J. *A history of Ebola in 24 outbreaks,* New York Times (Dec. 29, 2014).

Diallo B. *Ebola en Afrique de l'Ouest: "l'épidémie n'est pas hors de contrôle," selon l'OMS.* Africaguinee.com (July 10, 2014). French available at http://www.africaguinee.com/articles/2014/07/10/ebola-en-afrique-de-l-ouest-l-epidemie-n-est-pas-hors-de-controle-selon-l-oms.

———. *Ebola en Guinée: Quand Alpha Conde s'en prend à MSF, l'ONG de son "ami-jumeau" Bernard Kouchner.* Africaguinee.com (May 12, 2014). French available at http://www.africaguinee.com/articles/2014/05/12/ebola-en-guinee-quand-alpha-condes-enprend-msf-l-ong-de-son-ami-jumeau-bernard.

DuBois M, Wake C, Sturridge S, Bennett C. *The Ebola response in West Africa: exposing the politics and culture of international aid.* Working and Discussion Paper, ODI (Oct. 2015). Available at http://www.odi.org/publications/9956-ebola-response-west-africa-exposing-politics-culture-international-aid.

Ebola's legacy: UK deficits and their global lessons. 387(10017) Lancet 403 (Jan. 30, 2016).

Fink S. *Ebola crisis passes, but questions on quarantines persist.* New York Times (Dec. 2, 2015).

Fribault M. *Ebola in Guinea: historic violence and regimes of doubt.* 11 Anthropologie & Santé: Revue Internationale Francophone d'Anthropologie de la Santé (2015). French available at http://anthropologiesante.revues.org/1761.

Garrett L. *Ebola's lessons: how the WHO mishandled the crisis.* Foreign Affairs (Aug. 18, 2015).

Grünewald F. *Ebola: comment le virus est sorti de la clairière.* 40 Humanitaire 32–43 (2015). French available at http://humanitaire.revues.org/3135.

Henao-Restrepo AM, Longini IM, Egger M, Dean N, Edmunds J, Camacho A, et al. *Efficacy and effectiveness of an rVSV-vectored vaccine expressing Ebola surface glycoprotein: interim results from the Guinea ring vaccination cluster-randomised trial.* 386 Lancet 857–866 (2015).

Heymann D, Chen L, Takemi, K, Fidler P, Tappero J, Thomas M, et al. *Global health security: the wider lessons from the west African Ebola virus disease epidemic.* 385 Lancet 1884–1901 (2015).

Hickox K. *Caught between civil liberties and public safety fears: personal reflections from a healthcare provider treating Ebola.* 11 Journal of Health and Biomedical Law 9–23 (2015).

Higgins A. *Ebola fight in Africa is hurt by limits on ways to get out.* New York Times (Oct. 14, 2014).

ICG. *The politics behind the Ebola crisis.* Africa Report N°232 (Oct. 28, 2015). Available at http://www.crisisgroup.org/en/regions/africa/west-africa/232-the-politics-behind-the-ebola-crisis.aspx.

Kamradt-Scott A, Harman S, Wenham C, Smith F. *Civil-military cooperation in Ebola and beyond.* 387(10014) Lancet 104–105 (Jan. 9, 2016).

———. *Saving lives: the civil-military response to the 2014 Ebola outbreak in West Africa.* University of Sidney (Oct. 2015). Available at http://sydney.edu.au/mbi/news/2015/savinglives.php

Mari Saéz M, Weiss S, Nowak K, Lapeyre V, Zimmermann F, Düx A, et al. *Investigating the zoonotic origin of the West African Ebola epidemic.* 7(1) EMBO Molecular Medicine 17–23 (2014).

Moon S, Sridhar D, Pate M, Jha A, Clinton C, Delaunay S, et al. *Will Ebola change the game? Ten essential reforms before the next pandemic. The report of the Harvard-LSHTM Independent Panel on the Global Response to Ebola.* 386 Lancet 2204–2221 (2015).

MSF. *Ebola in West Africa: Epidemic requires massive deployment of resources.* (June 21, 2014). Available at http://www.msf.org/article/ebola-west-africa-epidemic- requires- massive-deployment-resources.

———. *Ebola response: where are we now?* (Dec. 2014). Available at https://www.doctorswithoutborders.org/sites/usa/files/ebola_briefing_paper_12.14.pdf.

———. Guinea: Mobilisation against an unprecedented Ebola epidemic (Mar. 31, 2014). Available at http://www.msf.org/article/guinea-mobilisation-against-unprecedented-ebola-epidemic.

———. MSF addresses UN Security Council emergency session on Ebola (Sept. 18, 2014). Available at http://www.msf.org/article/msf-addresses-un-security-council-emergency-session-ebola.

———. Pushed to the Limit and Beyond (2015). Available at http://www.msf.org.uk/article/ebola-pushed-to-the-limit-and-beyond-msf-report.

———. United Nations Special Briefing on Ebola (Sept. 2, 2014). Available at http://www.doctorswithoutborders.org/news-stories/speechopen-letter/united-nations-special-briefing-ebola.

National Academy of Medicine. The Neglected Dimension of Global Security: A Framework to Counter Infectious Disease Crises. Commission on a Global Health Risk Framework for the Future (2016).

Nossiter A. *Ebola now preoccupies once-skeptical leader in Guinea.* New York Times (Nov. 30, 2014).

Perache A. *"To put out this fire, we must run into the burning building": a review of MSF's call for biological containment teams in West Africa.* 64 Humanitarian Exchange (June 2015). Available at http://odihpn.org/magazine/to-put-out-this-fire-we-must-run-into-the-burning-building%C2%92-a-review-of-msf%C2%92s-call-for-biological-containment-teams-in-west-africa/.

Poncin M. *Ebola healthcare workers: a hazardous and isolating job.* HPN (June 8, 2015). Available at http://odihpn.org/blog/ebola-healthcare-workers-a-hazardous-and-isolating-job/.

Radio France International. *Ebola: à Macenta, un centre "quatre étoiles" contre l'épidémie* (Nov. 15, 2014). French available at http://www.rfi.fr/afrique/20141115-ebola-macenta-guinee-msf-croix-rouge-girardin.

Sack K, Fink S, Belluck P, Nossiter A. *How Ebola roared back.* New York Times (Dec. 29, 2014).

Samb S. *WHO says Guinea Ebola outbreak small as MSF slams international response.* Reuters (Apr. 1, 2014).

Schemm P. *WHO reduces Ebola death toll in Sierra Leone.* Yahoo.com (June 25, 2014).

WHO. Ebola Situation Report—3 February 2016. World Health Organization. Available at http://apps.who.int/ebola/current-situation/ebola-situation-report-3-february-2016.

———. Factors that contributed to undetected spread of the Ebola virus and impeded rapid containment (Jan. 2015). Available at http://www.who.int/csr/disease/ebola/one-year-report/factors/en/.

———. International Health Regulations. 2nd ed. Geneva: World Health Organization 44–46 (2005).

———. Report of the Ebola interim assessment panel—July 2015. World Health Organization (2015). Available at http://www.who.int/entity/csr/resources/publications/ebola/report-by-panel.pdf?ua=1.

3

The Effect of Ebola Virus Disease on Health Outcomes and Systems in Guinea, Liberia, and Sierra Leone

JOHN D. KRAEMER AND MARK J. SIEDNER

In March 2014, when the West African Ebola epidemic emerged, most global public health experts predicted a fairly quick resolution. Dozens of prior Ebola epidemics had instructed the public health community that, from a purely epidemiological perspective, Ebola is usually a readily controllable disease: transmission requires direct contact with bodily fluids of an infected individual and occurs only after the appearance of symptoms—which are often dramatic. To contain and overcome an epidemic, one need only isolate patients, ensure adequate clinical infection control, trace contacts, and enact safe burials.[1] In retrospect, these beliefs were naive, and they neglected to account for a number of features of the 2015 West African Ebola epidemic that set it apart in key, and ultimately disastrous, ways. That epidemic spun out of control because it emerged where it was not expected, it crossed national borders quickly and often, and its control required effective and coordinated action, which quickly outstripped the capacity of weak and unprepared health systems.

There is a great deal to be learned from the recent Ebola virus disease (EVD) epidemic. Preventing future calamities will require stronger and more resilient health systems, across the global to the subnational spectrum. Yet strengthening public health systems in resource-poor settings has been a long-sought goal, and this epidemic, more than anything, revealed how distant that goal remains. In West Africa specifically, the loss of health care workers (HCWs) and trust in the healthcare system will exacerbate the challenges facing health ministries in building public health resilience in the region.

This chapter proceeds in two steps. First, we seek to document the Ebola epidemic's effect on health outcomes and systems in Guinea, Liberia, and Sierra Leone.

---

[1] David L. Heymann, Control of communicable diseases manual (2008).

We do this by reviewing the existing literature—academic, news media, and other reports—to understand how Ebola caused short- and long-term harm to health that exceeds the direct consequences for those infected. Second, we identify opportunities for building stronger, more resilient health systems, with a particular focus on steps that would improve outcomes during both routine and emergency situations.

Immediate Health System Effects

The Ebola epidemic's health effects will likely never be fully quantified. The most apparent impacts are direct EVD infections and death, the number of which remains uncertain due to weak and overwhelmed surveillance systems. However, public health officials reported 28,638 cases and 11,316 deaths to the World Health Organization (WHO). These are likely an underestimate—as evidenced by the high proportion of cases without known exposures during the epidemic's height—though some probable and suspected reported cases were also likely manifestations of other diseases, especially early in the epidemic when confirmatory testing was rarely available.[2]

The epidemic's direct effects were extraordinary, particularly in Liberia and Sierra Leone. During the epidemic, it became fashionable in some global health circles to argue that Ebola is a minor killer and that focusing on it detract attention from greater public health concerns, like HIV/AIDS and malaria.[3] If one took a continent-wide perspective, this critique was understandable. However, the argument was akin to disclaiming the importance of HIV/AIDS in Haiti because it causes a relatively small percentage of deaths across the entire WHO region of the Americas.[4] Under reasonable assumptions, Ebola was Liberia's and Sierra Leone's leading cause of death in 2014 and a top-five killer in Guinea.[5]

Direct Ebola deaths were, however, only a fraction of the epidemic's total deaths, with most excess deaths resulting from health system disruptions. In Liberia, for example, more than half of the country's health facilities had closed at least temporarily by September 2014. That the Ebola epidemic rendered so many

---

[2] Martin Meltzer et al., *Estimating the future number of cases in the Ebola epidemic—Liberia and Sierra Leone, 2014–2015*, 26(63) MMWR Surveill Summ 1–14 (Sept. 26, 2014); World Health Organization, Ebola Situation Report—20 January 2016 (2016), available at http://apps.who.int/ebola/current-situation/ebola-situation-report-20-january-2016.

[3] Abby Phillip, *How Ebola is stealing attention from diseases that kill more people*, Washington Post (Sept. 5, 2014), available at https://www.washingtonpost.com/news/to-your-health/wp/2014/09/05/how-ebola-the-kardashian-of-diseases-is-stealing-attention-from-illnesses-that-kill-more-people/.

[4] Institute for Health Metrics and Evaluation, GBD Compare: Region of the Americas and Haiti (2015), available at http://ihmeuw.org/3qv6.

[5] Stephane Helleringer and Andrew Noymer, *Magnitude of Ebola relative to other causes of death in Liberia, Sierra Leone, and Guinea*, 3(5) Lancet Glob Health 255–256 (May 2015).

facilities inoperable underscores the extent to which health system vulnerabilities intersected in affected countries. Consider the principle reason for closure: that adequate infection control could not be maintained, leading to HCW or patient infections. These infections occurred not solely because of limited triage and diagnostic capacity, nor solely due to breakdowns in the personal protective equipment (PPE) supply chains, nor an inability to rapidly train and support providers on PPE use, nor challenges sterilizing the physical environment in which clinicians worked.[6] Rather, crosscutting limitations in health system capabilities combined to preclude adequate infection control. Importantly, the root causes of the failure of health systems to respond appropriately to the epidemic occurred at different levels of the health system, making it impossible for any one actor—a clinician, district health officer, or health ministry office—to separately solve infection control risks.

Facility closures caused dramatic direct impacts on health. Observational studies have documented the near cessation of facility-based services in heavily affected parts of Guinea, Liberia, and Sierra Leone at the epidemics' peaks. For example, one study found a 70% reduction in in-patient care across all Sierra Leonean facilities during the May–October phase of the epidemic compared with pre-Ebola baselines.[7] Similar reductions were reported in antenatal care, facility-based deliveries, and malaria intermittent presumptive therapy in two heavily affected Liberian counties.[8]

While facility closures were the most visible examples of health service interruption, the majority of facilities in affected countries remained open during the epidemic.[9] However, the Ebola epidemic also interfered with outreach- and community-based services. Outreach-based vaccination service essentially stopped during the epidemic in all three countries, leading to an estimated 200,000 additional children being unvaccinated against measles after 6 months' interruption.[10]

---

[6] Almea Matanock et al., *Ebola virus disease cases among health care workers not working in Ebola treatment units—Liberia, June–August, 2014,* 63(46) MMWR Morb Mortal Wkly Rep 1077–1081 (Nov. 21, 2014).

[7] Hakon Angell Bolkan et al., *Ebola and indirect effects on health service function in Sierra Leone,* PLoS Curr (Dec. 19, 2014), available at http://currents.plos.org/outbreaks/article/ebola-and-indirect-effects-on-health-service-function-in-sierra-leone/.

[8] Preetha Iyengar et al., *Services for mothers and newborns during the Ebola outbreak in Liberia: the need for improvement in emergencies,* PLoS Curr (Apr. 16, 2015), available at http://currents.plos.org/outbreaks/article/services-for-mothers-and-newborns-during-the-ebola-outbreak-in-liberia-the-need-for-improvement-in-emergencies/.

[9] Cathryn Streifel, How Did Ebola Impact Maternal and Child Health in Liberia and Sierra Leone?, 1–19 (2015), available at http://csis.org/files/publication/151019_Streifel_EbolaLiberiaSierraLeone_Web.pdf.

[10] Saki Takahashi et al., *Reduced vaccination and the risk of measles and other childhood infections post-Ebola,* 347(6227) Science 1240–1242 (Mar. 13, 2015).

As the epidemic waned, countries implemented catch-up vaccination campaigns,[11] but it is yet unclear to what extent they ameliorated under-vaccination.

Less discussed, but equally important, were the impacts of the epidemic on outreach-based family planning services that largely ceased in rural areas during the epidemic. In areas of low population density, oral contraceptives and injectables were often provided by clinicians during visits to rural villages, enabling substantial distance barriers to contraception access to be overcome.[12] Services stopped for several reasons, including reassignment of clinicians to Ebola-related tasks and injection-related blood-borne infection concerns. Interruptions also occurred for more pedestrian causes, such as having too few vehicles and insufficient fuel to permit both Ebola field activities and routine outreach services.

Simultaneously, demand for services fell dramatically during the epidemic, even in locations where facilities remained open. Most studies have focused on locales with intense transmission and, therefore, a relatively high risk of encountering EVD patients in clinical settings. A Guinean study, for example, found a 40% reduction in outpatient visits and a nearly 50% reduction in HIV care at a rural district hospital.[13] Similar reductions in HIV care were observed at the two largest hospitals in Monrovia.[14] In Bong County, a Liberian epicenter, facility-based delivery fell by two-thirds during the epidemic's peak.[15] A Sierra Leonean qualitative study found fear of facilities to be the primary explanation for why women avoided maternal services in a heavily affected location. Interestingly, over the course of the epidemic, the basis for fears converted from misconceptions about HCW malfeasance to perceived transmission risks.[16]

Limited evidence suggests that fear of facility-acquired infections also impacted care seeking in locations with few cases. For example, a study in Rivercess County,

---

[11] World Health Organization, Liberia Tackles Measles as the Ebola Epidemic Comes to an End (2015), available at http://www.who.int/features/2015/measles-vaccination-liberia/en/; World Health Organization Regional Office for Africa. Liberia Conducts First Polio, Measles Vaccination since Ebola Epidemic (2015), available at http://www.afro.who.int/en/liberia/press-materials/item/7654-joint-statement-from-the-ministry-of-health-and-social-welfare-liberia-the-cdc-unicef-and-the-who.html.

[12] Child Protection Working Group, Secondary Data Review: Child Protection Risks and Needs in Ebola Affected Countries (2015), available at http://cpwg.net/wp-content/uploads/sites/2/2015/02/SDR_ChildProtection_Ebola_2015.01.19_HJ1.docx; United Nations, The World Bank, European Union, and African Development Bank, Recovering from the Ebola Crisis 1–118 (2015).

[13] David Leuenberger et al., *Impact of the Ebola epidemic on general and HIV care in Macenta, Forest Guinea, 2014*, 29(14) AIDS 1883–1887 (Sep. 10, 2015).

[14] Paul Loubet et al., *Likely effect of the 2014 Ebola epidemic on HIV care in Monrovia, Liberia*, 29(17) AIDS 2347–2351 (Nov. 2015).

[15] Iyengar et al., *supra* note 8.

[16] Michelle Dynes et al., *Centers for Disease Control and Prevention (CDC). Perceptions of the risk for Ebola and health facility use among health workers and pregnant and lactating women—Kenema District, Sierra Leone, September 2014*, 63(51) MMWR Morb Mortal Wkly Rep 1226–1227 (Jan. 2, 2015).

Liberia, which had only a single EVD cluster, found that facility-based delivery dropped by almost 10% during the epidemic—reversing a trend toward greater facility-based delivery observed in previous years. Reductions in facility-based delivery were concentrated among those who believed health facilities posed an Ebola transmission risk.[17]

Several surveys of knowledge, attitudes, and practices (KAP) support the conclusion that the Ebola epidemic broadly worsened facility-based care seeking. A Liberian study conducted during the epidemic's peak found that about 55% of the public feared visiting treatment centers, though the majority reported that they would take a family member or go themselves if they developed Ebola symptoms. Fear of going to a treatment center if the respondent developed symptoms—which include symptoms of endemic diseases such as malaria—was about twice as high among respondents in locations with a low Ebola burden than in the most affected locales.[18] Indeed, in another Liberian study, the majority or respondents who reported they would not visit a health facility for suspected Ebola explained that they believed the facility would be contaminated.[19] Fear of health facilities was not unreasonable considering infection control challenges in the affected countries. In the United States, by contrast, where very few cases occurred, a nationally representative study conducted in December 2014 found that 13% of Americans intended to avoid health facilities to reduce their Ebola risk.[20]

Long-Term Health System Effects

Ebola's short-term collateral effects on the health systems of Guinea, Liberia, and Sierra Leone will likely continue. HCW deaths during the epidemic will challenge rebuilding and maintenance of essential health services. Liberia lost at least 5 of its estimated 90 physicians, 75 of its 1,800 nurses and midwives, and 9 of its 376 laboratory workers.[21] Similar losses were seen in Guinea and Sierra Leone. These

---

[17] John Ly et al., *Facility-based delivery during the Ebola virus disease epidemic in rural Liberia: analysis from a cross-sectional, population-based household survey*, Plos Med [forthcoming 2016].

[18] Miwako Kobayashi et al., *Community knowledge, attitudes, and practices regarding Ebola virus disease—five counties, Liberia, September-October, 2014*, 64(26) MMWR Morb Mortal Wkly Rep 714–718 (July 10, 2015).

[19] Liberia Ministry of Health and Social Welfare, National Knowledge, Attitudes, and Practices (KAP) Study on Ebola Virus Disease in Liberia 1–98 (2015).

[20] Bridget Kelly et al., *Perceptions and plans for prevention of Ebola: results from a national survey*, 15(1) BMC Public Health 1136-015-2441-7 (Nov. 16, 2015).

[21] World Health Organization Regional Office for Africa, Liberia: Health Workforce (2015), available at http://www.aho.afro.who.int/profiles_information/index.php/Liberia:Health_workforce_-_The_Health_System; World Health Organization, Health Worker Ebola Infections in Guinea, Liberia, and Sierra Leone 1–15 (2015).

figures likely underestimate actual numbers because EVD case registries incompletely recorded patients' status as HCWs.[22] It remains to be seen whether the epidemic will motivate HCW departures for safer, better-compensated positions in other countries. Anecdotal evidence suggests that EVD-related risks and the health system's inability to mitigate them for HCWs greatly contributed to worker dissatisfaction.[23] Before Ebola, the health workforce in all three countries was as sparse as anywhere in the world, that it was heavily concentrated in urban areas, and that capacity to train new skilled healthcare workers was limited. In Liberia, for example, there are currently 40 medical students—graduating 10 per year—and approximately 1,200 nursing and midwifery students.[24] Without substantial investments, it will take years for these three countries to resume their pre-Ebola health trajectories.

Health service interruptions will also have long-term ramifications, especially with respect to public health efforts with the most ameliorating effects, such as vaccine, bednet, and contraception provision. All three countries had pre-Ebola vaccination rates below levels necessary to maintain herd immunity against most vaccine-preventable illnesses.[25] Mathematical models suggest that vaccine disruptions were sufficient to enable large, generalized measles epidemics and increase the likelihood that they could affect bordering countries, which also have pockets with vaccination rates below those needed for herd immunity.[26] Similarly, bednet coverage was well below levels required for substantial community-level effects before the Ebola epidemic.[27] Lapses in community bednet distribution is expected to undermine the affected countries' malaria control initiatives, with mathematical

---

[22] *Id.*

[23] Agence France-Presse, *S. Leone Nurses Strike Over Ebola Hazard Pay Amid Lockdown.* (2015), available at http://reliefweb.int/report/sierra-leone/sleone-nurses-strike-over-ebola-hazard-pay-amid-lockdown, accessed Jan, 20, 2016; A. Look, Liberian Health Workers to Strike Over Ebola Hazard Pay (2014), available at http://www.voanews.com/content/liberian-health-workers-to-strike-over-ebola-hazard-pay/2476701.html, accessed Jan, 20, 2016.

[24] Liberia Ministry of Health and Social Welfare, Investment Plan for Building a Resilient Health System in Liberia 1–64 (2015).

[25] Liberia Institute of Statistics and Geo-Information Services (Monrovia), Liberia Demographic and Health Survey 2013 (2014); Statistics Sierra Leone, Sierra Leone Ministry of Health and Sanitation, and ICF Macro, Sierra Leone Demographic and Health Survey 2013 (2014); Institut National de la Statisique and ICF Macro, Guinea Enquete Demographique et de Sante et a Indicateurs Multiples (2013).

[26] Takahashi et al., *supra* note 10.

[27] Liberia Institute of Statistics and Geo-Information Services (Monrovia), Liberia Demographic and Health Survey 2013 (2014); Statistics Sierra Leone, Sierra Leone Ministry of Health and Sanitation, and ICF Macro, Sierra Leone Demographic and Health Survey 2013 (2014); Institut National de la Statisique and ICF Macro, Guinea Enquete Demographique et de Sante et a Indicateurs Multiples (2013); Folashade Agusto et al., *The impact of bed-net use on malaria prevalence*, 320 J Theor Biol 58–65 (Mar. 7, 2013).

models suggesting that an excess of 3.5 million malaria cases could be attributable to the epidemic in 2014 and 2015.[28] Emergency distribution, such as through a Global Fund emergency fund procurement of 400,000 bednets in Liberia,[29] may have reduced long-term risks. However, because distribution through mass gatherings was substituted for door-to-door campaigns, there is a risk of muted impact, particularly in rural areas with low population density.

The effects of interruptions in contraception outreach are currently unknown. Qualitative research suggests that adolescent pregnancy increased during the Ebola epidemic in Sierra Leone due to prolonged school closures and interruption of family planning services.[30] This is consistent with anecdotes from elsewhere in the region, which reported that pregnancy rates increased during the epidemic.[31] Over the long term, substantial increases in unintended pregnancies would be expected to increase maternal and child mortality. Equally important, pregnancy resulting in premature school cessation reduces women's autonomy and, secondarily, harms households' health and economic outcomes.[32] Future health surveys in the region will be required to quantify the full extent of maternal and child health fallout.

Finally, the Ebola epidemic caused dramatic macroeconomic disruptions across Guinea, Liberia, and Sierra Leone.[33] Economic losses across the three countries exceeded $500 million in 2014 and are estimated to be $1.6 billion in 2015. These correspond to 5% and 12% losses to combined GDP, respectively, with reverberating impacts expected to continue in the coming years. Substantial, sustained job loss, particularly among women, whose work as traders or small merchants was most disrupted by the epidemic, has been documented.[34] Epidemic-related food insecurity

---

[28] Patrick Walker et al., *Malaria morbidity and mortality in Ebola-affected countries caused by decreased health-care capacity, and the potential effect of mitigation strategies: a modelling analysis*, 15(7) Lancet Infect Dis 825–832 (Apr. 23, 2015).

[29] The Global Fund to Fight AIDS, Tuberculosis and Malaria, Global Fund News Flash: Bringing the Net Effect to Liberia (2015) available at http://www.theglobalfund.org/en/blog/2015-05-01_Global_Fund_News_Flash/; President's Malaria Initiative, Liberia Malaria Operational Plan FY 2016 (2015).

[30] Isabelle Risso-Gill, Children's Ebola Recovery Assessment: Sierra Leone (2015).

[31] Streifel, *supra* note 9; Jane Labous, *Ebola Shutdown Brings New Fears of Rape and Teenage Pregnancy*, available at http://news.trust.org//item/20141117091228-3n0cq/; Cinnatus Dumbaya, *Sierra Leone's First Lady: Ebola Has Increased Teenage Pregnancy Rates* (2015), available at http://archive.eboladeeply.org/articles/2015/01/7263/sierra-leones-lady-ebola-increased-teenage-pregnancy-rates/.

[32] Simon Appleton, Education and Health at the Household Level in Sub-Saharan Africa (2000); The World Bank Group, Voice and Agency: Empowering Women and Girls for Shared Prosperity (2014).

[33] Mark Siedner et al., *Strengthening the detection of and early response to public health emergencies: lessons from the West African Ebola epidemic*, 12(3) PLoS Med e1001804 (2015).

[34] The World Bank Group, The Economic Impact of Ebola on Sub-Saharan Africa: Updated Estimates for 2015 (2015).

increased in urban areas even though actual food shortages appeared to be rare; rather, economic disruption in urban areas appears to have increased the extent to which food became unaffordable in Liberia,[35] and there is some evidence that Ebola-related transport and market-gathering restrictions drove up prices in Sierra Leone.[36] The worst rural effects occurred where epidemic control measures prevented farmers from hiring laborers to help harvest or made crop sales impossible.[37]

Ebola's economic effects have also harmed national budgets. The Liberian government, for example, is expected to collect $100 million less in revenue in the first year after Ebola than pre-epidemic predictions—a 20% reduction in inflows. The need for national expenditures to combat Ebola and its effects, while partially offset by international funds, has caused a national budget deficit exceeding 10% of GDP, in contrast to a nearly balanced budget the year before. These shortfalls are projected to have major long-term implications for the sustainability of health system funding. In the short term, the country has sought to reduce its budget deficit by reducing funding for vehicle fuel by 25% and freezing the purchase of new vehicles and other "nonessential" goods.[38] This, unfortunately, can be expected to limit the resumption of health outreach activities—such as community contraception services—which the epidemic interrupted. As such, revenue reductions and austerity measures are likely to impact affected countries' health sectors for the coming years.

Restoring Health Systems and Building Resilience

For health systems, recovery from the Ebola epidemic will take years. Doing so will require the countries and their development partners to achieve two interrelated goals. First, health systems must be restored to their pre-Ebola levels and strengthened to the point where they can meet their populations' essential health needs—a challenge that requires substantial progress, especially in rural areas.[39] Second, health systems must be made more resilient, such that shocks like Ebola can be managed effectively and efficiently.[40] The challenge, of course, is how to tackle both

---

[35] Liberia Institute of Statistics and Geo-Information Services, the World Bank Group, and Gallup, The Socio-Economic Impact of Ebola in Liberia: Results From a High-Frequency Cell Phone Survey Round 5 (2015).

[36] Statistics Sierra Leone and the World Bank Group, The Socio-Economic Impacts of Ebola in Sierra Leone: Results of a High-Frequency Cell Phone Survey Round 3 (2015).

[37] Republic of Liberia, Economic Stabilization and Recovery Plan (2015).

[38] Id.

[39] Katherine Kentoffio et al., Charting Health System Reconstruction in Rural Liberia Prior to the Ebola Epidemic: A Comparison of Three Population-Based Surveys of Maternal and Child Healthcare Utilization, working paper [under review] (2016).

[40] David Heymann et al., *Global health security: the wider lessons from the West African Ebola virus disease epidemic*, 385(9980) Lancet 1884–1901 (May 9, 2015); Margaret Kruk et al., *What is a resilient health system? Lessons from Ebola*, 385(9980) Lancet 1910–1912 (May 9, 2015).

goals simultaneously and on timelines that will mitigate the pain attributable to the Ebola epidemic.

In the worst case, large-scale investments to protect against rare, high-consequence shocks can cause health systems to prioritize efforts to combat unlikely events over routine health needs.[41] On the other hand, there exist ample opportunities to build health system components that simultaneously strengthen the capabilities required for routine service delivery and make systems less fragile and more responsive to emergencies.[42] As a first step, strengthening rural health services, improving HCW protections, and better implementing the International Health Regulations would build stronger, more resilient health systems.

Strengthening Rural Health Services

Before the Ebola epidemic, rural-urban disparities in health outcomes and healthcare access were striking in Guinea, Liberia, and Sierra Leone. In Guinea, for example, rural women were 30% less likely to receive the recommended four antenatal checkups, and rural children with signs of pneumonia were less than half as likely to be treated in a health facility.[43] A study in rural Liberia found that more remote populations were less likely to access maternal and child health services and more likely to substitute informal and traditional providers for formal ones. In rural populations, accessing facility-based services tends to be more expensive than for urban dwellers because of substantial transportation costs and lost wages that accompany lengthy travel (when transport is even available).[44]

Strong community health systems reduce disparities between rural and urban health outcomes. Several systematic reviews have found evidence that community-health worker (CHW)-based programs are effective at reducing neonatal and child mortality, and improve maternal outcomes.[45] As a strategy for improving rural

---

[41] Gerald Markowitz and David Rosner, Emergency Preparedness, Bioterrorism, and the States: The First Two Years After September 11 (2004); Mike Stoto et al., *Lessons about the state and local public health system response to the 2009 H1N1 pandemic: a workshop summary*, 19(5) J Public Health Manag Pract 428–435 (Sept.–Oct. 2013).

[42] Kruk et al., *supra* note 40; Markowitz and Rosner, *supra* note 40; Stoto, et. al., *supra* note 40; Mike Stoto and Melissa Higdon, The Public Health Response to 2009 H1N1: A Systems Perspective (2015).

[43] Institut National de la Statisique and ICF Macro, Guinea Enquete Demographique et de Sante et a Indicateurs Multiples (2013).

[44] Avi Kenny et al., *Remoteness and maternal and child health service utilization in rural Liberia: a population-based survey*, 5(2) J Glob Health 020401 (Dec. 2015).

[45] Zohra Lassi and Zulfiqar Bhutta, *Community-based intervention packages for reducing maternal and neonatal morbidity and mortality and improving neonatal outcomes*, Cochrane Database Syst Rev 2015 Mar 23;3:CD007754; Simon Lewin et al., *Lay health workers in primary and community health care for maternal and child health and the management of infectious diseases*, Cochrane Database Syst Rev 2010 Mar 17;(3):CD004015. doi(3):CD004015; Agbessi Amouzou et al., *Assessing the impact of integrated community case management (iCCM) programs on child mortality: review of early results and lessons learned in sub-Saharan Africa*, 4(2) J Glob Health 020411 (Dec. 2014).

health, Liberia recently unveiled an ambitious plan to achieve a national CHW network as part of its integrated national strategy to rebuild a resilient health system.[46]

Community health programs work best when they are linked through adequate referral networks to higher-level facility-based care and integrated with national mechanisms for disease surveillance, health information management, and supply management.[47] These features also enhance resilience—enabling rapid identification of and response to emergencies while also continuing basic services even if facility-based care ceases. Increased community services can also support epidemic control measures by encouraging greater community buy-in.[48]

Protecting and Supporting Health Workers

Recognition of cases, triage and isolation, and provision of PPE were major challenges during the Ebola epidemic in all three countries.[49] These barriers were most apparent in preventable and tragic HCW infections and deaths, most of which appear to have occurred outside of Ebola-specific treatment sites.[50] HCW deaths will cause long-term harm to health systems in which worker scarcity was already severe. Less noticed, however, was the extent to which unsafe working conditions caused HCWs refrained from caring for patients and how these factors led to disruptions in routine care provision at health facilities.[51] There were multiple HCW strikes during the epidemic, as workers attempted to increase awareness about the lack of access to PPE and inadequate hazard pay.[52] Similarly, facilities with HCW

---

[46] Liberia Ministry of Health and Social Welfare, Investment Plan for Building a Resilient Health System in Liberia 1–64 (2015).

[47] World Health Organization, Global Health Workforce Alliance, Global Experience of Community Health Workers for Delivery of Health Related Millennium Development Goals: A Systematic Review, Country Case Studies, and Recommendations for Integration into National Health Systems (2010).

[48] Mosaka Fallah et al., *Interrupting Ebola transmission in Liberia through community-based initiatives*, 164(5) Ann Intern Med (Jan. 5, 2016); Aisha Yansaneh et al., *Determinants of utilization and community experiences with community health volunteers for treatment of childhood illnesses in rural Sierra Leone*, 41(2) J Community Health 376–386 (April 2016); Francis Kateh et al., *Rapid response to Ebola outbreaks in remote areas—Liberia, July–November 2014*, 64(7) MMWR Morb Mortal Wkly Rep 188–192 (Feb. 27, 2015).

[49] Peter Kilmarx et al., *Ebola virus disease in health care workers—Sierra Leone, 2014*, 63(49) MMWR Morb Mortal Wkly Rep 1168–1171 (Dec. 12, 2014); Ishani Pathmanathan et al., *Rapid assessment of Ebola infection prevention and control needs—six districts, Sierra Leone, October 2014*, 63(49) MMWR Morb Mortal Wkly Rep 1172–1174 (Dec. 12, 2014).

[50] Margaret Grinnell et al., *Ebola virus disease in health care workers—Guinea, 2014*, 64(38) MMWR Morb Mortal Wkly Rep 1083–1087 (Oct. 2, 2015); Olushayo Olu et al., *Epidemiology of Ebola virus disease transmission among health care workers in Sierra Leone, May to December 2014: a retrospective descriptive study*, 416 BMC Infect Dis (Oct. 13, 2015).

[51] Rony Zachariah et al., *Ebola, fragile health systems and tuberculosis care: a call for pre-emptive action and operational research*, 19(11) Int J Tuberc Lung Dis 1271–1275 (Nov. 2015).

[52] Agence France-Presse, S. Leone Nurses Strike over Ebola Hazard Pay Amid Lockdown 20, available at http://reliefweb.int/report/sierra-leone/sleone-nurses-strike-over-ebola-hazard-pay-amid-

infections—including facilities operated by international NGOs—generally ceased operations, sometimes for lengthy durations.[53] In other instances, inadequate infection control caused hospital-associated outbreaks.[54]

Inadequate infection control has long been recognized as a problem in many sub-Saharan African settings. While surveillance data are sparse, studies have repeatedly found clinicians to be at elevated risk for tuberculosis,[55] viral hepatitis,[56] HIV, and other infections.[57] Facility-acquired infections contribute to health system fragility even under non-epidemic conditions by leading to deaths and illness-related absences and by causing HCWs to emigrate for safer working conditions.[58] Poor infection control measures also contribute significantly to morbidity and mortality in the broader population,[59] with one Kenyan study estimating that 5% of in-hospital deaths were attributable to hospital-acquired bacteremia.[60]

Reducing nosocomial infection is a complicated challenge that must begin with routine incorporation of infection control into all healthcare settings. This

---

lockdown; A Look, Liberian Health Workers to Strike Over Ebola Hazard Pay (2014), available at http://www.voanews.com/content/liberian-health-workers-to-strike-over-ebola-hazard-pay/2476701.html, accessed Jan. 20, 2016.

[53] Pathmanathan et al., *supra* note 49; Grinnell et al., *supra* note 50; Olu et al., *supra* note 50; Zachariah et al., *supra* note 51; Joseph Forrester et al., *Cluster of Ebola cases among Liberian and U.S. health care workers in an Ebola treatment unit and adjacent hospital—Liberia, 2014*, 63(41) MMWR Morb Mortal Wkly Rep 925–929 (Oct. 17, 2014).

[54] Angela Dunn et al., *Nosocomial transmission of Ebola virus disease on pediatric and maternity wards: Bombali and Tonkolili, Sierra Leone*, 44(3) Am J Infect Control 269–272 (Mar. 1, 2016); Paul Shears and TJ O'Dempsey, *Ebola virus disease in Africa: epidemiology and nosocomial transmission*, 90(1) J Hosp Infect 1–9 (2015).

[55] Ntambwe Malangu and A Legothoane, *Analysis of occupational infections among health care workers in Limpopo Province of South Africa*, 5(1) Glob J Health Sci 44–51 (Nov. 2, 2012); Shahieda Adams et al., *Incidence of occupational latent tuberculosis infection in South African healthcare workers* 45(5) Eur Respir J 1364–1373 (May 2015); Anthony Harries et al., *Practical and affordable measures for the protection of health care workers from tuberculosis in low-income countries* 75(5) Bull World Health Organ 477–489 (1997).

[56] S. Rebaudet et al., *Risk of nosocomial infection in intertropical Africa—part 3: health care workers*, 67(3) Med Trop (Mars) 291–300 (2007).

[57] Elisabeth Rouveix et al., *Promoting the safety of healthcare workers in Africa: from HIV pandemic to Ebola epidemic*, 36(3) Infect Control Hosp Epidemiol 361–362 (Mar. 2015); TM Rossouw et al., *Blood-borne infections in healthcare workers in South Africa*, 104(11) S Afr Med J 732–735 (Nov. 2014); A. Dusé, *Infection control in developing countries with particular emphasis on South Africa*, 20(2) Southern African Journal of Epidemiology and Infection 37–41 (2005).

[58] Marko Vujicic et al., *The role of wages in the migration of health care professionals from developing countries*, 2(1) Hum Resour Health 3 (Apr. 28, 2004); World Health Organization, *The world health report: 2006: working together for health* (2006).

[59] Sepideh Bagheri Nejad et al., *Health-care-associated infection in Africa: a systematic review*, 89(10) Bull World Health Organ 757–765 Oct. 1, 2011).

[60] AM Aiken et al., *Risk and causes of paediatric hospital-acquired bacteraemia in Kilifi District Hospital, Kenya: a prospective cohort study*, 378(9808) Lancet 2021–2027 (Dec. 10, 2011).

requires adequate HCW training and supervision, appropriate facility construction and the maintenance of safe conditions, routinized infection identification and triage practices, and standard PPE provision and use. It has been argued that routine infection control practices would have greatly reduced the extent to which HCWs were infected during the epidemic's early stages.[61] However, while countries should ideally reserve an emergency supply of infection control materials, they likely cannot maintain adequate stocks of specialized equipment for large-scale epidemics without significantly trading off resources that could be used for routine health needs. During the Ebola epidemic, PPE stockouts were common, as procurement and supply chain systems were not able to rapidly deliver needed equipment to facilities.[62] As such, high-income countries must meet their International Health Regulations obligation to finance the WHO Contingency Fund for these needs.[63]

Strengthening IHR Implementation

The International Health Regulations form the backbone of collective global health security, but they remain incompletely implemented. Minimizing the potential for large-scale public health crises requires steps to be taken by both member states and the WHO. On one hand, the IHR obliges countries to build core domestic public health capacities—such as surveillance, emergency response, risk communication, and laboratory capacities—to identify and respond to emergencies before they cross national borders. It also requires the timely notification of potential emergencies to WHO. Although notification occurred promptly, initial identification of the epidemic was delayed in part by weak surveillance capacity in Guinea and weak response capacities in all three countries.[64] Simultaneously, the IHR charges WHO with declaring public health emergencies of international concern (PHEICs), issuing temporary recommendations, and supporting emergency response activities. High-income countries have IHR-based treaty obligations to

---

[61] World Health Organization, Health Worker Ebola Infections in Guinea, Liberia, and Sierra Leone 1–15 (2015).

[62] United Nations, The World Bank, European Union, and African Development Bank, Recovering from the Ebola Crisis 1–118 (2015); Olu et al., *supra* note 50; Janine Barden-O'Fallon et al., *Rapid assessment of Ebola-related implications for reproductive, maternal, newborn and child health service delivery and utilization in Guinea*, PLoS Curr (Aug. 4, 2015).

[63] Siedner et al., *supra* note 33; Suerie Moon et al, *Will Ebola change the game? Ten essential reforms before the next pandemic. The report of the Harvard-LSHTM Independent Panel on the Global Response to Ebola*, 386 (10009) Lancet 2204–2221 (Nov. 28, 2015).

[64] Siedner et al., *supra* note 33; Mark Siedner and John Kraemer, *The Global Response to the Ebola Fever Epidemic: What Took So Long?* (2014), available at http://blogs.plos.org/speakingofmedicine/2014/08/22/global-response-ebola-fever-epidemic-took-long/; Lawrence Gostin, Dan Lucey, and Alex Phelan, *The Ebola epidemic: a global health emergency*, 12(11) JAMA 1095–1096 (Sept. 17, 2014).

assist low-income countries to build capacities and to avoid unnecessarily restricting trade and travel in ways that might disincentivize countries from reporting potential PHEICs.[65]

When the epidemic began in 2014, all three principally affected countries had significant gaps in domestic IHR implementation. In contrast, counties that successfully handled Ebola cases during 2014, such as Nigeria, had more complete implementation.[66] This is not surprising, as achieving IHR capabilities requires a reasonably strong public health system, and Guinea, Liberia, and Sierra Leone have had very few resources to invest. These three countries made missteps during the epidemic—such as delaying calls for external assistance and, in some instances, enacting a cordon sanitaire that likely exacerbated economic harm and undermined public trust.[67] However, the failures by high-income countries before the epidemic to meet their capacity-building obligations were more egregious. Similarly, an independent expert panel led by the WHO determined that the delayed PHEIC declaration, a critical step in mobilizing global resources for the response, was a major contributor.[68] Nonetheless, the WHO Secretariat has continued to contest its role in the delay.[69]

A central paradox of the West African Ebola epidemic is that, eventually, high-income countries and international organizations—especially the governments of the United States, the United Kingdom, Germany, and France, as well as the World Bank[70]—expended enormous resources to control the epidemic. They should be commended for this. But those same resources are rarely made available to prevent epidemics, even though they would likely be more cost-effectively deployed then and could avert greater mortality. As an example, WHO's $100 million emergency fund, first proposed in 2011, was never funded by donors.[71] In contrast, the United States has appropriated over $6 billion to contain the Ebola epidemic.[72]

---

[65] Moon et al., *supra* note 63; John Kraemer, Mark Siedner, and Mike Stoto, *Analyzing variability in Ebola-related controls applied to returned travelers in the United States*, 13(5) Health Secur 295–306 (Sept.–Oct. 2015); World Health Organization, International Health Regulations (2005).

[66] World Health Organization, Global Health Observatory Data Repository: All Capacities Data by Country (2015), available at http://apps.who.int/gho/data/node.main-afro.IHR00ALLN?ang=en.

[67] Moon et al., *supra* note 63.

[68] World Health Organization, Report of the Ebola Interim Assessment Panel (2015).

[69] World Health Organization, WHO Secretariat Response to the Report of the Ebola Interim Assessment Panel (2015).

[70] Karen Grepin, *International donations to the Ebola virus outbreak: too little, too late?* 350 BMJ h376 (Feb. 3, 2015).

[71] Siedner et al., *supra* note 33.

[72] Jennifer Kates et al., The U.S. Response to Ebola: Status of the FY2015 Emergency Ebola Appropriation (2016), available at: http://kff.org/global-health-policy/issue-brief/the-u-s-response-to-ebola-status-of-the-fy2015-emergency-ebola-appropriation/

If, however, there is one positive outcome from the Ebola epidemic, it is that momentum may slowly be shifting toward pre-emergency commitments to build countries' capacity and strengthen the infrastructure for rapid global response. For example, theWHO formally created the Contingency Fund for Emergencies in 2015. Although China and Germany provided initial contributions, it remains woefully underfunded.[73] In addition to the WHO Contingency Fund, the nascent World Bank Pandemic Emergency Facility is designed to enable rapid disbursements of funds to curtail emergencies.[74] Similarly, the US-led Global Health Security Agenda is aimed in part at supporting countries to build IHR capabilities,[75] and the African Union's African Centres for Disease Control and Prevention, also supported by the US government, should facilitate regional collaboration to mitigate emergencies.[76] Finally, there are early signs that global partners, especially the World Bank, intend to fund major initiatives to strengthen health systems in the affected countries.[77]

Conclusion

The 2014–2015 West African Ebola epidemic underscored the importance of strong and resilient health systems. In the absence of such systems, the epidemic grew far larger and caused far more destruction in Guinea, Liberia, and Sierra Leone than would have occurred with a basic public health infrastructure in place. Fragile health systems also led to collateral health consequences, as routine services collapsed during the epidemic. The long-term consequences of the epidemic, stemming from healthcare worker deaths, degradation of herd immunity, undermined trust in the

---

[73] World Health Organization, The WHO Contingency Fund for Emergencies (2015); World Health Organization, Germany Provides US$1.1 million (EURO 1 million) to the WHO Contingency Fund for Emergencies (2015), available at http://www.who.int/about/who_reform/emergency-capacities/contingency-fund/germany-financing/en/; World Health Organization, WHO Contingency Fund for Emergencies Receives First Injection of Financing from China (2015), available at http://www.who.int/about/who_reform/emergency-capacities/contingency-fund/china-financing/en/.

[74] The World Bank, Pandemic Emergency Facility: Frequently Asked Questions (2016), available at http://www.worldbank.org/en/topic/pandemics/brief/pandemic-emergency-facility-frequently-asked-questions.

[75] Rebecca Katz et al., *Global health security agenda and the International Health Regulations: moving forward*, 12(5) Biosecur Bioterror 231–238 (Sept.–Oct. 2014); Lawrence Gostin and Alex Phelan, *The global health security agenda in an age of biosecurity*, 312(1) JAMA 27–28 (2014).

[76] Centers for Disease Control and Prevention, African Union and U.S. CDC Partner to Launch African CDC (2015), available at http://www.cdc.gov/media/releases/2015/p0413-african-union.html.

[77] Liberia Ministry of Health and Social Welfare, Investment Plan for Building a Resilient Health System in Liberia 1–64 (2015).

healthcare system, and economic devastation, will continue to worsen the health of the populations in the region. However, if global partners take seriously lessons gleaned from this epidemic, it remains possible that the necessary investments into the health infrastructure in this and similar regions can both improve the well-being of millions of people and prevent future epidemics from having similar disastrous effects. If so, the Ebola epidemic may provide a catalyst for sustained investments into a stronger, more resilient global public health system.

References

Adams S, Ehrlich R, Baatjies R, van Zyl-Smit RN, Said-Hartley Q, Dawson R, et al. *Incidence of occupational latent tuberculosis infection in South African healthcare workers.* 45(5) Eur Respir J 1364–1373 (2015).

Agence France-Presse. S. Leone Nurses Strike Over Ebola Hazard Pay Amid Lockdown (2015). Available at http://reliefweb.int/report/sierra-leone/sleone-nurses-strike-over-ebola-hazard-pay-amid-lockdown. Accessed Jan. 20, 2016.

Agusto FB, Del Valle SY, Blayneh KW, Ngonghala CN, Goncalves MJ, Li N, et al. *The impact of bed-net use on malaria prevalence.* 320 J Theor Biol 58–65 (Mar. 7, 2013).

Aiken AM, Mturi N, Njuguna P, Mohammed S, Berkley JA, Mwangi I, et al. *Risk and causes of paediatric hospital-acquired bacteraemia in Kilifi District Hospital, Kenya: a prospective cohort study.* 378(9808) Lancet 2021–2027 (Dec. 10, 2011).

Amouzou A, Morris S, Moulton LH, Mukanga D. *Assessing the impact of integrated community case management (iCCM) programs on child mortality: review of early results and lessons learned in sub-Saharan Africa* 4(2) J Glob Health 020411 (Dec. 2014).

Appleton S. Education and Health at the Household Level in Sub-Saharan Africa (2000).

Bagheri Nejad S, Allegranzi B, Syed SB, Ellis B, Pittet D. *Health-care-associated infection in Africa: a systematic review* 89(10) Bull World Health Organ 757–765 (Oct. 1, 2011).

Barden-O'Fallon J, Barry MA, Brodish P, Hazerjian J. *Rapid assessment of Ebola-related implications for reproductive, maternal, newborn and child health service delivery and utilization in guinea.* PLoS Curr 2015 Aug. 4;7:10.1371/currents.outbreaks.0b0ba06009dd091bc39ddb3c6d7b0826.

Bolkan HA, Bash-Taqi DA, Samai M, Gerdin M, von Schreeb J. *Ebola and indirect effects on health service function in Sierra Leone.* PLoS Curr (Dec. 19, 2014). Available at http://currents.plos.org/outbreaks/article/ebola-and-indirect-effects-on-health-service-function-in-sierra-leone/.

Centers for Disease Control and Prevention. African Union and U.S. CDC Partner to Launch African CDC (2015). Available at http://www.cdc.gov/media/releases/2015/p0413-african-union.html.

Child Protection Working Group. Secondary Data Review: Child Protection Risks and Needs in Ebola Affected Countries (2015). Available at http://cpwg.net/wp-content/uploads/sites/2/2015/02/SDR_ChildProtection_Ebola_2015.01.19_HJ1.docx.

Dumbaya C. Sierra Leone's First Lady: Ebola Has Increased Teenage Pregnancy Rates (2015). Available at http://archive.eboladeeply.org/articles/2015/01/7263/sierra-leones-lady-ebola-increased-teenage-pregnancy-rates/.

Dunn AC, Walker TA, Redd J, Sugerman D, McFadden J, Singh T, et al. *Nosocomial transmission of Ebola virus disease on pediatric and maternity wards: Bombali and Tonkolili, Sierra Leone.* 44(3) Am J Infect Control 269-272 (Mar. 1, 2016).

Dusé A. *Infection control in developing countries with particular emphasis on South Africa.* 20(2) Southern African Journal of Epidemiology and Infection 37–41 (2005).

Dynes MM, Miller L, Sam T, Vandi MA, Tomczyk B, Centers for Disease Control and Prevention (CDC). *Perceptions of the risk for Ebola and health facility use among health workers and pregnant and lactating women—Kenema District, Sierra Leone, September 2014.* 63(51) MMWR Morb Mortal Wkly Rep 1226–1227 (Jan. 2, 2015).

Fallah M, Dahn B, Nyenswah TG, Massaquoi M, Skrip LA, Yamin D, et al. *Interrupting Ebola transmission in Liberia through community-based initiatives.* 164(5) Ann Intern Med (Jan. 5, 2016).

Forrester JD, Hunter JC, Pillai SK, Arwady MA, Ayscue P, Matanock A, et al. *Cluster of Ebola cases among Liberian and U.S. health care workers in an Ebola treatment unit and adjacent hospital—Liberia, 2014.* 63(41) MMWR Morb Mortal Wkly Rep 925–929 (Oct. 17, 2014).

The Global Fund to Fight AIDS, Tuberculosis and Malaria. Global Fund News Flash: Bringing the Net Effect to Liberia (2015). Available at http://www.theglobalfund.org/en/blog/2015-05-01_Global_Fund_News_Flash/.

Gostin LO, Lucey D, Phelan A. *The Ebola epidemic: a global health emergency.* 12(11) JAMA 1095–1096 (Sept. 17, 2014).

Gostin LO, Phelan A. *The global health security agenda in an age of biosecurity.* 312(1) JAMA 27–28 (July 2, 2014).

Grepin KA. *International donations to the Ebola virus outbreak: too little, too late?* 350 BMJ h376 (Feb. 3, 2015).

Grinnell M, Dixon MG, Patton M, Fitter D, Bilivogui P, Johnson C, et al. *Ebola virus disease in health care workers—Guinea, 2014.* 64(38) MMWR Morb Mortal Wkly Rep 1083–1087 (Oct. 2, 2015).

Harries AD, Maher D, Nunn P. *Practical and affordable measures for the protection of health care workers from tuberculosis in low-income countries.* 75(5) Bull World Health Organ 477–489 (1997).

Helleringer S, Noymer A. *Magnitude of Ebola relative to other causes of death in Liberia, Sierra Leone, and Guinea.* 3(5) Lancet Glob Health e255–e256 (May 3, 2015).

Heymann, David L. Control of communicable diseases manual (2008).

Heymann DL, Chen L, Takemi K, Fidler DP, Tappero JW, Thomas MJ, et al., *Global health security: the wider lessons from the West African Ebola virus disease epidemic.* 385(9980) Lancet 1884–1901 (May 9, 2015).

Institute for Health Metrics and Evaluation. GBD Compare: Region of the Americas and Haiti (2015). Available at http://ihmeuw.org/3qv6.

Institut National de la Statisique and ICF Macro. Guinea Enquete Demographique et de Sante et a Indicateurs Multiples (2013).

Iyengar P, Kerber K, Howe CJ, Dahn B. *Services for mothers and newborns during the Ebola outbreak in Liberia: the need for improvement in emergencies.* PLoS Curr (Apr. 16, 2015). Available at http://currents.plos.org/outbreaks/article/services-for-mothers-and-newborns-during-the-ebola-outbreak-in-liberia-the-need-for-improvement-in-emergencies/.

Kateh F, Nagbe T, Kieta A, Barskey A, Gasasira AN, Driscoll A, et al. *Rapid response to Ebola outbreaks in remote areas—Liberia, July–November 2014.* 64(7) MMWR Morb Mortal Wkly Rep 188–192 (Feb. 27, 2015).

Kates J, Michaud J, Wexler A, Valentine A. *The U.S. Response to Ebola: Status of the FY2015 Emergency Ebola Appropriation* (2016). Available at http://kff.org/global-health-policy/issue-brief/the-u-s-response-to-ebola-status-of-the-fy2015-emergency-ebola-appropriation/.

Katz R, Sorrell EM, Kornblet SA, Fischer JE. *Global health security agenda and the International Health Regulations: moving forward.* 12(5) Biosecur Bioterror 231–238 (Sept.–Oct. 2014).

Kelly B, Squiers L, Bann C, Stine A, Hansen H, Lynch M. *Perceptions and plans for prevention of Ebola: results from a national survey.* 15(1) BMC Public Health 1136-015-2441-7 (Nov. 16, 2015).

Kenny A, Basu G, Ballard M, Griffiths T, Kentoffio K, Niyonzima JB, et al. *Remoteness and maternal and child health service utilization in rural Liberia: a population-based survey.* 5(2) J Glob Health 020401 (Dec. 2015).

Kentoffio KJ, Kraemer J, Griffiths T, Kenny A, Panjabi R, Sechler GA, et al. Charting Health System Reconstruction in Rural Liberia Prior to the Ebola Epidemic: A Comparison of Three

Population-Based Surveys of Maternal and Child Healthcare Utilization. Working Paper [under review] 2016.

Kilmarx PH, Clarke KR, Dietz PM, Hamel MJ, Husain F, McFadden JD, et al. *Ebola virus disease in health care workers—Sierra Leone, 2014*. 63(49) MMWR Morb Mortal Wkly Rep 1168–1171 (Dec. 12, 2014).

Kobayashi M, Beer KD, Bjork A, Chatham-Stephens K, Cherry CC, Arzoaquoi S, et al. *Community knowledge, attitudes, and practices regarding Ebola virus disease—five counties, Liberia, September–October, 2014*. 64(26) MMWR Morb Mortal Wkly Rep 714–718 (July 10, 2015).

Kraemer JD, Siedner MJ, Stoto MA. *Analyzing variability in Ebola-related controls applied to returned travelers in the United States*. 13(5) Health Secur 295–306 (Sept.–Oct. 2015).

Kruk ME,. Myers M, Varpilah ST, Dahn BT. *What is a resilient health system? Lessons from Ebola*, 385(9980) Lancet 1910–1912 (May 9, 2015).

Labous J. Ebola Shutdown Brings New Fears of Rape and Teenage Pregnancy (2014). Available at http://news.trust.org//item/20141117091228-3n0cq/.

Lassi ZS, Bhutta ZA. *Community-based intervention packages for reducing maternal and neonatal morbidity and mortality and improving neonatal outcomes*. 3 Cochrane Database Syst Rev CD007754 (Mar. 23, 2015).

Leuenberger D, Hebelamou J, Strahm S, De Rekeneire N, Balestre E, Wandeler G, et al. *Impact of the Ebola epidemic on general and HIV care in Macenta, Forest Guinea, 2014*. 29(14) AIDS 1883-1887 (Sep. 10, 2015).

Lewin S, Munabi-Babigumira S, Glenton C, Daniels K, Bosch-Capblanch X, van Wyk BE, et al. *Lay health workers in primary and community health care for maternal and child health and the management of infectious diseases*. 3 Cochrane Database Syst Rev CD004015 (Mar. 17, 2010).

Liberia Institute of Statistics and Geo-Information Services (Monrovia). Liberia Demographic and Health Survey 2013 (2014).

Liberia Institute of Statistics and Geo-Information Services, the World Bank Group, and Gallup. The Socio-economic Impact of Ebola in Liberia: Results from a High-Frequency Cell Phone Survey Round 5 (2015).

Liberia Ministry of Health and Social Welfare. Investment Plan for Building a Resilient Health System in Liberia 1–64 (2015).

———. National Knowledge, Attitudes, and Practices (KAP) Study on Ebola Virus Disease in Liberia 1–98 (2015).

Look A. Liberian Health Workers to Strike Over Ebola Hazard Pay (2014). Available at http://www.voanews.com/content/liberian-health-workers-to-strike-over-ebola-hazard-pay/2476701.html.

Loubet P, Mabileau G, Baysah M, Nuta C, Taylor M, Jusu H, et al. *Likely effect of the 2014 Ebola epidemic on HIV care in Monrovia, Liberia*. 29(17) AIDS 2347-2351 (2015).

Ly J, Sathananthan V, Griffiths T, Kanjee Z, Kenny A, Gordon N, et al. *Facility-based delivery during the Ebola virus disease epidemic in rural Liberia: analysis from a cross-sectional, population-based household survey*, Plos Med [forthcoming 2016].

Malangu N, Legothoane A. *Analysis of occupational infections among health care workers in Limpopo Province of South Africa* 5(1) Glob J Health Sci 44–51 (Nov. 2, 2012).

Markowitz G, Rosner D. Emergency Preparedness, Bioterrorism, and the States: The First Two Years After September 11 (2004).

Matanock A, Arwady MA, Ayscue P, Forrester JD, Gaddis B, Hunter JC, et al. *Ebola virus disease cases among health care workers not working in Ebola treatment units—Liberia, June-August, 2014*. 63(46) MMWR Morb Mortal Wkly Rep 1077–1081 (Nov. 21, 2014).

Meltzer MI, Atkins CY, Santibanez S, Knust B, Petersen BW, Ervin ED, et al. *Estimating the future number of cases in the Ebola epidemic—Liberia and Sierra Leone, 2014–2015*. 63 Suppl 3 MMWR Surveill Summ 1–14 (Sept. 26, 2014).

Moon S, Sridhar D, Pate M, Jha A, Clinton C, Delaunay S, et al. *Will Ebola change the game? Ten essential reforms before the next pandemic. The report of the Harvard-LSHTM Independent Panel on the*

Global Response to Ebola. 386 Lancet 2204–2221 (Nov. 28, 2015). Available at http://www.thelancet.com/journals/lancet/article/PIIS0140-6736%2815%2900946-0/abstract.

Olu O, Kargbo B, Kamara S, Wurie AH, Amone J, Ganda L, et al. *Epidemiology of Ebola virus disease transmission among health care workers in Sierra Leone, May to December 2014: a retrospective descriptive study*. 15 BMC Infect Dis 416-015-1166-7 (Oct. 13, 2015).

Pathmanathan I, O'Connor KA, Adams ML, Rao CY, Kilmarx PH, Park BJ, et al. *Rapid assessment of Ebola infection prevention and control needs—six districts, Sierra Leone, October 2014*. 63(49) MMWR Morb Mortal Wkly Rep 1172–1174 (Dec. 12, 2014).

Phillip A. *How Ebola is stealing attention from diseases that kill more people*. Washington Post (Sept. 5, 2014). Available at https://www.washingtonpost.com/news/to-your-health/wp/2014/09/05/how-ebola-the-kardashian-of-diseases-is-stealing-attention-from-illnesses-that-kill-more-people/.

President's Malaria Initiative. Liberia Malaria Operational Plan FY 2016 (2015).

Rebaudet S, Kraemer P, Savini H, De Pina JJ, Rapp C, Demortiere F, et al. *Risk of nosocomial infection in intertropical Africa—part 3: health care workers*. 67(3) Med Trop (Mars) 291–300 (2007).

Republic of Liberia. Economic Stabilization and Recovery Plan (2015).

Risso-Gill I, Finnegan L. Children's Ebola Recovery Assessment: Sierra Leone (2015).

Rossouw TM, van Rooyen M, Louw JM, Richter KL. *Blood-borne infections in healthcare workers in South Africa*. 104(11) S Afr Med J 732–735 (Nov. 2014).

Rouveix E, Madougou B, Pellissier G, Diaougah H, Saley SM, de Truchis P, et al. *Promoting the safety of healthcare workers in Africa: from HIV pandemic to Ebola epidemic*. 36(3) Infect Control Hosp Epidemiol 361–362 (Mar. 2015).

Shears P, O'Dempsey TJ. *Ebola virus disease in Africa: epidemiology and nosocomial transmission*. 90(1) J Hosp Infect 1–9 (2015).

Siedner MJ, Gostin LO, Cranmer HH, Kraemer JD. *Strengthening the detection of and early response to public health emergencies: lessons from the West African Ebola epidemic*. 12(3) PLoS Med e1001804 (2015).

Siedner MJ, Kraemer JD. *The Global Response to the Ebola Fever Epidemic: What Took So Long?* (2014). Available at http://blogs.plos.org/speakingofmedicine/2014/08/22/global-response-ebola-fever-epidemic-took-long/.

Statistics Sierra Leone, Sierra Leone Ministry of Health and Sanitation, and ICF Macro. Sierra Leone Demographic and Health Survey 2013 (2014).

Statistics Sierra Leone and the World Bank Group. The Socio-economic Impacts of Ebola in Sierra Leone: Results of a High-Frequency Cell Phone Survey Round 3 (2015).

Stoto MA, Higdon MA. The Public Health Response to 2009 H1N1: A Systems Perspective (2015).

Stoto MA, Nelson C, Higdon MA, Kraemer J, Hites L, Singleton CM. *Lessons about the state and local public health system response to the 2009 H1N1 pandemic: a workshop summary* 19(5) J Public Health Manag Pract 428–435 (Sept.–Oct. 2013).

Streifel C. How Did Ebola Impact Maternal and Child Health in Liberia and Sierra Leone? 1–19 (2015). Available at http://csis.org/files/publication/151019_Streifel_EbolaLiberiaSierraLeone_Web.pdf.

Takahashi S, Metcalf CJ, Ferrari MJ, Moss WJ, Truelove SA, Tatem AJ, et al. *Reduced vaccination and the risk of measles and other childhood infections post-Ebola*. 347(6227) Science 1240–1242 (Mar. 13, 2015).

Walker PG, White MT, Griffin JT, Reynolds A, Ferguson NM, Ghani AC. *Malaria morbidity and mortality in Ebola-affected countries caused by decreased health-care capacity, and the potential effect of mitigation strategies: a modelling analysis*. 15(7) Lancet Infect Dis 825–832 (Apr. 23, 2015).

United Nations, the World Bank, European Union, and African Development Bank. Recovering from the Ebola Crisis 1–118 (2015).

Vujicic M, Zurn P, Diallo K, Adams O, Dal Poz MR. *The role of wages in the migration of health care professionals from developing countries*. 2(1) Hum Resour Health 3 (Apr. 28, 2004).

The World Bank. Pandemic Emergency Facility: Frequently Asked Questions (2016). Available at http://www.worldbank.org/en/topic/pandemics/brief/pandemic-emergency-facility-frequently-asked-questions.

The World Bank Group. The Economic Impact of Ebola on Sub-Saharan Africa: Updated Estimates for 2015 (2015).

———. Voice and Agency: Empowering Women and Girls for Shared Prosperity (2014).

World Health Organization. Ebola Situation Report—20 January 2016 (2016). Available at http://apps.who.int/ebola/current-situation/ebola-situation-report-20-january-2016.

———. Germany Provides US$1.1 million (EURO 1 million) to the WHO Contingency Fund for Emergencies (2015). Available at http://www.who.int/about/who_reform/emergency-capacities/contingency-fund/germany-financing/en/.

———. Global Health Observatory Data Repository: All Capacities Data by Country (2015). Available at http://apps.who.int/gho/data/node.main-afro.IHR00ALLN?ang=en.

———. Health Worker Ebola Infections in Guinea, Liberia, and Sierra Leone 1–15 (2015).

———. International Health Regulations (2005) (2008).

———. Liberia Tackles Measles as the Ebola Epidemic Comes to an End (2015). Available at http://www.who.int/features/2015/measles-vaccination-liberia/en/.

———. Report of the Ebola Interim Assessment Panel (2015).

———. The WHO Contingency Fund for Emergencies (2015).

———. WHO Contingency Fund for Emergencies Receives First Injection of Financing from China (2015). Available at http://www.who.int/about/who_reform/emergency-capacities/contingency-fund/china-financing/en/.

———. WHO Secretariat Response to the Report of the Ebola Interim Assessment Panel (2015).

———. The World Health Report: 2006: Working Together for Health (2006).

World Health Organization Regional Office for Africa. Liberia Conducts First Polio, Measles Vaccination Since Ebola Epidemic (2015). Available at http://www.afro.who.int/en/liberia/press-materials/item/7654-joint-statement-from-the-ministry-of-health-and-social-welfare-liberia-the-cdc-unicef-and-the-who.html.

———. Liberia: Health Workforce (2015). Available at http://www.aho.afro.who.int/profiles_information/index.php/Liberia:Health_workforce_-_The_Health_System.

Yansaneh AI, George AS, Sharkey A, Brieger WR, Moulton LH, Yumkella F, et al. *Determinants of utilization and community experiences with community health volunteers for treatment of childhood illnesses in rural Sierra Leone*. 41(2) J Community Health 376-386 (April 2016).

Zachariah R, Ortuno N, Hermans V, Desalegn W, Rust S, Reid AJ, et al. *Ebola, fragile health systems and tuberculosis care: a call for pre-emptive action and operational research*. 19(11) Int J Tuberc Lung Dis 1271–1275 (Nov. 2015).

4

Infectious Disease Threats in High-Resource Settings

The MERS-CoV Outbreak in Korea

SUGY CHOI, JONG-KOO LEE, AND DANIEL R. LUCEY

While the Ebola outbreak was spreading out of control in Guinea, Liberia, and Sierra Leone, dramatically illustrating the global threat infectious diseases pose in low-resource countries, the Middle East respiratory syndrome (MERS) spread to the Republic of Korea (ROK), demonstrating that even in high-resource settings, failures in basic measures may result in substantial loss of life and economic well-being. ROK has experienced unprecedented economic progress since its independence in 1945. After the severe acute respiratory syndrome (SARS) epidemic in 2003 in other parts of Asia and Canada, ROK reformed its guidelines and public health measures to combat infectious diseases; however, the 2015 MERS outbreak demonstrates that these measures were inadequate. The MERS outbreak documented 186 laboratory-confirmed cases and 38 deaths (case fatality rate of 20.4%). This outbreak also resulted in 16,752 individuals being placed in isolation and incurred a national economic loss in the tourism industry of 3.4 trillion won.[1]

Patient zero's diagnosis in the MERS outbreak ("index patient") was laboratory confirmed on May 20, 2015. The last case of this MERS epidemic was on July 4, 2015. Within these 6 weeks, ROK successfully contained the outbreak within multiple hospitals and outside them, extending into the general community. Several important lessons were learned from this outbreak in ROK. As of this writing, the 2015 MERS outbreak was the largest outside of the Middle East and the second-largest outbreak after those occurring in Saudi Arabia in 2012–2015.

---

[1] *Tourism industry suffers 3.4 tln won loss from MERS outbreak: report,* Yonhap (Nov. 6, 2015).

This chapter examines the challenges of combating a sudden infectious disease outbreak in a high-income, high-resource country. The chapter will present the major stages of the MERS outbreak, provide details of the public health measures to share lessons learned and actions taken, and identify remaining challenges.

Details of the Infection and Transmission of the 2015 MERS Outbreak in the Republic of Korea

The outbreak spread unmanageably in the Republic of Korea, especially in Seoul, Gyeong-gi Province, and Daejeon Province. Figure 4.1 presents the epidemiological curve of the MERS outbreak reported by the Korea Centers for Disease Control and Prevention (KCDC). The figure illustrates all of the 178 patients of the 186 for whom complete data are known between May 11 and July 1, 2015, arranged according to the four associated hospital clusters of the outbreak.[2]

Epidemiological curve of 178 confirmed cases of MERS-CoV infection in the Republic of Korea, 2015. Panel A (integrated curve) depicts the overall epidemiological curve by date of symptom onset. Panel B shows the epidemic curve of each of the three main clusters. Stages of transmission are expressed by different patterns. An additional case in Hospital H whose stage of transmission is uncertain is excluded.

The nosocomial MERS outbreak in ROK began with a 68-year-old male index case who traveled frequently to the Middle East for business-related reasons. Although he was asymptomatic during his return to ROK in May 2015, he was not informed about control measures regarding MERS after his trip to the Middle East at the Incheon International Airport.[3] After he developed a fever on May 11, 2015, he sought care at a local clinic from May 12 to 14. He reported his visit to Bahrain, where no documented human cases of MERS had been reported. He sought additional care at two other hospitals after his conditions worsened from May 15 to 17. Finally, on May 20, he was diagnosed and confirmed to be infected with MERS-CoV at Samsung Medical Center, the main tertiary referral hospital in Seoul.

In total, this index patient visited four different hospitals before receiving his correct diagnosis of MERS-CoV. He eventually revealed his complete travel history in detail, including visits to Bahrain (April 18–29, April 30–May 1, May 2), the United Arab Emirates (April 29–30), Saudi Arabia (May 1–2), and Qatar (May 2–3). After the diagnosis, he was transferred to the National Medical Center in Seoul for isolation. The index case is known to have had direct or indirect contact with 38 patients within a month, as of June 23, 2015. A joint World Health Organization–ROK

---

[2] Moran Ki, *2015 MERS outbreak in Korea: hospital-to-hospital transmission*, 37 Epidemiol Health (July 21, 2015).

[3] World Health Organization, Summary of Current Situation, Literature Update and Risk Assessment (July 7, 2015).

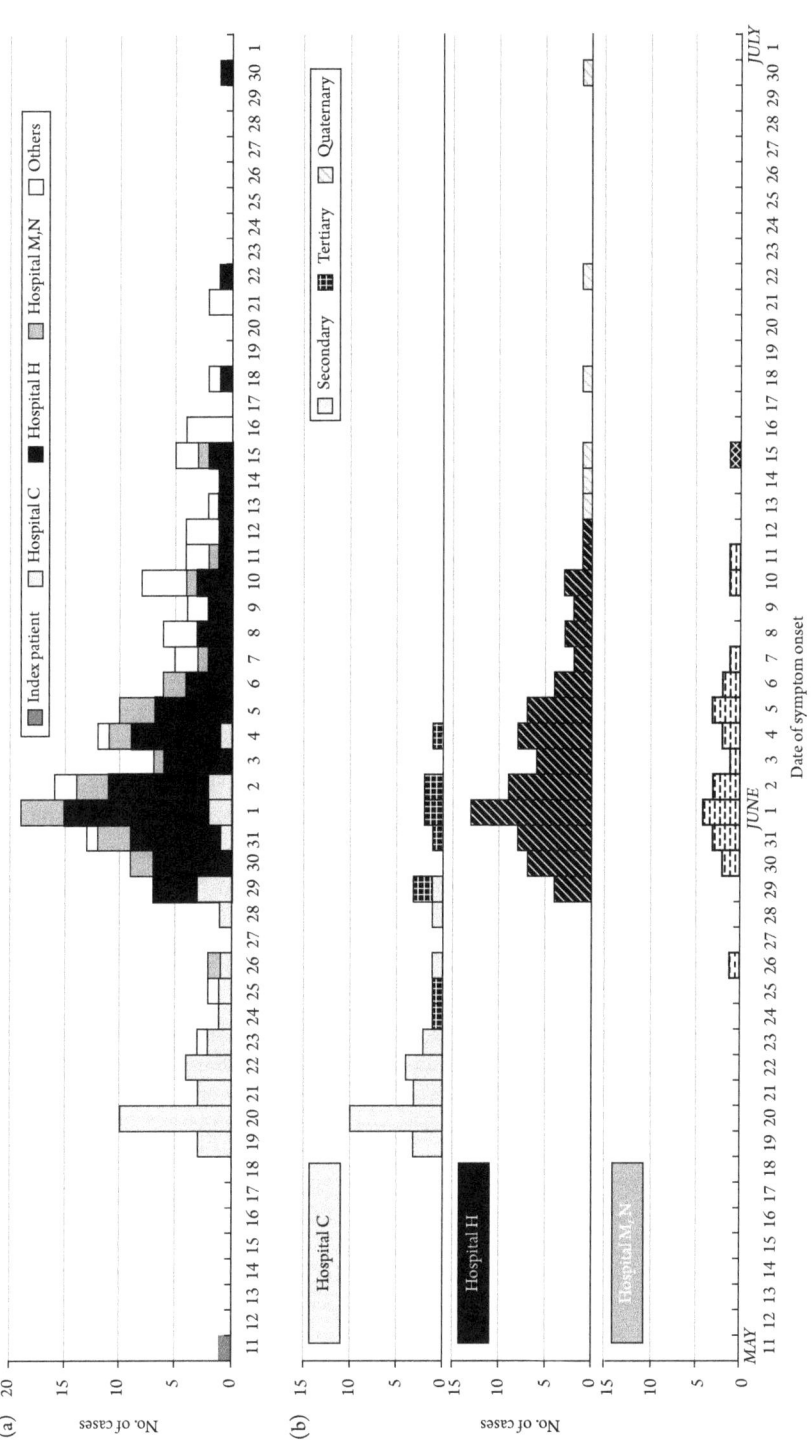

Figure 4.1 Epidemiological curve of the MERS outbreak (Korea Centers for Disease Control and Prevention).

Ministry of Health and Public Welfare commission has posted a detailed clinical course of the index patient as well.[4]

The index patient shared a hospital room with a patient who later infected his son, who in turn traveled to China. That patient did not comply with the recommended quarantine system and traveled by plane to Hong Kong on May 26, and then by bus to Huizhou in southern China. He was laboratory confirmed in Huizhou on May 29.[5]

The KCDC analyzed the demographic and epidemiological characteristics of all the laboratory-confirmed patients. The median age was 55 years, and 59.7% of the 186 confirmed cases were male. The majority of the confirmed cases were patients who had been exposed during admission or at clinics (44.1%) and caregivers (32.8%). The incubation period was 6.83 days (CI 95%: 6.31–7.36), and 95% of the infected patients had an onset of symptoms by day 13.48 (CI 95%: 12.23–14.37). When death occurred, it was by day 15 (CI 95%: 10–20) after illness onset.[6]

Among the most noteworthy aspects of the epidemic in ROK were the unprecedented four "superspreading"[7] events involving four patients (identified in the epidemiological chronicle as patients 1, 14, 16, and 76). Of the 186 total confirmed cases, 147 patients, or 79%, were infected by the four aforementioned superspreaders. In the Kingdom of Saudi Arabia, MERS-CoV transmission has not been reported in the literature to have been associated with even one superspreading event, if defined as for SARS, where 1 patient infects 10 or more other persons.

In sharp contrast, the Korean MERS epidemic was largely attributed to the role of these four superspreading events that occurred in hospital settings.[8] Adam Kucharski and Christian Althaus at the Centre for the Mathematical Modeling of Infectious Diseases, London School of Hygiene and Tropical Medicine, reported that an unprecedented outbreak like this one in ROK could be explained by the high probability of a single index case generating a transmission cluster of large numbers of other cases.[9] During the SARS outbreak, superspreading events led to

---

[4] World Health Organization, Middle East Respiratory Syndrome Coronavirus (MERS-CoV)-Republic of Korea (2015) [cited Jan. 5, 2016], available at http://www.who.int/mediacentre/news/mers/briefing-notes/update-15-06-2015/en/; Andrew Jack, *Why the panic? South Korea's MERS response questioned*, 350 BMJ (June 24, 2015), available at http://www.bmj.com/content/350/bmj.h3403.

[5] David Hui, Stanley Perlman, and Ali Zumla, *Spread of MERS to South Korea and China*, 3(7) Lancet Respir Med. 509–510 (2015), available at http://www.thelancet.com/journals/lanres/article/PIIS2213-2600(15)00238-6/abstract.

[6] Korea Centers for Disease Control and Prevention, *Middle East respiratory syndrome coronavirus outbreak in the Republic of Korea*, 6(4) Osong Public Health Res Perspect 269–278 (2015).

[7] The "superspreading" events refer to when "superspreaders" pass the virus on to many others; during the SARS outbreak in 2003, the term refers to cases when an individual had infected more than 10 individuals.

[8] Korea Centers for Disease Control and Prevention, *supra* note 6.

[9] Korean Society of Infectious Disease, Korean Society for Healthcare-Associated Infection Control Prevention, *An unexpected outbreak of Middle East respiratory syndrome coronavirus infection in*

the large-scale quarantine of persons who were exposed but not symptomatic.[10] The similarities between MERS-CoV superspreading events and SARS outbreaks in Guangzhou, Hong Kong, Singapore, Beijing, Toronto, and elsewhere informed the ROK's containment strategy. Unfortunately, it remains unknown why these four superspreading events were responsible for 79% of the 186 total cases.

Actions Taken: Public Health Measures

The KCDC was in charge of the epidemiological investigations. After determining the close contacts of infected persons, home isolation and monitoring of symptoms were implemented by jurisdictional health centers. Although at the beginning of the outbreak there were criticisms that the epidemiological investigations were not exhaustive, active identification of contacts and appropriate management processes followed. During the investigations, the role of technology in controlling the outbreak in ROK was crucial and may provide models for future outbreaks. For example, epidemiological teams utilized all necessary efforts to detect contacts via surveillance cameras located in hospitals, on public transportation, and elsewhere.[11]

The KCDC followed formal guidelines for outbreak containment ("Guidelines for Response to MERS") after ascertaining contacts. Because MERS spread primarily in hospital settings, the KCDC used both hospital isolation and home isolation approaches. Confirmed cases were isolated and treated at MERS-designated hospitals (policies similar to those adopted by the municipality of Toronto, Canada, during the second phase of its SARS outbreak in May through July 2003).[12] Exposed individuals were quarantined in their homes for 14 days after their last exposure.

The KCDC stated that the most effective outbreak containment processes included (1) early and complete identification and investigation of all contacts; (2) robust quarantine/isolation and monitoring of all contacts and suspected cases; (3) full implementation of infection prevention and control measures, including

---

the Republic of Korea, 2015, 47(2) Infect Chemother 120–122 (2015); Adam Kucharski and Christian Althaus, *The role of superspreading in Middle East respiratory syndrome coronavirus (MERS-CoV) transmission*, 20(25) Euro Surveill. 14–18 (2015).

[10] Gowri Gopalakrishna et al., *SARS transmission and hospital containment*, 10(3) Emerg. Infect. Dis. 395–400 (2004).

[11] World Health Organization, WHO Guidelines for Investigation of Cases of Human Infection with Middle East Respiratory Syndrome coronavirus (MERS-CoV) (2013), available at http://www.who.int/csr/disease/coronavirus_infections/MERS_CoV_investigation_guideline_Jul13.pdf; Centers for Disease Control and Prevention, Middle East Respiratory Syndrome—Interim Guidance for Healthcare Professionals (2015), available at http://www.cdc.gov/coronavirus/mers/interim-guidance.html.

[12] Tomislav Svoboda et al., *Public health measures to control the spread of severe acute respiratory syndrome during the outbreak in Toronto*, 350 N Engl J Med 2352–2361 (2004).

active surveillance and follow-up; and (4) prevention of travel, especially internationally, of infected persons and contacts.

Containing the outbreak involved taking steps to improve hospital infection prevention and control such as (1) obtaining mandatory travel histories from patients, (2) improving communication between healthcare facilities, and (3) requiring involvement and cooperation across all aspects of the society. Selected hospitals were designated to provide care for patients with severe respiratory failure and to optimize safety, triage, and assessment of suspected MERS cases. These hospitals required appropriately and sufficiently trained personnel, facility management, and communication with the public. Additionally, strengthening infection prevention and control was an essential part of the implementation strategy of hand hygiene, use of appropriate personal protective equipment, use of aerosol-generating procedures in negative-pressure isolation rooms, and monitoring of healthcare workers twice a day for 14 days after the last contact with a MERS patient.[13]

Lessons Learned

This case study in ROK demonstrates that even high-resource countries with robust compliance with the International Health Regulations must ensure the consistent application of measures intended to prevent, detect, and manage infectious disease. On June 8, 2015, the Joint Republic of Korea–World Health Organization mission, investigated the incidents leading to the outbreak and the success of measures taken to contain the outbreak once it had unfolded. This mission included 16 Korean and WHO experts, and the head of the ROK team is one of the authors (Jong-Koo Lee). The Joint ROK-WHO mission in the WHO Statement on the Ninth Meeting of the IHR Emergency Committee Regarding MERS-CoV, on June 17, 2015, identified five major factors that led to the outbreak:

1. A lack of awareness among healthcare workers and the general public about MERS
2. Suboptimal infection prevention and control measures in the hospitals
3. Close and prolonged contact of infected MERS patients in crowded emergency rooms and multibed rooms in hospitals
4. The practice of seeking care at multiple hospitals ("doctor shopping")
5. The custom of many visitors or family members staying with infected patients in the hospital rooms[14]

---

[13] MD Oh et al., *Middle East respiratory syndrome coronavirus superspreading event involving 81 persons, Korea 2015*, 30(11) J Korean Med Sci. 1701–1705 (2015).

[14] World Health Organization, *supra* note 4.

In high-resource settings including major metropoles where population density is high, the increasing movement of people and goods wrought by globalization increases the potential for rapid and explosive spread of infectious disease. Before the Korean outbreak, MERS-CoV was thought to afflict primarily states in the Middle Eastern region generally and the Arabian Peninsula specifically. It had not previously caused a large outbreak elsewhere in the world. Indeed, prior to May 2015, the ROK had never identified a single case of MERS-CoV. The realization that the disease had reached ROK caused widespread panic because, even during the SARS episode in 2003, it had largely escaped major outbreaks of the disease.

Attempting to change prevailing norms in the medical-professional context during an infectious disease crisis is exceedingly difficult. The joint mission noted the following:

> MERS CoV is difficult to diagnose, particularly in the early part of an outbreak when awareness is relatively low. The initial, or "index" case, did not report his recent travel history to the Middle East when he first sought treatment. MERS was not suspected, and the initial case exposed others for more than a week before he was isolated. Additionally early symptoms of MERS resemble other influenza-like illnesses making it difficult to recognize or suspect MERS. In the early stage of the disease when the upper respiratory track is infected, the virus may be more difficult to detect. The laboratory diagnosis is more robust with samples taken in the lower respiratory track usually in the later stage of the disease when the patient is hospitalized. Furthermore, samples taken from the upper respiratory system (e.g., nasal swabs) can sometimes provide negative test results when lower respiratory samples, which are difficult to collect, may be positive. . . . As has been seen in this and other outbreaks, lapses in early detection and isolation, and the tendency to refer patients to other facilities for testing or management, can facilitate rapid spread from a single infected person.[15]

Many front-line doctors who examined the MERS patients were unfamiliar with existing guidelines regarding infectious disease response in the beginning of the outbreak. Additionally, after health workers were quarantined, replacing those healthcare workers added other challenges.

The recent MERS outbreak in ROK is reminiscent of the emergence of the 2003 SARS epidemic and the 2012–2013 MERS outbreak in Saudi Arabia.[16] Outbreaks may spread rapidly, in days to weeks, and international travel means a risk of international spread. The aforementioned disease outbreaks were facilitated in and by

---

[15] World Health Organization, *supra* note 3.
[16] Abdullah Assiri et al., *Hospital outbreak of Middle East respiratory syndrome coronavirus*, 369(5) New Eng J Med 407 (2013), available at http://www.nejm.org/doi/pdf/10.1056/NEJMoa1306742.

hospital-based practices, and the MERS outbreak in ROK and SARS outbreaks in many cities have been fueled by superspreading events. Gerardo Chowell and his coauthors noted that a majority of the SARS cases occurred among healthcare workers in high-income locations such as Singapore and Toronto, Canada.[17] A majority of MERS cases in ROK were found among those who sought care in the same facilities as the patients.

The MERS outbreak in ROK also demonstrated that clear, early, and frequent communication with the public is essential for an effective response, including trust building, with both national citizens and the international public health community. ROK health authorities provided regular updates in both Korean and English on the epidemiological situation, investigations, and disease control measures. One of this chapter's authors (Sugy Choi) organized a team that provided translations from Korean to English every morning of the daily updates from the Ministry of Health. These translations were shared and posted each day on the website "Program for Monitoring Emerging Diseases (ProMED)," providing local and global access to information on the epidemic as it evolved and then ended over a six-week period.

When communication channels failed, panic resulted in policies that did little to help contain the outbreak and leveled indirect costs in the form of lost school or work days. In the early part of the outbreak, schools in Seoul and Gyeong-gi Province announced closings while the Ministry of Education and the Ministry of Health and Welfare held different views on school closures. More than 3,000 kindergartens, elementary schools, and secondary schools closed from 1 to 13 days.[18] As early as June 10, the joint ROK-WHO mission encouraged the schools to be reopened, noting that "schools have not been linked to transmission of (the virus) in the Republic of Korea or elsewhere."[19]

The MERS outbreak and response in ROK also illustrated weaknesses in the system for training emergency epidemiologists. Since 1999, Korea has trained Epidemic Intelligence Service (EIS) officers through the Field Epidemiology Training Program. Graduates of medical schools in Korea are selected and serve as public health doctors for their mandatory military service for a duration of 3 years. Some public health doctors are selected as EIS officers with 3 weeks basic training and work for central and provincial public health authorities conducting epidemiological investigations. As of 2013, there were a total of 31 EIS officers.[20] The central

---

[17] Gerardo Chowell et al., *Transmission characteristics of MERS and SARS in the healthcare setting: a comparative study*, 13 BMC Med 210 (2015).

[18] *Schools reopen after flawed MERS closures*, Korea Herald (June 15, 2015).

[19] Jack Kim and Ju-Min Park, *WHO team urges South Korea to reopen schools as more close in MERS crisis*, Reuters (June 10, 2015), available at http://www.reuters.com/article/us-health-mers-southkorea-idUSKBN0OQ0AY20150610.

[20] Geun-Yong Kwon et al., *Epidemic Intelligence Service officers and field epidemiology training program in Korea*, 4(4) Osong Public Health Res Perspect 215–221 (2013), available at http://www.ncbi.nlm.nih.gov/pmc/articles/PMC3767107/pdf/main.pdf.

EIS team included 12 officers at KCDC while each province had one or two province and local level epidemiological investigations in charge of approximately 250 public health centers. During the MERS outbreak, not only was the next cohort of field epidemiologists still in training, but EIS officers receive little additional training beyond that included in their mandatory military service. Additionally, there was confusion in commanding role of field epidemiology for infected patients and family members among local clinics, local governments and the central government.[21] ROK's system for implementation of the International Health Regulations focused on national implementation, with less emphasis on local capacity. This discrepancy between capacity to respond during the emergency response and isolation and quarantine at local and national levels may have contributed to some of the delays in coordination between governments, the central government, and KCDC.

Conclusion

Globalization exposes and connects the world via transportation, the internet and other technology, yet the world largely remains startlingly underprepared for the spread of emerging or re-emerging infectious diseases that accompany growing movements of goods and people. While the delayed and fragmented response to the Ebola outbreak in West Africa dramatically illustrated this lack of preparation, the MERS outbreak in ROK shows that preparedness is not only a matter of resources and broad commitment. Repeated training and global commitment and cooperation are essential.

Until ROK's experience, high-income countries outside the Middle East had not experienced MERS outbreaks. While the outbreak was brought under control in a relatively short 6-week window and was concentrated in hospitals, it also showed a potential for superspreading reminiscent of past infectious disease episodes with high fatality rates. Better preparation for nosocomial outbreaks such as training of relevant personnel and basic prevention control are key parts of preventing emergency situations like the ROK MERS episode. The MERS outbreak in ROK opened a political window for reform in national health system preparedness.

In addition to measures like those mentioned here, which are largely matters of local and national concern, the world must continue to strengthen the global framework for management of infectious disease largely embodied in the International Health Regulations but increasingly augmented by other international networks and organizations. In September 2015, ROK hosted the Global Health Security Agenda (GHSA) High Level Meeting in Seoul. The GHSA, which focuses exclusively on infectious diseases, includes 50 nations, as well as WHO and multiple governmental and nongovernmental organizations. ROK will also chair the GHSA

[21] *Id.*

Steering Group in 2017, as part of its commitment to better prepare for future outbreaks at the national and international levels. Another aspect of this effort involves the conceptions of infectious disease threats. The three-part "One Health" model of ecohealth, animal health, and human health emphasizes a broader and more comprehensive approach to fighting infectious disease.[22] The Korean MERS outbreak, like the recent Ebola outbreak in West Africa, reaffirms the need for better surveillance, training, analysis, coordination and appropriate responses. Although this outbreak has ended, the fight against infectious disease is perpetual and requires persistence, planning, and cooperation.

References

Butler, Declan. *South Korean MERS outbreak spotlights lack of research*. 522(7555) Nature 139–140 (2015).
Centers for Disease Control and Prevention. Middle East Respiratory Syndrome—Interim Guidance for Healthcare Professionals (2015). Available at http://www.cdc.gov/coronavirus/mers/interim-guidance.html.
Cho H-W. *Editorial*. 6(4) Osong Public Health and Research Perspectives 219–223 (2015).
Chowell G, Abdirizak F, Lee S, Lee J, Jung E, Nishiura H, et al. *Transmission dynamics and control of Ebola virus disease (EVD): a review*. 12 BMC Medicine 196 (2014).
Gostin LO, Lucey D. *Middle East respiratory syndrome: a global health challenge* 314(8) JAMA 771–772 (2015).
Hui DS, Perlman S, Zumla A. *Spread of MERS to South Korea and China*. 3(7) Lancet Respir Med 509–510 (2015). Available at http://www.thelancet.com/journals/lanres/article/PIIS2213-2600(15)00238-6/abstract.
International Symposium on MERS (2015). Available at www.ism2015.org.
Jack A. *Why the panic? South Korea's MERS response questioned*. 350 BMJ (June 24, 2015). Available at http://www.bmj.com/content/350/bmj.h3403.
Khan A, Farooqui A, Guan Y, Kelvin DJ. *Lessons to learn from MERS-CoV outbreak in South Korea*. 9(6) J Infect Dev Ctries 543–546 (2015).
Ki M. *2015 MERS outbreak in Korea: hospital-to-hospital transmission*, 37 Epidemiol Health (July 21, 2015).
Kim J, Park J. *WHO team urges South Korea to reopen schools as more close in MERS crisis*. Reuters (June 10, 2015). Available at http://www.reuters.com/article/us-health-mers-southkorea-idUSKBN0OQ0AY20150610.
Korea Centers for Disease Control and Prevention. *Middle East respiratory syndrome coronavirus outbreak in the Republic of Korea, 2015*. 6(4) Osong Public Health Res Perspect 269–278 (2015).
Korean Society of Infectious Disease, Korean Society for Healthcare-Associated Infection Control Prevention. *An unexpected outbreak of Middle East respiratory syndrome coronavirus infection in the Republic of Korea, 2015*. 47(2) Infect Chemother 120–122 (2015).
Kucharski AJ, Althaus CL. *The role of superspreading in Middle East respiratory syndrome coronavirus (MERS-CoV) transmission*. 20(25) Euro Surveill 14–18 (2015).
Kwon GY, Moon S, Kwak W, Gwack J, Chu C, Youn SK. *Epidemic Intelligence Service officers and field epidemiology training program in Korea*. 4(4) Osong Public Health Res Perspect 215–221 (2013). Available at http://www.ncbi.nlm.nih.gov/pmc/articles/PMC3767107/pdf/main.pdf.

---

[22] Lawrence Gostin and Daniel Lucey, *Middle East respiratory syndrome: a global health challenge*, 314(8) JAMA 771–772 (2015).

Oh MD, Choe PG, Oh HS, Park WB, Lee SM, Park J, et al. *Middle East respiratory syndrome coronavirus superspreading event involving 81 persons, Korea 2015*. 30(11) J Korean Med Sci. 1701–1705 (2015).

Shen Z, Ning F, Zhou W, He X, Lin C, Chin DP, et al. *Superspreading SARS events, Beijing, 2003*. 10(2) Emerg Infect Dis 256–260 (2004).

Tourism industry suffers 3.4 tln won loss from MERS outbreak: report. Yonhap (Nov. 6, 2015).

White House Joint Fact Sheet: The US-ROK Alliance (KOICA-USAID Cooperation) (2015). Available at http://www.koica.go.kr/english/board/focus_on/1321094_3563.html.

Wong G, Liu W, Liu Y, Zhou B, Bi Y, Gao GF. *MERS, SARS, and Ebola: the role of super-spreaders in infectious disease*. 18(4) Cell Host Microbe 398–401 (2015).

World Health Organization. MERS-CoV Joint Mission Findings Discussion (2015). Available at http://www.who.int/mediacentre/news/mers/briefing-notes/update-15-06-2015/en/.

———. Middle East Respiratory Syndrome Coronavirus (MERS-CoV)—Republic of Korea (2015). Available at http://www.who.int/mediacentre/news/mers/briefing-notes/update-15-06-2015/en/.

———. Summary of Current Situation, Literature Update and Risk Assessment (July 7, 2015).

———. WHO Guidelines for Investigation of Cases of Human Infection with Middle East Respiratory Syndrome Coronavirus (MERS-CoV) (2013).

5

Antibiotic Resistance

GAIL HANSEN

While infectious diseases are frequently characterized in ways that suggest they represent a pathogen-by-pathogen threat (e.g., Ebola, hepatitis, HIV, influenza, Middle East respiratory syndrome coronavirus [MERS-CoV], tuberculosis), one of the most important dimensions of fighting infectious disease is understanding all pathogens' capacity to adapt. That capacity is not only a natural process undertaken by virtually all living organisms; it may be accelerated and facilitated by human action (or inaction). Antimicrobial resistance has emerged as a key threat in the global effort against infectious diseases. Antimicrobial resistance renders current treatments for infectious diseases less effective or useless, endangering lives and raising the costs of medical treatment as infections from resistant pathogens often result in longer illnesses, more hospitalizations, and greater economic losses attributable to related morbidity and mortality. This chapter analyzes the scope and depth of the antimicrobial resistance problem; the principal factors contributing to increased antimicrobial resistance (emphasizing antibiotic resistance), including the role of industrial agricultural processes that promote the use of antibiotics in animal feed and water; physician prescription practices; and the evolutionary tendency for all organisms to adapt to environmental changes. It also assesses the relationship between increasing resistance and the human economic and health burden that resistance imposes. Finally, this chapter examines possible solutions to antibiotic resistance, with emphasis on the governmental and nongovernmental actors whose stewardship of antibiotic resources will play the most important role in preventing and managing the current problem. While the chapter is focused on the problem as it manifests in the United States, it also applies lessons from in the United States to the global problem of antimicrobial resistance.

Antimicrobial Resistance

Antimicrobial resistance is one of the most significant challenges facing public health systems today.[1] Antibiotics, (a subclass of antimicrobials), for example, are used to either kill bacteria that cause illness or suppress their ability to multiply, allowing the immune system to effectively respond to the bacteria's infective threat.[2] The phrase "antibiotic resistance" is used to describe the set of traits and genetic elements, developed and then disseminated, by which bacteria survive treatment by antibiotics, threatening not only the infected person but also the broader community, which collectively faces pathogenic bacteria that are more difficult to combat.[3] These drug-resistant bacteria, or "superbugs," present a serious and worsening threat to human health.[4] According to the Centers for Disease Control and Prevention (CDC), each year at least 2 million Americans acquire a serious infection caused by antibiotic-resistant bacteria, resulting in approximately 23,000 deaths.[5] Globally, drug resistant strains of HIV, malaria, and tuberculosis have been identified by the World Health Organization.

All antibiotic use may potentially contribute to the development of antibiotic-resistant bacteria.[6] This principle is an important one: even if more prudent and responsible policies were adopted tomorrow, the public health community would need to remain vigilant against the development of resistant pathogens. However, misuse of antibiotics in human and animal medicine has compounded the initial problem and favors the amplification and spread of antibiotic-resistant organisms. This misuse—"too short a time, or too small a dose, at inadequate strengths, or for the wrong disease"—allows resistant bacteria to survive and pass on resistant traits to other bacteria.[7] The consequences of antibiotic-resistant bacteria include infections that would not have otherwise occurred, infections that are more difficult to

---

[1] The Pew Charitable Trusts, *Tracking the Pipeline Development* (July 28, 2015), available at http://www.pewtrusts.org/en/research-and-analysis/issue-briefs/2014/03/12/tracking-the-pipeline-of-antibiotics-in-development (hereinafter *Tracking the Pipeline Development*).

[2] The Pew Charitable Trusts, *Antibiotic Resistance and the Industrial Animal Farm* (Feb. 8, 2010), available at http://www.pewtrusts.org/en/research-and-analysis/issue-briefs/2010/02/08/antibiotic-resistance-and-the-industrial-animal-farm.

[3] *Id.*

[4] *Tracking the Pipeline Development, supra* note 1.

[5] Centers for Disease Control and Prevention (CDC), *Antibiotic Resistance Threats to the United States* (2013), available at http://www.cdc.gov/drugresistance/threat-report-2013/index.html. The CDC concedes its estimates are conservative.

[6] Nicole Mahoney, *Getting Smart Is a Group Effort: Addressing the Crisis of Antibiotic Resistance* (Nov. 18, 2013), available at http://www.pewtrusts.org/en/about/news-room/opinion/2013/11/18/getting-smart-is-a-group-effort-addressing-the-crisis-of-antibiotic-resistance.

[7] The Pew Charitable Trusts, *How Antibiotic Resistance Happens* (Feb. 24, 2010), available at http://www.pewtrusts.org/en/research-and-analysis/issue-briefs/2010/02/24/how-antibiotic-resistance-happens (hereinafter *How Antibiotic Resistance Happens*).

treat, and increased severity of infections, which may include death.[8] Moreover, the multiplication of resistant bacteria is far outpacing the development of new antibiotic therapies.[9]

Sources of Antibiotic Resistance
Industrial Agriculture

Although there are multiple sources from which antibiotic-resistant bacteria may develop, one key source is industrial farming practices.[10] Large amounts of antibiotics have been used for growth promotion and treatment of infections among farm animals and in aquaculture.[11] "Routine, non-therapeutic use of antibiotics in food animal production [are commonly used]... to promote growth and to compensate for the effects of overcrowded and unsanitary conditions."[12] Industrial farm animals may excrete resistant bacteria in their feces, and some resistant bacteria can be released into the environment via the animal's feces-contaminated skin.[13] When manure is applied to farmland as fertilizer, it may contaminate crops with antibiotic-resistant bacteria.[14] Water runoff from industrial farms can carry resistant bacteria and unmetabolized antibiotics into the water supply and, as a result, contaminate drinking water.[15]

Resistant bacteria have been detected in the air more than 160 yards downwind from swine feedlots, multidrug-resistant bacteria have been detected in the topsoil of dairies, and resistant *E. coli* have been found in drinking water near hog facilities, as well as moving via vectors such as cockroaches and flies. Resistant bacteria of livestock origin are spread from the livestock to operators, who may then pass along the bacteria to their family, friends, and communities. Indirectly, resistant bacteria may spread through improperly handled or inadequately cooked contaminated meat.[16]

---

[8] *Id.*

[9] Mahoney, *supra* note 6.

[10] The Pew Charitable Trusts, *Latest Foodborne Illnesses Show Links Between Farm Antibiotic Use and Resistant Bacteria in U.S. Poultry Supply* (Oct. 16, 2013), available at http://www.pewtrusts.org/en/research-and-analysis/fact-sheets/2013/10/16/latest-foodborne-illnesses-show-links-between-farm-antibiotic-use-and-resistant-bacteria-in-us-poultry-supply; see also CDC, *supra* note 5, at 14.

[11] The Pew Charitable Trusts, *Avoiding Antibiotic Resistance: Denmark's Ban on Growth Promoting Antibiotics in Food Animals*, (2010) available at http://www.pewtrusts.org/~/media/legacy/uploadedfiles/phg/content_level_pages/issue_briefs/denmarkexperiencepdf.pdf.

[12] The Pew Charitable Trusts, *Health Care and the Antibiotic Resistance Crisis* (Jan. 21, 2011), available at http://www.pewtrusts.org/en/research-and-analysis/issue-briefs/2011/01/21/health-care-and-the-antibiotic-resistance-crisis.

[13] *How Antibiotic Resistance Happens, supra* note 7, at 2.

[14] *Id.*

[15] *Id.*

[16] *Id.*

The World Health Organization has noted the public threat posed by excessive antibiotic use in animals, declaring, "Widespread use of antimicrobials for disease control and growth with promotion in animals has been paralleled by an increase in resistance in those bacteria that can spread from animals, often through food, to cause infections in humans."[17] WHO has advocated that the use of "antimicrobial growth promoters . . . in humans and animals should be terminated or rapidly phased-out in the absence of risk-based evaluations."[18]

Currently, industrial agricultural firms in the United States are under few legal requirements to track, report, or disclose volumes of antibiotics used in raising food animals, so the full dimension of the problem is unknown.[19] Approximately 98% of medically important antibiotics sold for food animals are available over the counter rather than through prescription.[20] In 2013, drug makers sold over 25 million pounds of medically important antibiotics for use in food animals, the most ever reported and four times the amount sold to treat sick people.[21] Approximately 75% of antibiotics are used in feed and 20% in water; the remaining 5% are introduced through intramammary transmission, injection, and other modalities.[22] Although a few antibiotics have been banned or restricted for use in food animals, most are available, are used, and therefore continue to pose a threat to human health.[23]

Indeed, the overall therapeutic versus nontherapeutic legal authorizations for antibiotic use differ in important ways between animals and humans despite the relevance of practices for the former on the latter. While antibiotics must be prescribed for treatment, disease control, and prevention in humans, they are available over the counter for these indications in animals.[24] For purposes of growth promotion, there is no approved indication for prescribing antibiotics to humans, but animals may be given antibiotics for that purpose over the counter. Development and acceptance of alternatives to nontherapeutic dosing of animals have become politically sensitive issues, complicating regulatory approaches to the industrial agriculture context specifically.

---

[17] *Id.*

[18] *Id.*

[19] The Pew Charitable Trusts, *Antibiotic-Resistant Bacteria in Animals and Unnecessary Human Health Risks* (Feb. 8, 2010), available at http://www.pewtrusts.org/en/research-and-analysis/issue-briefs/2010/02/08/antibioticresistant-bacteria-in-animals-and-unnecessary-human-health-risks.

[20] Food and Drug Administration, 2013 Summary Report on Antimicrobials Sold or Distributed for Use in Food-Producing Animals 6 (Apr. 2015), available at http://www.fda.gov/downloads/ForIndustry/UserFees/AnimalDrugUserFeeActADUFA/UCM440584.pdf (hereinafter FDA Summary).

[21] FDA Summary at p. 16.

[22] FDA Summary at 10, 18.

[23] *Antibiotic-Resistant Bacteria in Animals and Unnecessary Human Health Risks*, *supra* note 18.

[24] Some antibiotics for treatment and disease control in animals do require a prescription.

Misuse of Antibiotics in the Modern Healthcare System

Overprescription of antibiotics by medical professionals is a second factor that has influenced the rise of antibiotic-resistant bacteria.[25] Antibiotics are "among the most commonly prescribed drugs used in human medicine."[26] The more antibiotics are used, the less effective they become.[27] On average, about half of patients admitted to hospitals receive antibiotics during their stay.[28] Approximately 60% of dollars spent on antibiotics are spent in the outpatient setting and for viral illnesses such as the common cold and influenza that do not respond to antibiotic treatment.[29] Up to 50% of antibiotic use in humans is unnecessary or inappropriate as prescribed.[30] Roughly 63% of doctors have treated patients with infections that did not respond to any antibiotics.[31] As a result, increased awareness among medical professionals is a key component of any strategy to slow or prevent the evolution of antibiotic-resistant pathogens.

The Biological Mechanisms of Antibiotic Resistance

Whether through agricultural or healthcare systems, the mechanism is the same: "Bacteria develop ways to fight off antibiotics by: preventing antibiotics from reaching their target cell (e.g., changing the permeability of cell walls or pumping drugs out of the cells), changing the structure of target cells or entirely replacing them; or producing enzymes that destroy antibiotics."[32] Resistance to antibiotics develops "through a process of genetic exchange or mutation, where acquisition of a resistance gene or changes to the bacteria's genetic code provide a mechanism for a given bacterium to survive in the presence of a given antimicrobial or group of antimicrobial drugs."[33] Resistance genes "encode proteins that allow bacteria to

---

[25] Brad Spellberg et al., *The epidemic of antibiotic-resistant infections: a call to action for the medical community from the Infectious Diseases Society of America*, 46 Clinical Infectious Diseases 155, 156 (2008), available at http://cid.oxfordjournals.org/content/46/2/155.full.pdf+html.

[26] CDC, *supra* note 5, at 11.

[27] The Pew Charitable Trusts, *Antibiotic Use in Human Healthcare* (Feb. 2015), available at http://www.pewtrusts.org/~/media/Assets/2015/02/AntibioticOveruseInfographic_2pgs.pdf?la=en (hereinafter *Antibiotic Use in Human Healthcare*).

[28] Scott Fridkin et al., *Vital signs: improving antibiotic use among hospitalized patients*, 63 Morbidity and Mortality Weekly Report 181, 195 (Mar. 7, 2014), available at http://www.cdc.gov/mmwr/pdf/wk/mm6309.pdf.

[29] *Antibiotic Use in Human Healthcare*, *supra* note 26.

[30] *Id.*

[31] *Id.*

[32] *How Antibiotic Resistance Happens*, *supra* note 7, at 1.

[33] Meghan F. Davis and Lainie Rutkow, *Regulatory strategies to combat microbial resistance of animal origin: recommendations for a science-based U.S. approach*, 25 Tul. Envtl. L.J. 327, 335 (Summer

evade attack, typically by providing target-specific evasion from the antimicrobial, by inactivating the drug, or by removing the drug from the bacterium."[34] Multiple mutations endow the bacteria with resistance to those antibiotics that are prescribed for treatment. These bacteria can acquire genes for microbial resistance via a process called "horizontal gene transfer."[35] Furthermore, when a gene that provides resistance to a particular antibiotic, and is positioned next to another gene that provides resistance to a different antibiotic, multidrug resistance can result resulting in multidrug resistance.[36] Therefore, when antimicrobials are added to an ecosystem (e.g., by administering drugs to sick humans or by feeding antimicrobials to broiler chickens in a poultry facility), they facilitate resistance.[37]

Bacteria share these adaptations with other bacteria. As Davis and Rutkow describe it, "Microorganisms join together and transfer DNA to each other; free-floating DNA pieces are picked up, which can carry resistance to a number of antibiotics; small pieces of DNA jump from one DNA molecule to another, and then are incorporated; and DNA remnants are scavenged from dead or degraded bacteria."[38] The persistent exposure to antibiotics allows those bacteria to replicate and successfully share genetic information, which leads to the expansion of resistance until a majority of the species becomes resistant to a given antibiotic.[39] When bacteria pass on the resistance traits to other bacteria, the resistance results in more virulent infections, increased illness, and even death.[40]

Stagnation in the Antibiotic Drug Development Pipeline

Aside from the general problems associated with antibiotic-resistant bacteria, there are a dwindling number of effective antibiotics to successfully combat infections.[41] Unfortunately, there are not enough new antibiotics being researched or developed to solve the resistance problem.[42] Most pharmaceutical firms have retreated from

---

2012), available at http://www.jhsph.edu/research/centers-and-institutes/johns-hopkins-center-for-a-livable-future/_pdf/research/clf_reports/Davis%20Regulatory%20Strategies.pdf.

[34] *Id.*
[35] Davis and Rutkow, *supra* note 32, at 336.
[36] *Antibiotic Resistance and the Industrial Animal Farm, supra* note 2.
[37] Davis and Rutkow, *supra* note 32, at 336–337.
[38] *Id.* at 1.
[39] CDC, *supra* note 5.
[40] The Pew Charitable Trusts, *supra* note 11.
[41] The Pew Charitable Trusts, *Getting Smart About Antibiotic Resistance* (Nov. 15, 2010), available at http://www.pewtrusts.org/en/research-and-analysis/issue-briefs/2010/11/15/getting-smart-about-antibiotic-resistance.
[42] *Id.*

antibiotic research, leaving an accelerating trend of resistance against declining investments in research and development of new antibiotic therapies.[43] Antibiotics are a "societal drug" in that even though a decision to treat disease with an antibiotic might be individualized, it has inevitable ramifications for the entire ecosystem of agricultural production and human health, which relies on the availability of antibiotics to remain secure.[44]

The Public Health Response

Awareness is the first step in slowing the growing epidemic of antibiotic resistance. Awareness will lead to citizens, government, healthcare providers, and other organizations working together and independently to reduce the overuse and misuse of antibiotics.[45] The influence of awareness has already manifested in common end-use outlets. Grocery stores and restaurants, for example, contribute to spreading awareness by advertising, selling, and serving meat and poultry from animals that are raised without antibiotics.[46]

The healthcare system has also made some important gains in adopting stewardship programs aimed at making conscientious and attentive decisions about antibiotic prescription practices.[47] The CDC has set guidelines for stewardship programs, such as "dedicating necessary resources, tracking prescribing and drug-resistance patterns, appointing a single leader responsible for program outcomes, and educating clinicians on appropriate use."[48] Through disease-by-disease analysis of clinical guidelines, educational outreach, and tracking prescribing practices, it is possible to slow the development of antibiotic resistance and lengthen the time available for new antibiotic treatments to be developed.

For aforementioned reasons, as well as others, reforming the use of antibiotics in food animals requires a wider response engaging the broadest cast of players, including traditional agriculture sector advocacy groups. Relatively straightforward

---

[43] Carl Nathan and Otto Cars, *Antibiotic resistance—problems, progress, and prospects*, 371 New Eng. J. Med. 1761, 1762 (Nov. 2014), available at http://www.nejm.org/doi/pdf/10.1056/NEJMp1408040.

[44] Pew Charitable Trusts, *Antibiotics and Industrial Farming 101* (May 5, 2014), available at http://www.pewtrusts.org/en/research-and-analysis/fact-sheets/2014/05/05/antibiotics-and-industrial-farming-101.

[45] The Pew Charitable Trusts, *Food Animal Production and Antibiotic Resistance* 2 (July 16, 2012), available at http://www.pewtrusts.org/~/media/legacy/uploadedfiles/phg/supporting_items/IBSaveAntibioticsTheSolutionpdf.pdf.

[46] Id.

[47] CDC, Antibiotic Resistance Threats in the United States, 2013, http://www.cdc.gov/drugresistance/pdf/ar-threats-2013-508.pdf.

[48] Id.

first steps include agreeing on definitions, such as "nontherapeutic," to facilitate clear policies and improve drug use estimates.[49] To reduce the risk of microbial resistance, antibiotics being used for nontherapeutic indications should be phased out and prohibited.[50] Following the phaseout of these antibiotics, an improved monitoring and reporting system should be implemented to track antimicrobials sold and used for food animals.[51] Procedures to easily monitor antibiotic use and resistance in food supplies, the environment, animals, and humans are urgently needed.[52] More oversight, monitoring, and reporting are necessary to increase responsible antibiotic use and evaluate steps taken to reduce antibiotic resistance.

On September 18, 2014, President Barack Obama signed Executive Order 13676, the National Action Plan for Combating Antibiotic-Resistant Bacteria, which was adopted to "guide action by public health, healthcare, and veterinary partners in a common effort to address urgent and serious drug-resistant threats that affect people in the U.S. and around the world."[53] The National Action Plan explicitly acknowledges that antibiotic resistance had become a national security priority at the highest level. It sets forth measures, such as a stewardship program to promote responsible antibiotic use, and review and reform of regulations currently in place concerning antibiotics.[54] The National Action Plan adopted nine objectives to combat antibiotic resistance:

> minimize the emergence of antibiotic-resistant bacteria; preserve the efficacy of new and existing antibacterial drugs; advance research to develop improved methods for combating antibiotic resistance and conducting antibiotic stewardship; strengthen surveillance efforts in public health and agriculture; develop and promote the use of new, rapid diagnostic technologies; accelerate scientific research and facilitate the development of new antibacterial drugs, vaccines, diagnostics, and other novel therapeutics; maximize the dissemination of the most up-to-date information on the appropriate and proper use of antibiotics to the general public and healthcare providers; work with the pharmaceutical industry to include information on the proper use of over-the-counter and prescription antibiotic medications for humans and animals; and improve international

---

[49] The Pew Charitable Trusts, *Industrial Animal Farms and Antibiotic Resistance* (Feb. 2010), available at http://www.pewtrusts.org/~/media/legacy/uploadedfiles/phg/content_level_pages/issue_briefs/HHIFIBIndustrialFarmsAntibioticResistancepdf.pdf.

[50] *Id.*

[51] *Id.*

[52] *Id.*

[53] White House, National Action Plan for Combating Antibiotic-Resistant Bacteria 4 (Mar. 2015), available at https://www.whitehouse.gov/sites/default/files/docs/national_action_plan_for_combating_antibotic-resistant_bacteria.pdf; Exec. Order 13676, 184 Fed. Reg. 56931 (Sept. 23, 2014), available at http://www.gpo.gov/fdsys/pkg/FR-2014-09-23/pdf/2014-22805.pdf.

[54] *Combating antibiotic-resistant bacteria*, 184 Fed. Reg. at 56933.

collaboration and capabilities for prevention, surveillance, stewardship, basic research, and drug and diagnostics development.[55]

These objectives are aimed at achieving detection, prevention, and control of illness and death "related to antibiotic-resistant infections by implementing measures that reduce the emergence and spread of antibiotic-resistant bacteria and [to] help ensure the continued availability of effective therapeutics for the treatment of bacterial infections."[56] The executive order established coordinating mechanisms across federal agencies, a forum that includes all relevant stakeholders, and processes for facilitating international cooperation on the antibiotic resistance issue. Targets and goals were set for the use of antibiotics in human inpatient and outpatient settings, but timelines and explicit goals were conspicuously absent from the discussions of animal uses of antibiotics. In the absence of clear targets, it is unlikely that progress will be made to decrease the amount of antibiotics used in food animal production.

To be sure, not all constituencies view the correct approach to the problem, or even the existence of a problem, in the same way. The American Farm Bureau Federation, for example, argues that "antibiotic use in animals has not been scientifically linked to increases in human antibiotic resistance."[57] The Animal Health Institute asserts that "the main problems in human medicine are with bacterial infections that do not originate in food animals."[58] Similar sentiments are expressed by advocacy groups for poultry and meat production firms. Yet a small and growing number of farms are raising livestock on organic feed and without antibiotics in response to awareness of the relationship between antibiotics used for food animals and human health.[59] The National Action Plan explicitly calls for an inclusive approach to the antibiotic resistance problem, including all stakeholders and acknowledging that all constituencies, including the medical community, the government, farmers, and private and public advocacy organizations, need to be good stewards of antibiotic resources in order to slow the progression of antibiotic resistance.

Conclusion

Antimicrobial resistance begins in environments that allow bacteria to survive in the presence of antibiotics. Administering antibiotics frequently, excessively, and with

---

[55] White House, *supra* note 52, at 2.

[56] *Combating antibiotic-resistant bacteria*, 184 Fed. Reg. at 56931.

[57] American Farm Bureau Federation, *Preserving Antibiotic Access*, available at http://www.fb.org/issues/docs/antibiotics15.pdf.

[58] Animal Health Institute, *Antibiotics in Livestock: Frequently Asked Questions*, available at http://www.ahi.org/issues-advocacy/animal-antibiotics/antibiotics-in-livestock-frequently-asked-questions/#05.

[59] *Industrial Animal Farms and Antibiotic Resistance*, *supra* note 48.

minimal judgment allows these bacteria to thrive and replicate. Once the bacteria begin to survive antibiotic treatment, those bacteria pass along survival genes to other bacteria. This process breeds bacteria that are able to withstand the best antibiotics available. For understandable economic reasons, pharmaceutical firms have curtailed research and development of new and improved antibiotics. However, it is possible to create incentives to spur innovation in the sector as part of a broader campaign raising awareness of the threat that resistance poses to the community. The president's National Action Plan, wholly consistent with the World Health Organization's Plan on Combating Antibiotic Resistance, makes clear the urgency of addressing microbial resistance. By heeding the concerns raised by the public health community and adopting common-sense and relatively low-cost measures now in all sectors using antibiotics, a much greater threat to public health may be averted.

References

American Farm Bureau Federation. *Preserving Antibiotic Access.* Available at http://www.fb.org/issues/docs/antibiotics15.pdf.

Animal Health Institute. *Antibiotics in Livestock: Frequently Asked Questions.* Available at http://www.ahi.org/issues-advocacy/animal-antibiotics/antibiotics-in-livestock-frequently-asked-questions/#05.

Centers for Disease Control and Prevention. *Antibiotic Resistance Threats to the United States* (2013). Available at http://www.cdc.gov/drugresistance/threat-report-2013/index.html.

Davis, M., and Lainie Rutkow. *Regulatory strategies to combat microbial resistance of animal origin: recommendations for a science-based U.S. approach.* 25 Tul. Envtl. L.J. 327, 335 (Summer 2012). Available at http://www.jhsph.edu/research/centers-and-institutes/johns-hopkins-center-for-a-livable-future/_pdf/research/clf_reports/Davis%20Regulatory%20Strategies.pdf.

Food and Drug Administration. 2013 Summary Report on Antimicrobials Sold or Distributed for Use in Food-Producing Animals (April 2015). Available at http://www.fda.gov/downloads/ForIndustry/UserFees/AnimalDrugUserFeeActADUFA/UCM440584.pdf.

Fridkin, S., et al. *Vital signs: improving antibiotic use among hospitalized patients.* 63 Morbidity and Mortality Weekly Report 181, 195 (Mar. 7, 2014). Available at http://www.cdc.gov/mmwr/pdf/wk/mm6309.pdf.

Mahoney, Nicole. *Getting Smart Is a Group Effort: Addressing the Crisis of Antibiotic Resistance* (Nov. 18, 2013). Available at http://www.pewtrusts.org/en/about/news-room/opinion/2013/11/18/getting-smart-is-a-group-effort-addressing-the-crisis-of-antibiotic-resistance.

Nathan C., and Otto Cars. *Antibiotic resistance—problems, progress, and prospects.* 371 New Eng. J. Med. 1761, 1762 (Nov. 2014). Available at http://www.nejm.org/doi/pdf/10.1056/NEJMp1408040.

The Pew Charitable Trusts. *Antibiotic Resistance and the Industrial Animal Farm* (Feb. 8, 2010). Available at http://www.pewtrusts.org/en/research-and-analysis/issue-briefs/2010/02/08/antibiotic-resistance-and-the-industrial-animal-farm.

———. *Antibiotic Use in Human Healthcare* (Feb. 2015). Available at http://www.pewtrusts.org/~/media/Assets/2015/02/AntibioticOveruseInfographic_2pgs.pdf?la=en.

———. *Antibiotics and Industrial Farming 101* (May 5, 2014). Available at http://www.pewtrusts.org/en/research-and-analysis/fact-sheets/2014/05/05/antibiotics-and-industrial-farming-101.

———. *Antibiotic-Resistant Bacteria in Animals and Unnecessary Human Health Risks* (Feb. 8, 2010). Available at http://www.pewtrusts.org/en/research-and-analysis/issue-briefs/2010/02/08/antibioticresistant-bacteria-in-animals-and-unnecessary-human-health-risks.

———. *Avoiding Antibiotic Resistance: Denmark's Ban on Growth Promoting Antibiotics in Food Animals.* (2010) Available at http://www.pewtrusts.org/~/media/legacy/uploadedfiles/phg/content_level_pages/issue_briefs/denmarkexperiencepdf.pdf.

———. *Getting Smart About Antibiotic Resistance* (Nov. 15, 2010). Available at http://www.pewtrusts.org/en/research-and-analysis/issue-briefs/2010/11/15/getting-smart-about-antibiotic-resistance.

———. *Health Care and the Antibiotic Resistance Crisis* (Jan. 21, 2011). Available at http://www.pewtrusts.org/en/research-and-analysis/issue-briefs/2011/01/21/health-care-and-the-antibiotic-resistance-crisis.

———. *How Antibiotic Resistance Happens* (Feb. 24, 2010). Available at http://www.pewtrusts.org/en/research-and-analysis/issue-briefs/2010/02/24/how-antibiotic-resistance-happens.

———. *Tracking the Pipeline Development* (July 28, 2015). Available at http://www.pewtrusts.org/en/research-and-analysis/issue-briefs/2014/03/12/tracking-the-pipeline-of-antibiotics-in-development.

Spellberg, B., et al. *The epidemic of antibiotic-resistant infections: a call to action for the medical community from the infectious diseases society of America.* 46 Clinical Infectious Diseases 155, 156 (2008). Available at http://cid.oxfordjournals.org/content/46/2/155.full.pdf+html.

PART II

GLOBAL SYSTEMS FOR PREVENTION AND MANAGEMENT OF INFECTIOUS DISEASE THREATS

6

The International Health Regulations*
The Governing Framework for Global Health Security

LAWRENCE O. GOSTIN AND REBECCA KATZ

In 2005, the World Health Assembly (WHA) fundamentally revised the International Health Regulations (IHR),[1] a treaty meant to herald a new era of global cooperation to make the world more secure. Yet in the aftermath of the West African Ebola epidemic, the IHR faces critical scrutiny, with the World Health Organization (WHO),[2] the Harvard/London School of Hygiene and Tropical Medicine,[3] the National Academy of Medicine,[4] and the United Nations[5] all urging major reforms.

Frustration with lack of progress on IHR implementation has led member states to launch independent programs with strikingly similar aims. The United States

---

* The majority of this chapter was first published as: Lawrence O. Gostin and Rebecca Katz, The International Health Regulations: The Governing Framework for Global Health Security © 2016 The Milbank Memorial Fund.

[1] WHO, International Health Regulations (2005), available at http://whqlibdoc.who.int/publications/2008/9789241580410_eng.pdf.

[2] WHO, Report of the Ebola Interim Assessment Panel (July 2015), available at http://who.int/csr/resources/publications/ebola/report-by-panel.pdf.; WHO, 2014 Ebola virus disease outbreak and follow-up to the Special Session of the Executive Board on Ebola (May 23, 2015), available at http://apps.who.int/gb/ebwha/pdf_files/WHA68/A68_ACONF5-en.pdf.

[3] Suerie Moon et al., *Will Ebola change the game? Ten essential reforms before the next pandemic. The report of the Harvard-LSHTM Independent Panel on the Global Response to Ebola*, 386 (10009) Lancet 2204–2221 (Nov. 28, 2015).

[4] Commission on a Global Health Risk Framework for the Future, The Neglected Dimension of Global Security: A Framework to Counter Infectious Disease Crises (2016), available at www.nam.edu/GHRF.

[5] UN Secretary General Press Release, Secretary-General Appoints High-Level Panel on Global Response to Health Crises (Apr. 2015), available at http://www.un.org/press/en/2015/sga1558.doc.htm.

established the Global Health Security Agenda (GHSA), partnering with approximately 50 countries to accelerate progress toward global capacity to prevent, detect, and respond to biological threats.[6] The United States has committed to support up to 31 countries in developing these capacities,[7] and the 2015 G7 Summit pledged to double that number.[8] As the IHR faces probing questions and parallel initiatives are developed, we review its historical origins, its performance, and its future.

A Brief History

The IHR's origins can be traced to a series of Sanitary Conferences, beginning in 1851, to forge an international agreement to curb the spread of infectious diseases (originally cholera, followed by plague and yellow fever) entering Europe from Asia, particularly from India and the Levant.[9] At that time, the concept of global health security meant protecting Europe without unduly hindering trade. The Sanitary Conferences led to a binding agreement in 1892—the International Sanitary Convention (ISC)—focused on quarantine for cholera. European states subsequently adopted additional conventions, which were incorporated into a single ISC. By 1926, the ISC covered primarily cholera, yellow fever, and plague.

In 1907, the Rome Agreement created the Office International d'Hygiène Publique (OIHP), an agency that was entrusted with overseeing the international health agreements.[10] At its creation in 1948, WHO assumed OIHP's mandate and oversight of the ISC. The WHO constitution empowered the organization to adopt regulations to prevent the international spread of disease. Its power to adopt regulations is far-reaching—binding on member states unless they affirmatively opt out.[11] In 1951, the WHA exercised this authority to replace the ISC with the International Sanitary Regulations (ISR), covering six diseases. In 1969, the WHA revised the ISR, changed its name to the International Health Regulations (IHR), and removed typhus and relapsing fever. The WHA removed smallpox in 1981 after the disease's global eradication. By 1995, the treaty applied only to the same three diseases as the original ISC—cholera, plague, and yellow fever.

---

[6] White House, Global Health Security Agenda: Toward a World Safe and Secure From Infectious Disease Threats (2014), available at http://www.globalhealth.gov/global-health-topics/global-health-security/GHS%20Agenda.pdf.

[7] White House, Fact Sheet: The U.S. Commitment to the Global Health Security Agenda (Nov. 16, 2015), available at https://www.whitehouse.gov/the-press-office/2015/11/16/fact-sheet-us-commitment-global-health-security-agenda.

[8] G7, G-7 Leaders' Declaration (June 8, 2015), available at http://www.interaction.org/document/2015-g7-leaders-declaration.

[9] Norman Howard-Jones, The scientific background of the International Sanitary Conferences 1851–1938 (1975), available at http://whqlibdoc.who.int/publications/1975/14549_eng.pdf.

[10] Lawrence O. Gostin, Global health law (2014).

[11] WHO, WHO Constitution (1946), available at http://whqlibdoc.who.int/hist/official_records/constitution.pdf.

The IHR (2005): International Responsibilities of WHO and States Parties

With the emergence and pandemic potential of HIV/AIDS, the spread of endemic diseases to new parts of the world, and outbreaks of viral hemorrhagic fever, it became clear that the IHR was insufficiently flexible to respond to new infectious disease threats. The WHA called for the IHR's revision in 1995, and subsequent resolutions in 2001 and 2002 brought attention to the early detection of, and rapid response to, public health threats; yet the WHA took little action to shore up this obvious weakness in the IHR.[12]

The imperative for global health governance took on fresh urgency with the advent of severe acute respiratory syndrome (SARS). Although SARS cases emerged in November 2002, China delayed notifying WHO until February 2003. Later, Beijing conceded it had experienced hundreds more cases than previously reported.[13] WHO director-general Gro Harlem Brundtland criticized China's delays,[14] catalyzing a political shift toward a norm of transparency and prompt reporting, further driving IHR reform.[15] The WHA adopted the revised IHR in 2005, and it entered into force in 2007. The IHR has 196 State Parties—every WHO member plus Liechtenstein and the Holy See.[16]

Scope

The revised IHR aims "to prevent, protect against, control and provide a public health response to the international spread of disease" (Article 2). The IHR broke from a disease-specific model, embracing an "all-hazards" strategy. It defines "disease" as including all illnesses or medical conditions, irrespective of origin or source, that could present significant harm to humans. The drafters intended to incorporate

---

[12] World Health Assembly (hereinafter WHA), Revision and updating of the International Health Regulations, WHA48.7 (1995); WHA, Global health security: epidemic alert and response, WHA 54.14 (2001); WHA, Global public health response to natural occurrence accidental release or deliberate use of biological and chemical agents or radionuclear material that affect health, WHA55.16 (2002).

[13] David Heymann, *The international response to the outbreak of SARS in 2003*, 359(1447) Philosophical Transactions of the Royal Society B 1127–1129 (2004), available at http://rstb.royalsocietypublishing.org/content/royptb/359/1447/1127.full.pdf.

[14] Fiona Fleck, *How SARS changed the world in less than six months* 81(8) Bulletin of the World Health Organization 625–626 (2003), available at http://www.who.int/bulletin/volumes/81/8/News0803.pdf?ua=1.

[15] David Heymann, John Mackenzie, and Malik Peiris, *SARS legacy: outbreak reporting is expected and respected*, 381(9869) Lancet 779–781 (2013).

[16] WHO, States Parties to the International Health Regulations (2005), available at http://www.who.int/ihr/legal_issues/states_parties/en/.

biological, chemical, and radionuclear events, as well as zoonotic diseases and threats to food safety.

Recognizing the importance of travel and commerce, the IHR contains a "balancing dynamic," comprising public health, trade, and human rights. This balance informs health measures a State Party may take for international travelers upon arrival and departure and for keeping ships and aircraft free of contamination and disease vectors. States Parties must, though, have sufficient scientific evidence of the risk posed and whether the measure adopted is likely to ameliorate that risk before instituting restrictive travel or trade measures or impinging on human rights.

The IHR obligates States Parties to develop core capacities to detect, assess, report, and respond to potential public health emergencies of international concern. The IHR prescribes explicit capacities for surveillance and response, and for controlling/containing disease at points of entry. The IHR identifies minimum core capacities required at the local, intermediate, and national levels to detect unexpected morbidity and mortality, report information, confirm and assess the status of reported events, notify WHO when required, and respond effectively to contain and mitigate the event.

To guide States Parties in developing IHR core capacities, WHO published the IHR Core Capacity Monitoring Framework in 2010 (subsequently updated).[17] The IHR Monitoring Framework and accompanying IHR Monitoring Tool (IHRMT) identified eight specific core capacities, as well as points of entry and four specific hazards. For each of these 13 core capacities, WHO identified attributes and actions, asking states to use these attributes to assess their compliance (Table 6.1).

The concept of core capacities embraced an "upstream" public health strategy to prevent and contain outbreaks at their source. States Parties agreed "to collaborate with each other to the extent possible" to develop and maintain core capacities (Article 44). States Parties were required to develop and maintain core capacities by 2012, with a possible extension to 2014 and an additional extension to 2016. In 2015, the 68th WHA extended the deadline to 2016 for *all* 81 States Parties that requested extensions. The WHA also decided to support 60 priority countries, including those in West and Central Africa, to meet core capacities by June 2019 (Figure 6.1).[18] Still, the organization's pattern has been to accept continual delays in State Party compliance.

The IHR contains rules regarding points of entry, as well as health measures for conveyances, goods, containers, and travelers. States Parties must apply health measures in a nondiscriminatory manner, justify additional measures, collaborate with other states, and treat personal data confidentially. States Parties must report to

---

[17] World Health Organization, IHR Core Capacity Monitoring Framework: Checklist and indicators for monitoring progress in the development of IHR core capacities in States Parties (2013), available at http://www.who.int/ihr/checklist/en/.

[18] WHO, *supra* note 3.

Table 6.1 **IHR Monitoring Framework: Core Capacities**

Core Capacities to Detect, Assess, Report, and Respond
- Laboratories
- Human resources
- Surveillance
- Preparedness
- Response
- Risk communication
- Coordination and NFP
- National legislation, policy, and financing

Other hazards
- Zoonotic events
- Food safety
- Radiation emergencies Chemical events

Points of entry

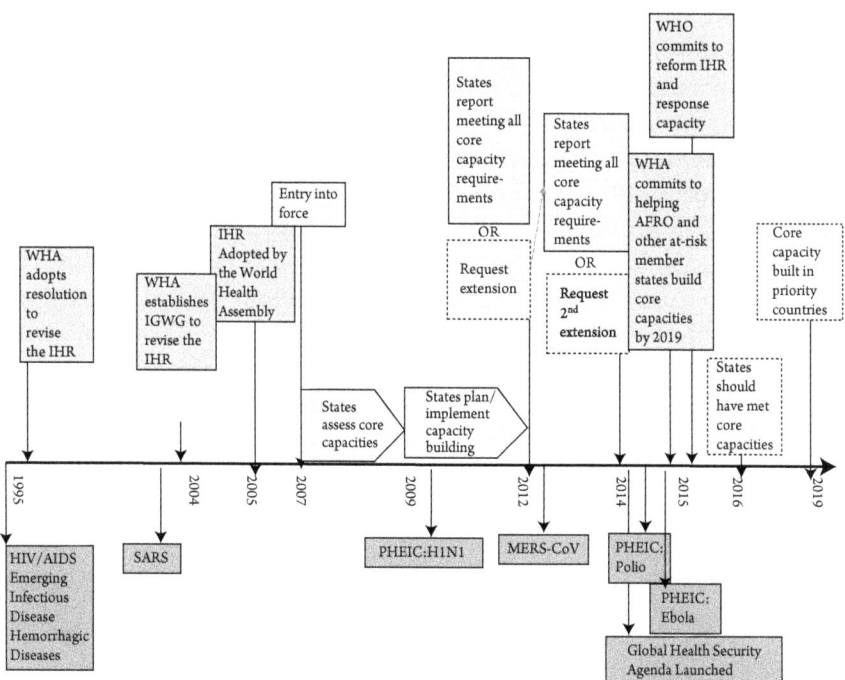

Figure 6.1 IHR timeline.

WHO on their IHR implementation and comply with prescribed dispute resolution procedures. Importantly, the IHR also set up new mechanisms for communication and information sharing between WHO and States Parties. The IHR mandates that each State Party appoint a National IHR Focal Point (NFP) for routine information sharing and coordination during health crises (Figure 6.2). All states have NFPs, at least on paper, but many NFPs are either not well trained in IHR implementation or not properly tasked to routinely communicate with WHO.

Notifications and Declarations of PHEICs

The IHR requires States Parties to promptly notify WHO of events that may constitute a public health emergency of international concern (PHEIC), with an ongoing obligation to inform and respond to subsequent requests. Notifications alert the world to unfolding public health events, as well as marshal resources and coordinate global response efforts. To guide notifications, Annex 2 of the IHR contains a decision instrument requiring State Parties to always notify WHO of four specific diseases: smallpox, wild poliomyelitis, novel human influenza, and SARS. The algorithm also lists pandemic-prone diseases that trigger further assessment, including cholera, yellow fever, and viral hemorrhagic fevers. Beyond listed diseases, States Parties must utilize the instrument to assess any event of potential international public health concern, including from unknown causes, to determine if it is unusual or unexpected, may cross boarders, or may require travel or trade restrictions. The IHR authorizes WHO to consider reports from unofficial sources, such as scientists, nongovernmental organizations, and social media platforms. WHO seeks verification from States Parties in whose territory the event occurs.

The Director-General (D-G) has sole power to declare a PHEIC. In determining whether to declare a PHEIC, the D-G considers (1) information provided by the State Party; (2) the decision instrument; (3) the advice of the Emergency Committee, which the D-G also has sole discretion to convene; (4) scientific principles and evidence; and (5) a risk assessment regarding human health, international spread, and interference with international traffic. If the D-G declares a PHEIC, he or she must issue temporary, nonbinding recommendations describing health measures States Parties should take. The D-G is also empowered to terminate a PHEIC, which automatically expires after 3 months unless extended, modified, or terminated earlier.

Declared PHEICs

In 2009, The D-G declared the first-ever PHEIC (pandemic influenza H1N1) after consultation with Mexico and the United States.[19] WHO was later criticized for

---

[19] Rebecca Katz, *Use of revised International Health Regulations during influenza A (H1N1) epidemic, 2009*, 15(8) Emerging Infectious Diseases (2009).

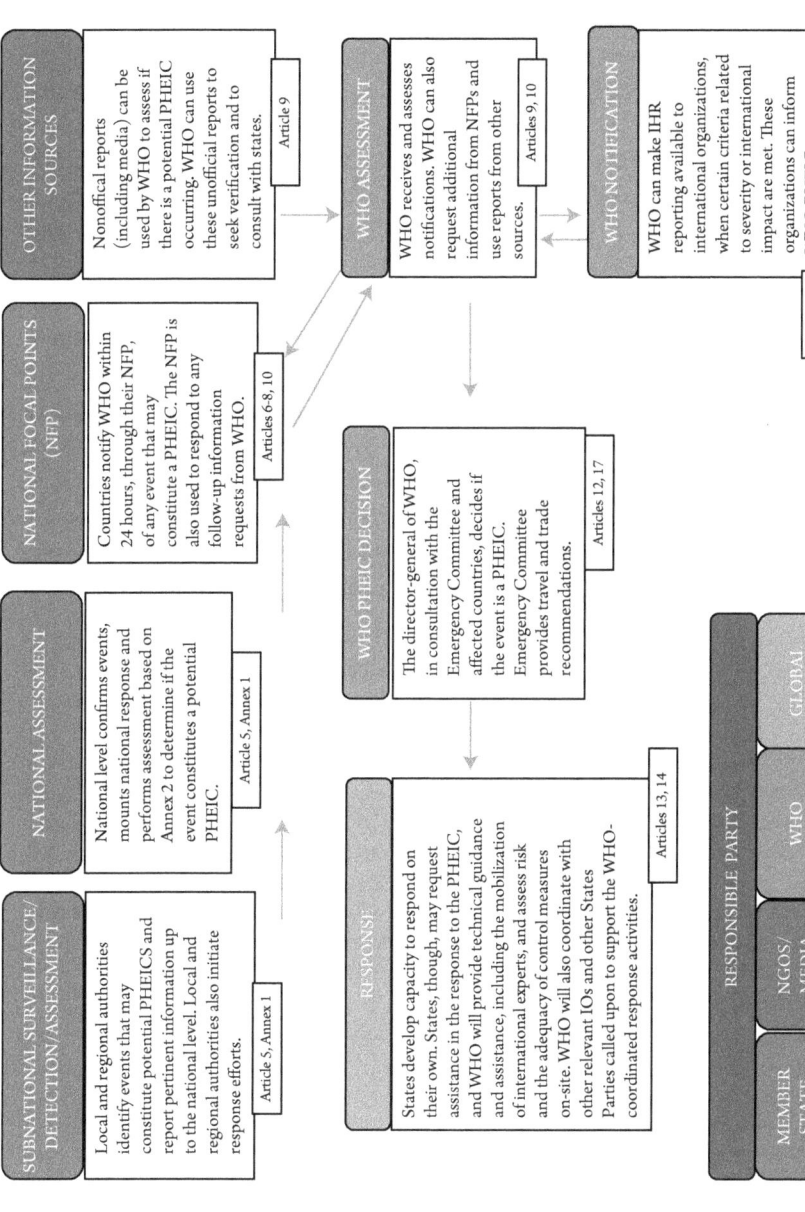

Figure 6.2 IHR process for global governance of disease.

fueling public fear when it became clear the virus was not highly pathogenic,[20] but that criticism was aimed primarily at the classification scheme that WHO used at that time for pandemic phases. Many States Parties also disregarded WHO's temporary recommendations against travel and trade restrictions; several states banned pork imports, while others instituted travel restrictions and advisories.[21] In 2011, the WHO Review Committee charged with reviewing IHR functioning during the H1N1 pandemic cautioned, "The world is ill-prepared to respond to a severe influenza pandemic."[22]

In 2014, the D-G declared two further PHEICs, for polio and for Ebola. The designation for polio appeared counterintuitive given that there were only a handful of cases. Yet small pockets of polio in Afghanistan, Pakistan, and Nigeria jeopardized global eradication. The following year, the WHA endorsed extension of the PHEIC given political instability in the regions with ongoing outbreaks.[23]

In the case of Ebola, the D-G waited 4 months after announcing an "unprecedented outbreak" in April 2014 before declaring a PHEIC on August 8, 2014.[24] The delay looked worse with time, as leaked WHO documents revealed that its decisions were politicized and lacked transparency.[25] WHO's Ebola Interim Assessment Panel stated that urgent warnings "either did not reach senior leaders or senior leaders did not recognize their significance."[26] The temporary recommendations also suffered major flaws of their own, asking states with limited infrastructure to ensure health system capacities without adequate international assistance.[27]

---

[20] Donald McNeilJr, *W.H.O. estimate of swine flu deaths in 2009 rises sharply*, New York Times (Nov. 27, 2013), available at http://www.nytimes.com/2013/11/27/health/who-revises-estimate-of-swine-flu-deaths.html.

[21] WHO, Swine influenza: statement by WHO Director-General, Dr. Margaret Chan (Apr. 27, 2009), http://www.who.int/mediacentre/news/statements/2009/h1n1_20090427/en/; WHO, Implementation of the International Health Regulations (2005): responding to public health emergencies: report by the Director-General, para. 10 (May 15, 2015), available at http://apps.who.int/gb/ebwha/pdf_files/WHA68/A68_22-en.pdf.

[22] WHO, Implementation of the International Health Regulations (2005): report of the Review Committee on the Functioning of the International Health Regulations (2005) in Relation to Pandemic (H1N1) 2009, Doc. A64/10 (May 5, 2011), available at http://apps.who.int/gb/ebwha/pdf_files/WHA64/A64_10-en.pdf.

[23] WHO, Statement on the 5th IHR Emergency Committee meeting regarding the international spread of wild poliovirus (May 5, 2015), available at http://www.who.int/mediacentre/news/statements/2015/polio-5th-statement/en/.

[24] Richard Horton, *A plan to protect the world—and save WHO* 386(9989) Lancet 103 (2015).

[25] Maria Cheng and Raphael Satter, *Emails: UN health agency resisted declaring Ebola emergency*, AP (Mar. 20 2015), available at http://bigstory.ap.org/article/2489c78bff86463589b41f3faaea5ab2/emails-un-health-agency-resisted-declaring-ebola-emergency.

[26] WHO, *supra* note 2.

[27] WHO, Statement on the meeting of the International Health Regulations Emergency Committee regarding the 2014 Ebola outbreak in West Africa (Aug. 8, 2014), available at http://www.who.int/mediacentre/news/statements/2014/ebola-20140808/en/.

The Ebola PHEIC declaration did rally the international community, but not before the disease claimed more than 11,300 lives.[28] President Barack Obama sent in military assets to build treatment facilities and provide logistical support; the United Nations Security Council adopted a resolution calling Ebola a threat to international peace; and the UN secretary-general created the UN Mission for Ebola Emergency Response (UNMEER). Although the D-G continued the PHEIC on December 18, 2015, human-to-human transmission had virtually ended in the three most affected countries.

On February 1, 2016, the D-G declared the fourth, and most recent, PHEIC, in response to the Zika epidemic.[29] Since Brazil reported Zika in May 2015, an estimated 1 million infections have occurred in 25 countries in the Americas. IHR NFPs throughout the Americas have been reporting laboratory-confirmed cases of Zika to the Pan American Health Organization (PAHO).[30] Most concerning is the Zika virus's role in causing neurological disease (Guillain-Barré syndrome) and fetal abnormalities (microcephaly). Curbing the Zika epidemic will require effective vector control, mosquito and human surveillance, and research for reliable diagnostic tests and a vaccine. In 2016, the US Centers for Disease Control and Prevention advised pregnant women to postpone travel to Zika-affected countries.[31]

This is the first time the D-G has declared a PHEIC for a mosquito-borne disease, but the scope of the declaration was narrower than for other PHEICs. Dr. Chan said, "I am now declaring that the recent cluster of microcephaly cases and other neurological disorders reported in Brazil, following a similar cluster in French Polynesia in 2014, constitutes a Public Health Emergency of International Concern."[32] In other words, the PHEIC was for the cluster of microcephaly and Guillain-Barré syndrome rather than for the Zika virus itself. From a legal perspective, the wording of the PHEIC introduces confusion because neither microcephaly

---

[28] WHO, *supra* note 3.

[29] Anthony S. Fauci and David Morens, *Zika virus in the Americas—yet another arbovirus threat*, 106 New England Journal of Medicine (Jan. 13, 2016); Daniel Lucey and Lawrence Gostin, *The emerging Zika pandemic: enhancing preparedness*. JAMA.

[30] WHO and PAHO, Epidemiological alert: Neurological syndrome, congenital malformations, and Zika virus infection: implications for public health in the Americas (Dec. 1, 2015), available at http://www.paho.org/hq/index.php?option=com_content&view=article&id=11599&Itemid=41691&lang=en.

[31] Emily Petersen et al., *Interim guidelines for pregnant women during a Zika virus outbreak—United States, 2016*, 65(2) MMWR Morb Mortal Wkly Rep. 30–33 (2016).

[32] WHO director-general summarizes the outcome of the Emergency Committee regarding clusters of microcephaly and Guillain-Barré syndrome, available at http://www.who.int/mediacentre/news/statements/2016/emergency-committee-zika-microcephaly/en/; WHO statement on the first meeting of the International Health Regulations (2005) (IHR 2005) Emergency Committee on Zika virus and observed increase in neurological disorders and neonatal malformations (Feb. 1, 2016), available at http://www.who.int/mediacentre/news/statements/2016/1st-emergency-committee-zika/en/.

nor Guillain-Barré syndrome is an infectious disease. These neurological and congenital conditions per se do not appear to be hazards that could cross borders under the meaning of Annex 2.

Undeclared and Potential PHEICs

The world is now closely watching outbreaks of Middle East respiratory syndrome (MERS), which originated in Saudi Arabia in 2012.[33] MERS has yet to trigger a PHEIC declaration despite reaching more than two dozen countries and accounting for at least 1,621 laboratory-confirmed cases and 584 deaths by December 2015.[34] By September 2015, the D-G had convened 10 Emergency Committee meetings,[35] with the last 2 occurring during and after the virus spread from Saudi Arabia to the Republic of Korea, sparking a large outbreak.[36] Most MERS cases were linked to hospital settings, and absent sustained community transmission, the committee concluded the conditions to declare a PHEIC had not been met.[37]

For many global health crises, the D-G chose not to convene an Emergency Committee, including cholera in Haiti, the Fukushima nuclear disaster in Japan, and chemical weapons use in Syria. Each event would have required notification under Annex 2, as have the several hundred events that have been reported to WHO as *potential* PHEICs. Confusion still exists as to what events warrant consideration by an Emergency Committee and potentially a PHEIC declaration. What steps can and should WHO take to ensure prompt notification and information sharing, and how can the D-G improve the transparency and scientific rigor for declaring a PHEIC?

Operationalizing the IHR: Widespread Noncompliance

The IHR affords a vital governing framework to limit the international spread of disease. Yet, 10 years of experience has shed light on the critical challenges in

---

[33] WHO, Middle East respiratory syndrome—Saudi Arabia (Dec. 4, 2015), available at http://www.who.int/csr/don/4-december-2015-mers-saudi-arabia/en/.

[34] Daniel R. Lucey, MERS in Korea: why this outbreak can be stopped soon (June 7, 2015), available at http://csis.org/files/publication/150608_MERS%20in%20Korea%20Why%20This%20Outbreak%20Can%20Be%20Stopped%20Soon.pdf.

[35] WHO, Emergency Committee—9th meeting summary: briefing notes on MERS-CoV (June 22, 2015), available at http://www.who.int/mediacentre/news/mers/briefing-notes/update-22-june-2015/en/.

[36] Gostin and Lucey, *supra* note 24.

[37] WHO, WHO statement on the eighth meeting of the IHR Emergency Committee regarding MERS-CoV (Feb. 5, 2015), available at http://www.who.int/mediacentre/news/statements/2015/8th-mers-emergency-committee/en/.

implementing the IHR, as well as major omissions in the regulations. These challenges and gaps have become politically salient, with deepening concern that the IHR, and WHO itself, failed to fulfill the promises of sound governance and leadership. States Parties, in particular, have undermined the IHR's effectiveness by failing to fully comply with their international obligations. In the following, we explain the gaps and features of noncompliance.

National Core Capacities

National capacities for preparedness, detection, and response form the bedrock of global health security (Table 6.2).[38] Yet most States Parties have yet to fully establish core capacities. In 2014, only 64 States Parties reported meeting core capacities, while 48 failed even to respond to WHO (Figure 6.3).[39] Governments have not properly funded and implemented required capacities, and international assistance has been limited.[40] Achieving IHR core capacities by all states remains an indisputable baseline for global health security. Every WHO IHR Review Committee and all the major commissions have demanded that State Parties build and strengthen core capacities—all to no avail.[41]

Finding the resources to support health system capacity building has been challenging. Although States Parties committed to providing domestic resources to build core capacities, national budgets often neglect this commitment under the IHR. Many countries lack the resources to build systems for unknown threats as they have struggled to meet the everyday health needs of their populations. Similarly, WHO and higher-income States Parties agreed to provide technical and financial assistance to countries in need, but with some exceptions, very few have funded projects explicitly for building IHR core capacities.[42] The bulwark of international financing has been in the form of vertical funding streams, such as for AIDS, tuberculosis, and malaria. All in all, sustainable funding commensurate with the need for IHR core capacities has come neither from national governments nor from donors.

---

[38] Lawrence O. Gostin and Eric A. Friedman, *A retrospective and prospective analysis of the West African Ebola virus disease epidemic: robust national health systems at the foundation and an empowered WHO at the apex*, 385 Lancet 1902–1909 (2015).

[39] WHO, Implementation of the International Health Regulations (2005): report of the Review Committee on Second Extensions for Establishing National Public Health Capacities and on IHR Implementation: report by the director-general, para. 17 (Mar. 27, 2015), available at http://apps.who.int/gb/ebwha/pdf_files/WHA68/A68_22Add1-en.pdf.

[40] *Id.*

[41] *Id.* at paras. 45–49; WHO, *supra* note 2, at 6.

[42] Dac Phu Tran et al., *Strengthening global health security capacity—Vietnam demonstration project, 2013*, 63(4) MMWR Morb Mortal Wkly Rep 77–80 (Jan. 31, 2014); Andres Lescano et al., *Outbreak investigation and response training*, 318(5850) Science 574–575 (Oct. 26, 2007).

Table 6.2 **Panels, Committees, and Reports Related to IHR Reform**

Ebola Interim Assessment Panel	WHO
Review Committee on the Role of the IHR in the Ebola Outbreak and Response	WHO
Roadmap for Action on Ebola	WHO
Advisory Group on Reform of WHO's Work in Outbreaks and Emergencies With Health and Humanitarian Consequences	WHO
Review Committee on the Functioning of IHR in Relation to the Pandemic (H1N1)	WHO
UN Secretary General High Level Panel on Global Response to Health Crises	UN
Commission on a Global Health Risk Framework for the Future	US National Academy of Medicine
Harvard-LSHTM Independent Panel on the Global Response to Ebola	Academia

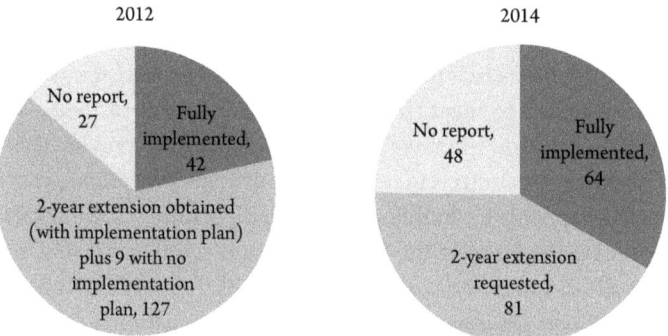

Figure 6.3 IHR implementation, 2012–2014.

Meaningful Metrics

Through the IHR Monitoring Tool, WHO expects States Parties to conduct annual self-assessments on IHR implementation, focusing on the 13 core capacities. States were supposed to issue formal reports in 2012 (with additional reports in 2014 and 2016 for governments that requested extensions) to declare if they have fully implemented the regulations. If they have not, countries are supposed to submit a concrete plan to reach full implementation.

Even if States Parties had reported accurately and in a timely manner, national self-assessments are unacceptable and cannot ensure uniformly high-quality

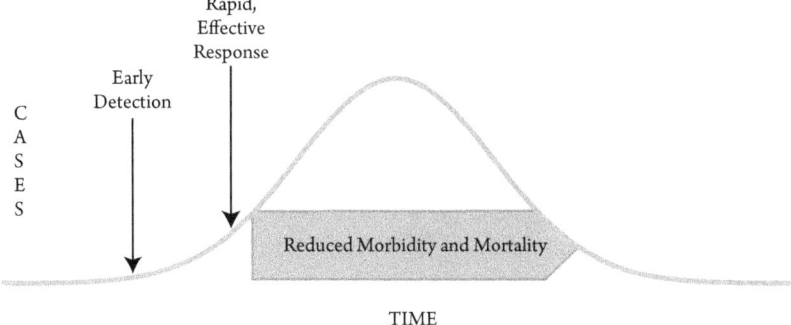

Figure 6.4 Theoretical framework: Early detection leads to rapid response, leads to reduced morbidity and mortality.

national preparedness. States Parties have not collected sufficient or the right kinds of data to produce quantitative assessments of what are predominantly qualitative questions. Governments, moreover, do not use a consistent set of evidence-based metrics to measure their compliance. Most important, self-assessments are inherently self-interested and unreliable, absent rigorous independent validation. These deficiencies undermine the integrity and utility of self-assessments.[43]

Timely and Full Notification

Although the IHR called for robust information sharing through reporting of potential PHEICs, countries continue to delay notifications and/or limit the information reported. Delayed reporting and/or lack of transparency and cooperation, for example, occurred in West Africa during Ebola and in Saudi Arabia during MERS. Additionally, governments have failed to share pertinent information about international travelers, either ignoring their international obligations or simply due to confusion about patient privacy.

The IHR cannot effectively govern global health security unless governments promptly report novel infections. This follows the simple pattern of the epidemiological curve: the faster health authorities know about a novel event, the faster they can mount an effective response (Figure 6.4). But governments have economic reasons to withhold or delay transparent information sharing. They fear that once they have disclosed an outbreak of a novel infection, governments and private parties may impose travel and trade restrictions, with severe economic consequences. Once they have honestly disclosed, the IHR Emergency Committee could conclude that travel and trade restrictions are warranted; more likely, governments or the private sector may simply take action, disregarding WHO recommendations.

[43] WHO, *supra* note 41.

Given previous patterns, national concern about the economic repercussions of prompt reporting appears fully justified. Guinea, Sierra Leone, and Liberia, for example, experienced aggregate cumulative losses of more than 10% of GDP as a result of the Ebola outbreak.[44] Canada during SARS as well as Mexico and the United States during H1N1 suffered major loses from precipitous reductions in tourism and trade. Yet the failure to raise the global alert ultimately can be even more impactful in terms of human life and national treasure. The Commission on a Global Health Risk Framework for the Future concluded, "The global community has massively underestimated the risks that pandemics present to human life and livelihoods. . . . There are very few risks facing mankind that threaten loss of life on the scale of pandemics . . . [and] that have the potential for such catastrophic economic impact." The commission estimates that a pandemic in the 21st century could cost in excess of $6 trillion.[45]

Despite the severe health and economic repercussions of unnecessary travel and trade restrictions, WHO has not had the political authority or capacity to prevent States Parties from disregarding its recommendations. WHO is not a policing agency, and the IHR offers scant inducements to ensure consistent State Party compliance. When countries balance their IHR obligation to report against the risk of economic sanctions, they may wait as long as possible before sharing vital information.

WHO Governance

The Ebola epidemic highlighted major deficiencies in mobilizing a large-scale, coordinated response to health emergencies. The IHR provides a framework for global health security, but it functions only if WHO is an effective leader and governments build strong health systems. WHO erred on multiple levels during the Ebola epidemic. The D-G waited 5 months after cross-border spread before declaring an emergency. The WHO Regional Office for Africa and country offices impeded deployment of international aid workers and equipment. Most important, WHO failed to mobilize adequate fiscal and human resources until the epidemic was spinning out of control. The organization eventually corrected these mistakes, but the delay probably cost thousands of lives. In fairness, the fault lies not only with the WHO Secretariat but also with member states that have starved the agency of resources for many years.

---

[44] United Nations Development Group (UNDG)—Western and Central Africa, Socio-economic Impact of Ebola Virus Disease in West African Countries (2015), available at http://www.africa.undp.org/content/dam/rba/docs/Reports/ebola-west-africa.pdf.

[45] Commission on a Global Health Risk Framework for the Future, The Neglected Dimension of Global Security: A Framework to Counter Infectious Disease Crises; National Academy of Medicine (2016), available at www.nam.edu/GHRF.

The reasons for WHO's failures are well understood but remain resistant to change. In 2011, the agency cut its budget by nearly US$600 million due to a severe fiscal deficit, notably its epidemic response capabilities.[46] Its regional structures also have been long-standing problems, with significant variability among regional organizations. The D-G has called on governments and donors to build core capacities and has asked for State Party compliance with the IHR, but without impact.[47] All the Ebola commissions have exhibited an implicit distrust in the organization to make the necessary reforms. Instead, each panel has proposed a well-funded and accountable WHO Center for Global Health Preparedness and Response. The Harvard-LSHTM panel, for example, insisted that a new center should be quasi-independent, with a separate governing board.

WHO is the agency charged with overseeing the IHR. Without effective leadership, the IHR's security framework breaks down. In other words, a strong treaty text is insufficient without a well-funded and robust operational response.

Major Gaps in the IHR

When the revised IHR was negotiated, member states aimed to be as inclusive of all public health threats as possible. However, there remained major omissions in the text, notably sample sharing and zoonotic threats.

Sample Sharing: Inequitable Distribution of Benefits

Indonesia sent shock waves around the world in December 2006, when its minister for health, Siti Fadila Supari, refused to share samples of avian influenza A (H5N1) with WHO. Indonesia's decision revealed fissures within the international community. Developing countries backed Indonesia's claim that it was unfair to share viruses without any reciprocal obligation to make vaccines and medicines affordable.

WHO led a 5-year negotiation that resulted in the 2011 Pandemic Influenza Preparedness (PIP) Framework.[48] This PIP Framework, however, applies only to pandemic influenza and not to other novel pathogens such as SARS, MERS, and Zika. The framework stands entirely outside the IHR. The regulations, moreover, are silent on the health security issues of sample sharing and equitable access to medical countermeasures.

---

[46] Lawrence Gostin and Eric Friedman, *Ebola: a crisis in global health leadership*, 384 Lancet 1323–1325 (2014).

[47] World Health Organization, Report by the director-general to the Executive Board at its 138th session, Geneva (Jan. 25, 2016), EB 138/2.

[48] David Fidler and Lawrence Gostin, *The WHO Pandemic Influenza Preparedness Framework: a milestone in global governance for health*, 306(2) JAMA 200–201 (2011).

Neither international agreement, moreover, addresses a modern biosecurity hazard. In the not-too-distant future, scientists will be able to sequence the genetic composition of pathogens, which will enable them to recreate novel viruses and to manipulate their genetic makeup. Although, for example, smallpox has been eradicated, scientists can sequence its genome, synthesize a real smallpox virus using the genetic code, and potentially enhance the virus's ability for airborne transmission. These capabilities pose major biosecurity threats, which the IHR and PIP Framework do not govern. Harmonizing the IHR and the PIP Framework, and closing major coverage gaps, would markedly improve health security.

Zoonotic Threats

Approximately 70% of all emerging infectious diseases have a zoological origin, yet negotiators intentionally did not explicitly include animal diseases in the IHR. The drafters were perhaps too deferential to existing regimes, such as the World Organization for Animal Health (OIE) and the UN Food and Agriculture Organization (FAO). Although the IHR broadly defines "disease," its practical scope is narrow, and the regulations do not incorporate a "one-health" approach. The failure to integrate animal health could become a particularly salient omission for diseases such as Zika, with large animal reservoirs and with the primary mode of transmission through an insect source.

The IHR Monitoring Framework sought to include zoonotic diseases as "other hazards," but the regulations fail to govern multisectoral engagement and coordination on zoonotic diseases, or the laboratory or surveillance capacities required to identify disease in animals. As the world faces the peril of novel zoonotic diseases and the overuse of antibiotics in both humans and agriculture (exacerbating the global antimicrobial-resistance crisis), it appears anomalous that the IHR does not facilitate and guide research and practice at the intersection of human and animal health.

The Future of IHR: Recommendations for Reform

The IHR is the governing framework for global health security, yet it requires textual and operational reforms. The WHO Secretariat is engaged in an internal reform process, ranging from the WHO Roadmap for Action on Ebola[49] to the Advisory Group on Reform of WHO's Work in Outbreaks and Emergencies with Health and

---

[49] WHO, Follow up to the World Health Assembly decision on the Ebola virus disease outbreak and the Special Session of the Executive Board on Ebola: Roadmap for Action (Sept. 2015), available at http://www.who.int/about/who_reform/emergency-capacities/WHO-outbreasks-emergencies-Roadmap.pdf.

Humanitarian Consequences.[50] In addition to the Ebola Interim Assessment Panel,[51] the agency established the WHO Review Committee on the Role of the IHR in the Ebola Outbreak and Response.[52] On January 30, 2016, the D-G announced internal reforms, including a single program and incident management to oversee all health emergencies. The D-G stressed yet again, however, that the program required sustainable funding from member states.[53]

The proliferation of internal and external reform processes could be transformative. This is "the defining moment for the health of the global community."[54] Yet it is just as likely that the maze of recommendations will lead to weak or muddled reforms. Here we offer proposals for fundamental reform of IHR implementation, WHO oversight, and State Party conformance. We propose politically feasible pathways to reform to avoid a long history of bureaucratic stagnation. Thus, our proposals balance the ideal with the politically possible.

Build Robust IHR Core Capacities: Link Capacities to Metrics and Financing

Meeting IHR core capacities requires mutual responsibility and accountability. It starts with governments dedicating resources to build and sustain health systems. Every State Party should undergo independent, rigorous review of IHR core capacities, using measurable metrics and targets. Shared responsibilities also require technical assistance and international financing to close capacity gaps. Collective security is assured only by fulfilling these mutual obligations to sustainably build, measure, and finance health systems.

Building sustainable core capacities requires fresh thinking both by donors and by recipient countries. Too often, countries that are heavily dependent on external funding follow the priorities of donors, agreeing to erect vertical programs, yet meeting IHR core capacities requires the development of horizontal programs, including diagnostic laboratories that can be used for more than just one pathogen or condition, specimen transport systems that are applicable to all samples, and event-based surveillance systems designed to pick up unusual or unexpected public health events. Building core capacity also requires integrating these systems into annual budgeting for health system strengthening.

---

[50] WHO, Advisory Group on Reform of WHO's Work in Outbreaks and Emergencies with Health and Humanitarian Consequences, available at http://www.who.int/about/who_reform/emergency-capacities/advisory-group/en/.

[51] WHO, *supra* note 2.

[52] WHO, Review Committee on the Role of the International Health Regulations (2005) in the Ebola outbreak and response, available at http://www.who.int/ihr/review-committee-2016/en/.

[53] WHO, Global Policy Group Statement on reforms of WHO work in outbreaks and emergencies (Jan. 30, 2016), available at http://www.who.int/dg/speeches/2016/reform-statement/en/.

[54] WHO, *supra* note 2.

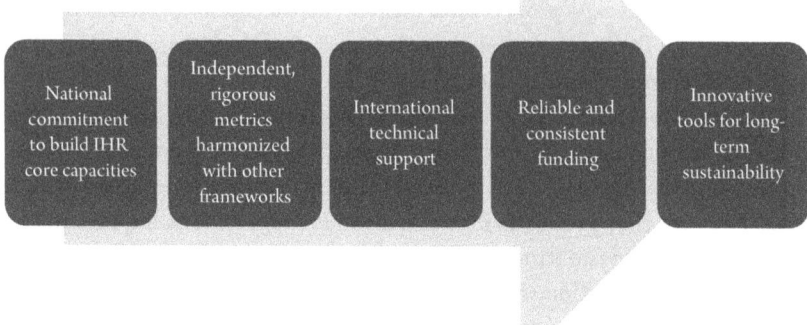

Figure 6.5 Pathway to strong, measured, funded, and sustained IHR core capacities.

Develop Metrics and Rigorous Assessments

For IHR metrics to be meaningful, valued, and utilized, they must undergo rigorous external evaluations. WHO should establish an independent evaluation system, with a feedback loop and continuous quality improvement. Independent assessments would use evidence-based metrics and indicators. Unless assessment criteria are clear, transparent, and valid, they will not be fully trusted. The measurable benchmarks for the external assessment process, moreover, should be integrated directly into the IHR, Annex 1, which contains the core capacity requirements for surveillance and response. It may be necessary either to amend Annex 1 or to adjust its operationalization.

Parallel initiatives such as the GHSA and OIE's PVS Pathways (measuring compliance with OIE standards on Veterinary Services) should be harmonized with the IHR. The IHR is the only agreement with the international legal and political legitimacy to set global security standards. Harmonizing extant multiple standards within the IHR would be more holistic, ensuring a One Health strategy and reducing redundancies for governments exposed to multiple evaluations. WHO recently took such steps and released the Joint External Evaluation Tool, an assessment tool that integrates IHR core capacities and GHSA action packages into a single document. The intent is that the JEE will be used both for self assessment and for occasional external assessments.

States, however, often resist external assessment due to sovereignty concerns, but the new system could be designed to foster cooperation. Evaluation teams would comprise both domestic and external experts, so national governments would be fully involved in the process. WHO, regional, and country offices would play a strategic role. Civil society should be fully engaged, much like the UNAIDS monitoring mechanisms. Expert panels would work constructively and collaboratively to identify capacity gaps, develop a roadmap, and identify funding sources to achieve measurable benchmarks for success. The mandate, therefore, would be not to give a passing or failing grade but to continuously improve health infrastructure with strategic plans and adequate financing.

The World Bank's Pandemic Emergency Facility (PEF) should tie funding to country cooperation with IHR assessments. Additionally, international donors such as Regional Development Banks, the Global Fund, and philanthropies could create funding streams for national IHR core capacities, also conditioned upon rigorous assessments. All these measures would reinforce national commitments to build robust health systems, which align well with the UN Sustainable Development Target of Universal Health Coverage (UHC).[55] These possibilities are mapped at Figure 6.5.

"What gets measured gets done." But Laud Boateng, a GHSA Next Generation Fellow from Ghana, shifts this discourse to better reflect national experiences, noting, "What gets measured gets done, but only what gets political support gets measured, and only that which is funded gets political support."[56] Thus, tying independent evaluations to external funding would foster cooperation and marshal resources for building core capacities. The World Bank has started the process of exploring mechanisms for tying strengthening of public health infrastructure to external funding, but the metrics and details are still being developed.

Create Reliable and Consistent Financing Mechanisms

Robust financing is required not only to build national health systems but also to support WHO's own capacities and to ensure a surge in resources in a health emergency. Several financing models could operate separately or in concert. Increasing WHO member state assessed contributions would be the most logical funding source. Mandatory dues are more predictable and sustainable than discretionary funding for targeted projects. Moreover, as the treaty oversight agency, WHO holds the legal obligation to implement the regulations, including ensuring adequate financing.

Assessed dues, however, are politically fraught. Several member states do not have sufficient confidence in the agency to increase their dues, and they want discretion to direct the destination of the assistance. Consequently, it will be necessary to create alternative financing mechanisms. The GHSA Action Packages and the PEF are realistic funding sources, but they should be synchronized with the IHR. The Global Fund offers another model, whereby WHO and the World Bank could host

---

[55] Ashish Jha et al., *Accelerating achievement of the sustainable development goals: a game changer in global health*, 352 BMJ (Jan. 29, 2016).

[56] Laud Boateng, Perspectives in Global Health Security: Effective prevention, detection and response to global pandemics, CRDF Global Sponsored Briefing (Oct. 2015).

a donors' conference to boost international support and cooperation.[57] Ensuring sustainable resources to develop and maintain core capacities would benefit both low- and high-income countries by strengthening security for all.

Invest in Human Resources

The Ebola outbreak demonstrated that a well-trained, well-equipped health workforce is crucial to an effective response, including doctors, nurses, community health workers, lab technicians, infection control practitioners, and public health experts. If there are insufficient health personnel and their numbers are depleted even further by exposure to infection, the health system will fail to control outbreaks. Educating, training, supporting, and protecting health workers is a defining issue for global health security.

Even a well-prepared workforce may not be able to cope in a public health emergency. In such cases, WHO must make provisions for a surge in human resources, such as through the Global Outbreak Alert and Response Network (GOARN). The 2015 WHA endorsed a Global Health Reserve Workforce but failed to guarantee funding. WHO, however, is continuing to try to build this emergency response workforce.

Civil Society: Holding States Parties to Account

AIDS advocates demonstrated the power of civil society to demand global health equity.[58] Civil Society Organizations (CSOs) care for their communities, monitor governments, and hold stakeholders to account. As with other spheres of international law, such as in human rights or climate change, civil society could offer "shadow" reports and advocate for funding national capacities and fulfilling IHR and human rights obligations. Harnessing the power of civil society requires more than incorporating CSOs into existing or new IHR functions. Borrowing from the Framework Convention on Tobacco Control, WHO could regularly host a Conference of the Parties (COP) where civil society representatives could meet with governments to advance IHR implementation. The Framework Convention Alliance (CSOs committed to effective implementation of the Framework Convention on Tobacco Control) has propelled tobacco control reforms. A similar CSO network for IHR implementation could be transformative.

---

[57] WHO, *supra* note 2; *What lessons for the International Health Regulations?*, 384(9951) Lancet 1321 (2014).

[58] Kent Buse, Lawrence Gostin, and Eric Friedman, *Pathways towards a framework convention on global health: political mobilization for the human right to health*, in Michael Freeman, Sarah Hawkes, and Belinda Bennett (eds.), Law and Global Health (2014).

Emergency Committees: Independence and Scientific Expertise

After facing criticism for disclosing Emergency Committee members only after the H1N1 PHEIC was terminated, WHO improved public trust by releasing member names for subsequent Emergency and Review Committees.[59] WHO also pledged transparency on expert committee members' conflicts of interest.[60] Concerns still persist, however, that Emergency Committees are influenced by politics rather than strictly by scientific evidence. The D-G and Emergency Committee offered no evidence for their decisions regarding H1N1,[61] very little for the first Emergency Committee meeting on Ebola,[62] and little during the initial meetings on MERS.[63] They gave more transparent explanations for polio[64] and recent MERS and Zika Emergency Committees.[65] The D-G and Emergency Committee should publicly disclose their evidence and decision-making processes. Transparency would include full minutes of Emergency Committee meetings, web access to relevant documents, and live updates through social media platforms.

Independent and transparent Emergency Committee decision-making would build public confidence, but these reforms are of little value if the D-G fails to convene an Emergency Committee. Outside WHO's governing structure and drawing on civil society shadow reports, a committee of independent experts, particularly from academia and civil society, could coalesce to regularly review data on disease outbreaks and recommend actions, including recommending the D-G to convene an Emergency Committee.

---

[59] WHO, *supra* note 23, at 16.

[60] WHO, Frequently asked questions on IHR Emergency Committee (2015), available at http://www.who.int/ihr/procedures/en_ihr_ec_faq.pdf.

[61] WHO, Swine influenza: statement by WHO director-general, Dr. Margaret Chan (Apr. 25, 2009), available at http://www.who.int/mediacentre/news/statements/2009/h1n1_20090425/en/.

[62] WHO, WHO statement on the meeting of the International Health Regulations Emergency Committee regarding the 2014 Ebola outbreak in West Africa (Aug. 8, 2014), available at http://www.who.int/mediacentre/news/statements/2014/ebola-20140808/en/.

[63] WHO, WHO statement on the second meeting of the IHR Emergency Committee concerning MERS-CoV (July 17, 2013), available at http://www.who.int/mediacentre/news/statements/2013/mers_cov_20130717/en/.

[64] WHO, WHO statement on the meeting of the International Health Regulations Emergency Committee concerning the international spread of wild poliovirus (May 5, 2014), available at http://www.who.int/entity/mediacentre/news/statements/2014/polio-20140505/en/index.html.

[65] WHO, WHO statement on the ninth meeting of the IHR Emergency Committee regarding MERS-CoV (June 17, 2015), available at http://www.who.int/mediacentre/news/statements/2015/ihr-ec-mers/en/.

Reliable and Timely PHEIC Declarations

The declaration of a PHEIC is the public face of WHO's outbreak response, but the agency must respond long before an outbreak becomes an international emergency. Beyond the IHR, WHO has multiple instruments that support early action. For example, WHO utilizes the Emergency Response Framework (ERF) to measure the level of risk and inform the international community of an outbreak's severity in a graduated manner.[66] As evidenced during the Ebola epidemic, using two distinct sets of governing rules (the ERF and the IHR) confused first responders and the public. Similar confusion arose during the H1N1 pandemic, where WHO did not coordinate the six pandemic phases in the Pandemic Influenza Preparedness and Response Framework (since revised)[67] with the PHEIC. Given the public symbolism of a PHEIC, multiple emergency response frameworks must be integrated with IHR processes.

The WHO Ebola Interim Assessment Panel recommended introducing an intermediate-level emergency—allowing gradation while retaining the power of a PHEIC.[68] A gradient system would not necessarily require a textual amendment to the IHR, as many diplomats fear. WHO could develop informal guidelines through Article 11, which allows that agency to share information with States Parties, alerting them to potential emergencies in a graduated fashion. Alternatively, the WHA could adopt a new IHR annex illustrating the risk gradient, limiting negotiations only to the new annex. To maintain credibility, different grades should trigger clear operational and financial strategies. For example, an intermediate-level emergency could allow WHO to access resources from the Contingency Fund. Similarly, the World Bank could release PEF funds based on graded emergency declarations by WHO.[69] The promise of international assistance with adequate funding, even at an early stage, could provide additional incentives for States Parties to report a potential PHEIC through the Annex 2 algorithm. A full PHEIC declaration, however, would still be needed to raise the global alert, stiffen political resolve, and mobilize major resources.

Fostering a Culture of Compliance: Carrots and the Sticks

State disregard for Article 43's "Additional Health Measures" and Emergency Committee temporary recommendations (e.g., travel and trade restrictions and

---

[66] WHO, Emergency response framework 19 (2013), available at http://apps.who.int/iris/bitstream/10665/89529/1/9789241504973_eng.pdf?ua=1.

[67] WHO, Current WHO phases of pandemic alert for pandemic (H1N1) (20090, available at http://www.who.int/csr/disease/swineflu/phase/en/.

[68] WHO, *supra* note 2.

[69] CJ Standley et al., *New framework for global public health emergency reporting and response* 348(6236) Science 762–763 (May 15, 2015).

injudicious quarantines) undermines the IHR. During the H1N1 and Ebola outbreaks, States Parties disregarded WHO recommendations and imposed additional measures, impeding deployment of critical medical supplies and health workers. Regional and international carriers suspended flights; States Parties banned travel to and from, or trade with, affected countries; and quarantines of health workers returning from the region dampened the charitable instinct to help.

WHO is not a policing agency that can readily impose sanctions on States Parties for noncompliance with their legal obligations, but it does have means at its disposal to enhance compliance. The D-G should publicly request clear rationales for and reconsideration of additional measures, while working with States Parties to dismantle harmful policies. The D-G could more actively encourage States Parties to pursue available dispute mediation and arbitration under Article 56(3). He or she could similarly steer States Parties toward the Permanent Court of Arbitration Optional Rules for Arbitrating Disputes Between Two States. WHO and World Trade Organization could similarly encourage use of the WTO Dispute Resolution procedures by States Parties harmed by additional measures. Although the WTO is primarily constituted to adjudicate WTO treaties, it could intervene in cases where state action adversely impacts both public health and international trade—such as a poultry ban during influenza H5N1 outbreaks.

Beyond WTO, other institutions could encourage IHR compliance. For example, at various points during the H1N1 pandemic, the FAO, OIE, and WTO joined WHO in issuing joint statements discouraging trade restrictions on pork and pigs.[70] It also may be possible to look to the International Court of Justice (ICJ) when one country's active violation of the IHR causes specific damage to either the population or the economy of a second country.

The WHO could do still more to signal strong political commitment to IHR compliance. The WHA, for example, could amend Article 48 to elevate temporary recommendations from the Emergency Committee during a PHEIC to a binding status. Even though States Parties could still disregard their international obligations, more obligatory treaty language could increase pressure to comply.

Realpolitik: Making IHR Reform Politically Possible

Textual reforms are more difficult to achieve than operational reforms. Reopening the full text of the IHR for revision would result in a multiyear negotiating process,

---

[70] FAO, WHO, OIE, and WTO, Joint FAO/WHO/OIE/WTO statement on influenza A(H1N1) and the safety of pork (May 2, 2009), available at http://www.who.int/mediacentre/news/statements/2009/h1n1_20090502/en/.

would require considerable resources, and could result in weaker IHR norms and human right safeguards. Our proposals for reform, therefore, should be achieved, wherever possible, by textual interpretation, understandings, and amendments to specific annexes rather than the main text.

There is precedent for amending an IHR annex without reopening the entire text to negotiation (2014 Resolution regarding Annex 7 and Yellow Fever).[71] States Parties could find consensus on new language or understandings focused only on particular annexes. Revisions to the main text through textual interpretations or understandings would be politically feasible. In arms control treaties, for example, States Parties use the mechanism of Review Conferences to agree on a series of understandings to guide treaty implementation and State Party compliance. The States Parties decide specifically not to reopen the original text to revision. IHR States Parties could adopt similarly effective political strategies, fully consistent with international law. "Smart" global health diplomacy could enhance IHR functioning without bureaucratic hurdles standing in the way of sensible reform (Table 6.3).

The Way Forward

Ten years after its adoption, it is time to realize the promise of the IHR. The unconscionable Ebola epidemic in West Africa opened a window of opportunity for fundamental reform—both for the IHR and for the organization that oversees the treaty. That political window, however, is rapidly closing. Donor fatigue, fading memories, and competing priorities (e.g., climate change, the Paris bombings, and fighting the Islamic State) are diverting political attention. The promising results of the vaccine trial *Ebola ça Suffit* (Ebola that's enough),[72] although transformative, could further weaken political resolve. Empowering WHO and realizing the IHR's potential would shore up global health security—a vital investment in human and animal health—while reducing the vast economic consequences of the next global health emergency.

---

[71] WHO, Implementation of the International Health Regulations (2005), WHA67.13 (May 24, 2914), available at http://apps.who.int/gb/ebwha/pdf_files/WHA67/A67_R13-en.pdf.

[72] Ana Maria Henao-Restrepo et al., *Efficacy and effectiveness of an rVSV-vectored vaccine expressing Ebola surface glycoprotein: interim results from the Guinea ring vaccination cluster-randomised trial*, 386 (9996) Lancet, 857–866 (Aug. 29, 2015), available at http://www.thelancet.com/pdfs/journals/lancet/PIIS0140-6736(15)61117-5.pdf.

Table 6.3 Compilation of Our Recommended Reforms of the IHR and its Implementation

	Recommended Reform	Who and Why	Political Mechanism
IHR core capacities	National and global commitment to build, strengthen, and maintain IHR core capacities, linked directly to independent assessments and financing.	*Who*: National governments, international organizations, bilateral donors, and funding organizations. *Why*: Global health security is dependent on every nation having the ability to detect, assess, report and respond to public health emergencies.	No textual change to IHR required for commitment to core capacities. Political and financial commitment to support process required by WHO and other funding entities, such as the World Bank and regional development banks.
Independently assessed metrics	Rigorous metrics assessed by independent evaluators to identify capacity gaps, develop a roadmap, and identify funding sources to achieve core capacities.	*Who*: Independent evaluation teams of domestic and external experts, with WHO, regional and country offices and civil society participation. *Why*: Independently assessed vigorous metrics will provide accurate analysis of national core capacities that can then be used by funding entities to invest in core capacities or for use in insurance mechanisms.	Amend Annex 1 of IHR to include measurable benchmarks. Task WHO, working with funding entities, to create rigorous metrics and organize assessments.
Harmonization	Independent assessments and metrics harmonized with GHSA and PVS.	*Who*: WHO, working collaboratively with GHSA and OIE. *Why*: To ensure a One Health strategy and reduce redundancies for governments exposed to multiple evaluations.	Harmonization incorporated into Annex 1 amendment. WHO, GHSA, and OIE enhanced communication and collaboration.

(*continued*)

Table 6.3 Continued

	Recommended Reform	Who and Why	Political Mechanism
New financing mechanisms	Robust financing to build core capacities, as well as to support WHO's capacity (including surge capacity in emergencies) and building human resources.	*Who*: WHO member states, World Bank PEF, GHSA, WHO Contingency Fund, WHO Global Workforce Reserve, including GOARN. *Why*: Core capacities cannot be built or sustained without reliable funding. For funding agencies, the return on investment for building core capacities (as opposed to experiencing a large-scale, uncontrolled outbreak) is significant.	Existing IHR text under Article 44. Increase WHO member states' assessed contributions; GHSA Action Packages in support of IHR implementation; World Bank PEF; and/or raising resources support through donors' conferences, modeled on the Global Fund.
Workforce development	National assessments and career plans for a robust clinical and public health workforce, and commitment to developing and maintaining the workforce. Ready international emergency workforce to respond when national systems are overwhelmed.	*Who*: National governments, with international funding and assistance. WHO coordination for emergency workforce. *Why*: Achieving IHR core capacities, and universal health coverage in general, will require developing (and sustaining) a well-trained, well-equipped national workforce. In times of emergency, when even a well-prepared workforce cannot cope, the international community must provide surge capacity.	Domestic workforce supported through national commitment and assessment, with funding assistance from WHO, World Bank, and other funding agencies. WHO commitment to GOARN, the Global Health Reserve Workforce, and Foreign Medical Teams, including major CSOs such as Médecins Sans Frontières.
Emergency Committee Transparency	Independent and transparent Emergency Committee decision-making, supported by civil society shadow reporting.	*Who*: WHO, working collaboratively with civil society. *Why*: Independent and transparent Emergency Committees will build public trust.	Administrative action by WHO.

Tiered PHEIC process for early action	Institute a gradient or tiered process for declarations of a PHEIC. Harmonize diverse WHO global alert frameworks with the IHR.	*Who*: WHO *Why*: A tiered PHEIC declaration process would allow for formal action prior to a full declaration. It could also trigger clear operational and financial strategies, such as access to the Contingency Fund.	WHO could develop informal guidelines through Article 11 with an understanding by WHA; or WHA could adopt a new IHR annex illustrating the risk gradient without opening the full text for negotiation.
Enhanced compliance	Enhance IHR compliance through a series of carrots and sticks to encourage development of core capacities, and keep member states from taking action inconsistent with the Emergency Committee travel and trade recommendations.	*Who*: WHO, in consultation with other arbitration bodies, such as the WTO, FAO, and ICJ. *Why*: States Parties' disregard for travel and trade recommendations and insufficient devotion of resources to building core capacity undermine the IHR and weaken global health security.	WHO should publicly request clear rationales from States Parties that take additional measures outside Emergency Committee recommendations. Actively pursue dispute mediation and arbitration under the IHR; use the Permanent Court of Arbitration Optional Rules for Arbitrating Disputes; encourage challenges through the WTO or even ICJ. WHA could amend the IHR to elevate temporary recommendations to a binding status.
Role of civil society organizations	Engage civil society in IHR governance and implementation, including shadow reports, inputs to the Emergency Committee, and participation in independent assessments of core capacities.	*Who*: Civil society organizations, academics, and other interested partners working in close collaboration with WHO. *Why*: Civil society organizations are already deeply engaged in care for communities, monitoring governments, and holding stakeholders to account. They should be engaged as productive partners.	WHO administrative action.

(continued)

Table 6.3 Continued

	Recommended Reform	Who and Why	Political Mechanism
Link IHR with PIP Framework, and close gaps in governing sample sharing and equitable access to vaccines and treatments	Harmonize IHR and PIP Framework; enhance governance of sample sharing and equitable access, and integrate mechanisms to address biosecurity challenges associated with genomic sequencing.	*Who*: WHA member states. *Why*: IHR does not address sample sharing, PIP does not apply to any agent beyond novel influenzas, and neither agreement addresses genomic sequencing. This leaves major gaps in global governance of disease.	WHA understandings or addition of an annex to the IHR.
One Health approach	Adapt the IHR to take an explicit One Health approach to addressing global health security challenges.	*Who*: WHO and WHA member states, in collaboration with FAO and OIE. *Why*: Most emerging infectious disease threats are zoonotic, and effectively addressing them requires a One Health approach that fully integrates animal and human health systems. The benefits include better detection and response, as well as addressing major challenge of antimicrobial resistance.	WHA understandings and operational guidance from WHO, OIE, and FAO.

References

Boateng L. Perspectives in Global Health Security: Effective prevention, detection and response to global pandemics. CRDF Global Sponsored Briefing. October 2015. Washington, DC.

Buse K, Gostin LO, Friedman EA. *Pathways towards a framework convention on global health: political mobilization for the human right to health*, in Michael Freeman, Sarah Hawkes, Belinda Bennett (eds.), Law and Global Health (2014).

Cheng M, Satter F. 2015. *Emails: UN health agency resisted declaring Ebola emergency.* AP. (Mar. 20, 2015). Available at http://bigstory.ap.org/article/2489c78bff86463589b41f3faaea5ab2/emails-un-health-agency-resisted-declaring-ebola-emergency.

Commission on a Global Health Risk Framework for the Future. The Neglected Dimension of Global Security: A Framework to Counter Infectious Disease Crises. National Academy of Medicine (2016).

FAO, WHO, and OIE. Joint FAO/WHO/OIE statement on influenza A(H1N1) and the safety of pork (May 7, 2009). Available at http://www.who.int/mediacentre/news/statements/2009/h1n1_20090430/en/.

Fauci AS, Morens DM. Zika virus in the Americas: yet another arbovirus threat. *N Engl J Med.* Published online January 13, 2016. doi:10.1056/NEJMp1600297.

Fidler DP, Gostin LO. *The WHO Pandemic Influenza Preparedness Framework: A milestone in global governance for health.* 306(2) JAMA 200–201 (2011).

Fleck F. *How SARS changed the world in less than six months.* 81(8) Bulletin of the World Health Organization 625–626 (2003). Available at http://www.who.int/bulletin/volumes/81/8/News0803.pdf?ua=1.

Gostin LO. Global health law (2014).

Gostin LO, Friedman EA. *Ebola: a crisis in global health leadership.* 384 Lancet 1323–1325 (2014).

———. *A retrospective and prospective analysis of the West African Ebola virus disease epidemic: robust national health systems at the foundation and an empowered WHO at the apex.* 385 Lancet 1902–1909 (2015).

Gostin LO, Lucey D. *Middle East respiratory syndrome: a global health challenge.* 314(8) JAMA 771–772 (2015).

Henao-Restrepo AM, Longini IM, Egger M, Dean N, Edmunds J, Camacho A, et al. *Efficacy and effectiveness of an rVSV-vectored vaccine expressing Ebola surface glycoprotein: interim results from the Guinea ring vaccination cluster-randomised trial.* 386 Lancet 857–866 (2015). Available at http://lancet.com/pb/assets/raw/Lancet/pdfs/S0140673615611175.pdf.

Heymann DL. *The international response to the outbreak of SARS in 2003.* 359(1447) Philosophical Transactions of the Royal Society B 1127–1129 (2004). Available at http://rstb.royalsocietypublishing.org/content/royptb/359/1447/1127.full.pdf.

Heymann DL, Mackenzie JS, Peiris M. *SARS legacy: outbreak reporting is expected and respected.* 381(9869) Lancet 779–781 (2013).

Horton R. *A plan to protect the world—and save WHO.* 386(9989) Lancet 103 (2015).

Howard-Jones N. The scientific background of the International Sanitary Conferences 1851–1938 (1975). Available at http://whqlibdoc.who.int/publications/1975/14549_eng.pdf.

Jha A, Kickbusch I, Taylor P, Abbasi K. Accelerating achievement of the sustainable development goals: a game changer in global health. *BMJ.* 2016;352:i409. doi:10.1136/bmj.i409.

Katz R. Use of revised International Health Regulations dur- ing influenza A (H1N1) epidemic, 2009. *Emerg Infect Dis.* 2009;15(8):1165–1170.

Lescano AG, et al. *Outbreak investigation and response training.* 318(5850) Science 574–575 (Oct. 26, 2007).

Lucey DR. MERS in Korea: why this outbreak can be stopped soon (June 7, 2015). Available at http://csis.org/files/publication/150608_MERS%20in%20Korea%20Why%20This%20Outbreak%20Can%20Be%20Stopped%20Soon.pdf.

Lucey DR, Gostin LO. The emerging Zika pandemic: Enhancing preparedness. *JAMA*. 2016 Mar 1;315(9):865-6. doi: 10.1001/jama.2016.0904.

McNeil DG Jr. *W.H.O. estimate of swine flu deaths in 2009 rises sharply*. New York Times (Nov. 27, 2013). Available at http://www.nytimes.com/2013/11/27/health/who-revises-estimate-of-swine-flu-deaths.html.

Moon S, Sridhar D, Pate M, Jha A, Clinton C, Delaunay S, et al. 2015. *Will Ebola change the game? Ten essential reforms before the next pandemic. The report of the Harvard-LSHTM Independent Panel on the Global Response to Ebola*. 386 Lancet 2204–2221 (2015).

Petersen EE, Staples JE, Meaney-Delman D, et al. *Interim guidelines for pregnant women during a Zika virus outbreak—United States, 2016*. 65(2) MMWR Morb Mortal Wkly Rep. 30–33 (2016).

Report of the Ebola Interim Assessment Panel (July 2015). Available at http://www.who.int/csr/resources/publications/ebola/ebola-panel-report/en/.

Standley CJ, Sorrell EM, Kornblet S, Vaught A, Fischer JE, Katz R. *New framework for global public health emergency reporting and response*. 348(6236) Science 762–763 (May 15, 2015).

Tran PD, et al. *Strengthening global health security capacity—Vietnam demonstration project, 2013*. 63(4) MMWR Morb Mortal Wkly Rep 77–80 (Jan. 31, 2014).

United Nations Development Group (UNDG)—Western and Central Africa. Socio-economic Impact of Ebola Virus Disease in West African Countries (2015). Available at http://www.africa.undp.org/content/dam/rba/docs/Reports/ebola-west-africa.pdf.

UN Secretary General Press Release. Secretary-General Appoints High-Level Panel on Global Response to Health Crises (Apr. 2015). Available at http://www.un.org/press/en/2015/sga1558.doc.htm.

What lessons for the International Health Regulations? 384(9951) Lancet 1321 (2014).

White House. Fact Sheet: The U.S. Commitment to the Global Health Security Agenda. (Nov. 16, 2015). Available at https://www.whitehouse.gov/the-press-office/2015/11/16/fact-sheet-us-commitment-global-health-security-agenda.

———. Global Health Security Agenda: Toward a World Safe and Secure From Infectious Disease Threats (2014). Available at http://www.globalhealth.gov/global-health-topics/global-health-security/GHS%20Agenda.pdf.

World Health Assembly. Global health security: epidemic alert and response. WHA 54.14 (2001).

———. Global public health response to natural occurrence, accidental release or deliberate use of biological and chemical agents or radionuclear material that affect health. WHA55.16 (2002).).

———. Revision and updating of the International Health Regulations. WHA48.7 (1995).

WHO. Advisory Group on Reform of WHO's Work in Outbreaks and Emergencies with Health and Humanitarian Consequences. Available at http://www.who.int/about/who_reform/emergency-capacities/advisory-group/en/.

———. Current WHO phases of pandemic alert for pandemic (H1N1) (2009). Available at http://www.who.int/csr/disease/swineflu/phase/en/.

———. Director-general summarizes the outcome of the Emergency Committee regarding clusters of microcephaly and Guillain-Barré syndrome. Available at http://www.who.int/mediacentre/news/statements/2016/emergency-committee-zika-microcephaly/en/.

———. Ebola virus disease outbreak. Available at www.who.int/csr/disease/ebola/en/.

———. 2014 Ebola virus disease outbreak and follow-up to the Special Session of the Executive Board on Ebola (May 23, 2015). Available at http://apps.who.int/gb/ebwha/pdf_files/WHA68/A68_ACONF5-en.pdf.

———. Emergency Committee—9th meeting summary: briefing notes on MERS-CoV (June 22, 2015). Available at http://www.who.int/mediacentre/news/mers/briefing-notes/update-22-june-2015/en/.

———. Emergency response framework 19 (2013). Available at http://apps.who.int/iris/bitstream/10665/89529/1/9789241504973_eng.pdf?ua=1.

———. Follow up to the World Health Assembly decision on the Ebola virus disease outbreak and the Special Session of the Executive Board on Ebola: Roadmap for Action (Sept. 2015).

Available at http://www.who.int/about/who_reform/emergency-capacities/WHO-outbreasks-emergencies-Roadmap.pdf.

———. Frequently asked questions on IHR Emergency Committee. Available at http://www.who.int/ihr/procedures/en_ihr_ec_faq.pdf.

———. Global Policy Group Statement on reforms of WHO work in outbreaks and emergencies (Jan. 30, 2016). Available at htt://www.who.int/dg/speeches/2016/reform-statement/en/.

———. IHR Core Capacity Monitoring Framework: Checklist and indicators for monitoring progress in the development of IHR core capacities in States Parties (2013). Available at http://www.who.int/ihr/checklist/en/.

———. Implementation of the International Health Regulations (2005). WHA67.13 (May 24, 2014). Available at http://apps.who.int/gb/ebwha/pdf_files/WHA67/A67_R13-en.pdf.

———. Implementation of the International Health Regulations (2005): report of the Review Committee on Second Extensions for Establishing National Public Health Capacities and on IHR Implementation: report by the director-general para. 17, 45–49 (Mar. 27, 2015). Available at http://apps.who.int/gb/ebwha/pdf_files/WHA68/A68_22Add1-en.pdf.

———. Implementation of the International Health Regulations (2005): report of the Review Committee on the Functioning of the International Health Regulations (2005) in Relation to Pandemic (H1N1) 2009, Doc. A64/10 (May 5, 2011). Available at http://apps.who.int/gb/ebwha/pdf_files/WHA64/A64_10-en.pdf.

——— Implementation of the International Health Regulations (2005): report of the Review Committee on Second Extensions for Establishing National Public Health Capacities and on IHR Implementation. A68/22 Add 1. (Mar. 2015). Available at http://apps.who.int/gb/ebwha/pdf_files/WHA68/A68_22Add1-en.pdf?ua=1.

———. Implementation of the International Health Regulations (2005): responding to public health emergencies: report by the director-general para. 10 (May 15, 2015). Available at http://apps.who.int/gb/ebwha/pdf_files/WHA68/A68_22-en.pdf.

———. International Health Regulations (2005) (2008). Available at http://whqlibdoc.who.int/publications/2008/9789241580410_eng.pdf.

———. Middle East respiratory syndrome—Saudi Arabia (Dec. 4, 2015). Available at http://www.who.int/csr/don/4-december-2015-mers-saudi-arabia/en/.

———. Report of the Ebola Interim Assessment Panel 6 (July 2015). Available at http://www.who.int/csr/resources/publications/ebola/report-by-panel.pdf.

———. Review Committee on the role of the International Health Regulations (2005) in the Ebola outbreak and response. Available at http://www.who.int/ihr/review-committee-2016/en/. Accessed Dec. 10, 2015.

———. Statement on the 5th IHR Emergency Committee meeting regarding the international spread of wild poliovirus (May 5, 2015). Available at http://www.who.int/mediacentre/news/statements/2015/polio-5th-statement/en/.

———. Statement on the first meeting of the International Health Regulations (2005) (IHR 2005) Emergency Committee on Zika virus and observed increase in neurological disorders and neonatal malformations (Feb. 1, 2016). Available at http://www.who.int/mediacentre/news/statements/2016/1st-emergency-committee-zika/en/.

———. Statement on the meeting of the International Health Regulations Emergency Committee regarding the 2014 Ebola outbreak in West Africa (Aug. 8, 2014). Available at http://www.who.int/mediacentre/news/statements/2014/ebola-20140808/en/.

———. States Parties to the International Health Regulations (2005). Available at http://www.who.int/ihr/legal_issues/states_parties/en/.

———. Swine influenza: statement by WHO director-general, Dr. Margaret Chan (Apr. 27, 2009). Available at http://www.who.int/mediacentre/news/statements/2009/h1n1_20090427/en/. Accessed July 1, 2015.

———. WHO Constitution (1946). Available at http://whqlibdoc.who.int/hist/official_records/constitution.pdf.

———. WHO statement on the second meeting of the IHR Emergency Committee concerning MERS-CoV (July 17, 2013). Available at http://www.who.int/mediacentre/news/statements/2013/mers_cov_20130717/en/.

———. WHO statement on the eighth meeting of the IHR Emergency Committee regarding MERS-CoV (Feb. 5, 2015). Available at http://www.who.int/mediacentre/news/statements/2015/8th-mers-emergency-committee/en/. Accessed July 1, 2015.

———. WHO statement on the Ninth Meeting of the IHR Emergency Committee regarding MERS-CoV (June 17, 2015). Available at http://www.who.int/mediacentre/news/statements/2015/ihr-ec-mers/en/. Accessed July 3, 2015.

WHO and PAHO. Epidemiological alert: neurological syndrome, congenital malformations, and Zika virus infection: implications for public health in the Americas (Dec. 1, 2015). Available at http://www.paho.org/hq/index.php?option=com_content&view=article&id=11599&Itemid=41691&lang=en.

7

Global Health Diplomacy and the Ebola Outbreak

DAVID P. FIDLER

The outbreak of Ebola virus disease in West Africa, the health and humanitarian emergencies it caused, and problems with the international response came as a shock to global health officials, experts, and advocates. What happened in West Africa, at the World Health Organization (WHO), and in countries around the world ran roughshod over concepts, strategies, initiatives, and rules crafted over 20 years of global health efforts. As post-outbreak reviews of what went wrong attest, this event was more than another "wake-up call" to the international community concerning microbial threats. It was a disaster for global health politics, governance, and international law concerning infectious diseases.

This political, governance, and legal disaster casts a particularly harsh spotlight on global health diplomacy, a topic of great interest in the years leading up to the Ebola outbreak.[1] This chapter focuses on what the Ebola outbreak means for global health diplomacy in efforts to manage infectious disease threats. The outbreak and the responses to it reveal a disturbing failure of global health diplomacy not only during the crisis but also before it. What diplomatic efforts achieved prior to Ebola's appearance in West Africa proved gossamer, leaving populations, civil society organizations, governments, and international institutions to cobble together desperate, ad hoc responses using means and methods found nowhere in the global strategies previously designed for managing serious infectious disease events.

The Ebola outbreak triggered a flood of reform proposals that form part of an endeavor to ensure a similar debacle does not happen again.[2] To move forward,

---

[1] Kelley Lee and Richard Smith, *What is "global health diplomacy?" A conceptual Review*, 5(1) Global Health Governance (2011), available at http://blogs.shu.edu/ghg/files/2011/11/Lee-and-Smith_What-is-Global-Health-Diplomacy_Fall-2011.pdf.

[2] The problems experienced with the Ebola outbreak produced 5 formal efforts to review what happened and make recommendations (in alphabetical order): Commission on Global Health Risk

these proposals would require negotiations on many topics in multiple venues, and this need for extensive diplomacy raises questions about whether suggested reforms align with the political interests of states and whether reforms that are turned into collective action will address the range of problems the outbreak exposed. Not enough time has passed to determine whether states, international organizations, and nonstate actors will answer through effective diplomacy the challenges the Ebola crisis has presented. However, early signs are not promising. Potentially making things worse is the occurrence of another serious infectious disease event that is dramatically different from the Ebola epidemic—the spread of the mosquito-borne Zika virus and its role in causing microcephaly in newborn infants and neurological disorders.[3]

The Concept of "Global Health Diplomacy"

The more prominent profile that global health achieved in international relations and foreign policy over the past two decades increased interest in how governance, law, and diplomacy function in this once-neglected area of world politics.[4] In the diplomatic sphere, practitioners and professors produced diverse perspectives on "global health diplomacy," "health diplomacy," and "medical diplomacy." This literature did not reach consensus about the diplomatic dimensions of global health, but keen interest in this topic and the proliferation of analyses reflected not only the newness of global health as a topic of serious political attention but also broader perceptions that diplomacy, across many policy areas, was changing in ways not fully understood.[5]

Framework for the Future; Harvard University–London School of Hygiene and Tropical Medicine Independent Panel on the Global Response to Ebola; Review Committee on the Role of the International Health Regulations (2005) in the Ebola Outbreak and Response; UN Secretary-General's High-Level Panel on Global Response to Health Crises; and WHO Ebola Interim Assessment Panel. As of this writing, four of the review efforts have issued their reports (in chronological order of when the reports appeared): the WHO Ebola Interim Assessment Panel (July 2015); the Harvard University–London School of Hygiene and Tropical Medicine Independent Panel (November 2015); the Commission on Global Health Risk Framework for the Future (January 2016); and the UN Secretary-General's High-Level Panel on the Global Response to Health Crises (January 2016).

[3] Laurie Garrett, *The Zika virus isn't just an epidemic, it's here to stay*, Foreign Policy (Jan. 28, 2016), available at http://foreignpolicy.com/2016/01/28/the-zika-virus-isnt-just-an-epidemic-its-here-to-stay-world-health-organization/.

[4] Kelley Lee and Adam Kamradt-Scott, *The multiple meanings of global health governance: a call for conceptual clarity*, Globalization and Health (2014), available at https://globalizationandhealth.biomedcentral.com/articles/10.1186/1744-8603-10-28; Lawrence O. Gostin, Global Health Law (2014); and Sara E. Davies, Adam Kamradt-Scott, and Simon Rushton, Disease Diplomacy: International Norms and Global Health Security (2015).

[5] Andrew F. Cooper, Jorge Heine, and Ramesh Thakur, *Introduction: the challenges of 21st-century diplomacy*, in Andrew F. Cooper, Jorge Heine, and Ramesh Thakur (eds.) Oxford Handbook of Modern Diplomacy 1–31 (2013).

One striking difference in approaches to explaining global health diplomacy was disagreement about what happens with diplomacy when health is the focus. For some, the objective of improving health provided a means to transform diplomacy from an instrumental process of negotiations among states to a normative endeavor that could improve health outcomes and generate foreign policy "spillover" supporting better collective action in other areas of international relations.[6] For others, putting "global health" in front of "diplomacy" did not change the nature of diplomacy or the difficult political problems negotiations on international health issues face.[7]

The gap between these two perspectives reflects different understandings of health as a political issue and diplomacy as a political process. When health is seen as a paramount objective, the necessity of negotiating among states and nonstate actors to support and promote it becomes imbued with political purpose and ethical energy. Here, diplomacy is malleable, and the imperative of improving health can shape and expand it. By contrast, when health struggles to compete for priority with other political interests, negotiations involving health raise questions about the substance and sustainability of commitments made. In this view, diplomacy is inelastic and no more accommodating to health than other political or ethical objectives.

Although they reach different conclusions, both perspectives perceive diplomacy as a process through which states and nonstate actors negotiate to translate political interests into collective action in the form of governance regimes and/or international law (Figure 7.1). Collective-action regimes and rules then structure and guide ongoing diplomatic activities on the issues in question in particular ways. For example, agreement to cooperate on infectious disease surveillance and response in WHO and through the International Health Regulations (IHR) means that continuing diplomacy on these issues occurs within this governance regime under those rules of international law. Anchoring diplomacy in governance regimes and/or international law also affects diplomacy in related contexts and the politics associated with such interrelated issues. Under this two-way dynamic, diplomacy is the channel through which political interests produce governance regimes and international law, the means of sustaining these collective-action strategies, and the conduit for disseminating collective-action benefits back to the realm of politics.

This simplified model proves useful in analyzing what happened with global health diplomacy before and during the Ebola outbreak. It also provides a way to peer, however cautiously, into the post-Ebola future of diplomacy on infectious diseases. Prior to Ebola, states and nonstate actors reconceptualized infectious diseases as threats to national and international security, producing foreign policy

---

[6] Lee and Smith, *supra* note 1.

[7] David P. Fidler, *Health diplomacy* in Andrew F. Cooper, Jorge Heine, and Ramesh Thakur (eds.) Oxford Handbook of Modern Diplomacy 691–707, at 691–693 (2013).

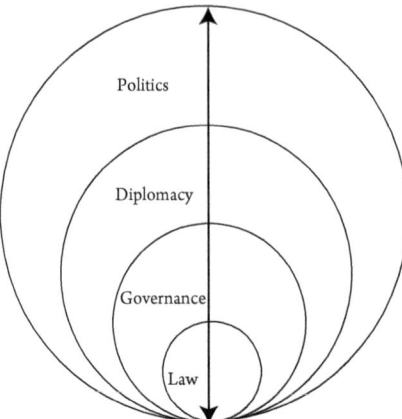

Figure 7.1 Global Health Diplomacy in Context.

interest in "health security" and "global health security."[8] These political interests informed negotiations that produced reinvigorated activities on infectious disease threats within WHO (governance regime)[9] and through the revised IHR adopted in 2005 (international law).[10] These governance and legal commitments became focal points for ongoing diplomacy concerning infectious diseases and the catalyst for other diplomatic and political activities in related contexts.

In the Ebola outbreak, what global health diplomacy achieved in governance and international legal terms proved fragile and did not guide global responses to the outbreak and the crises it caused. This fragility revealed weaknesses not only in what diplomacy produced but also in the diplomatic activities meant to sustain WHO's governance efforts and compliance with the IHR in the face of infectious disease challenges. As explored in this chapter, the Ebola outbreak exposed a comprehensive failure of global health diplomacy.

The Ebola Outbreak and Global Health Diplomacy

Commentary during and after the outbreak harshly criticized WHO's performance and identified widespread noncompliance with the IHR before and during the crisis.[11] WHO's credibility took a massive hit because the organization failed

---

[8] David L. Heymann, *The true scope of health security*, 385 Lancet 1884–1887 (2015); Simon Rushton and Jeremy Youde, eds., *Routledge Handbook of Global Health Security* (2015).

[9] For example, WHO established the Global Outbreak Alert and Response Network in the early 2000s to address more effectively various infectious disease threats. WHO, Global Outbreak and Response: Report of a WHO Meeting, WHO.CDS/CSR/2000.3 (Apr. 28-29, 2000).

[10] World Health Organization, International Health Regulations (2005), available at http://www.who.int/ihr/publications/9789241596664/en/.

[11] For example, the WHO Ebola Interim Assessment Panel argued that the "Ebola crisis not only exposed organizational failings in the functioning of WHO, but it also demonstrated shortcomings in

to respond appropriately to what was happening in West Africa. Indeed, WHO's response was considered so slow and ineffective that the Secretary-General of the United Nations (UN) intervened, displaced WHO as the lead agency, and created the UN Mission for Ebola Emergency Response (UNMEER).[12] The outbreak's consequences became so severe that the UN Security Council declared it a threat to international peace and security.[13] These facts and decisions revealed significant weaknesses with the long-standing strategies of expecting WHO to be the primary governance regime for addressing infectious disease threats, empowering WHO for this purpose through the IHR, and regulating state behavior through the IHR.

This strategy emerged in the 1990s after two shocks to WHO's role in global governance of infectious diseases. First, UN leaders perceived that WHO had not been effective in responding to the HIV/AIDS pandemic and, as a result, created the Joint UN Programme on HIV/AIDS (UNAIDS) in 1996 to be the central global governance mechanism for addressing this threat.[14] Second, experts concerned about the emergence and re-emergence of infectious diseases (including, but not limited to, HIV/AIDS) did not believe WHO was equipped to cope with this problem.[15] These concerns produced efforts to frame infectious diseases as threats to national and international security, strengthen WHO's surveillance and response capabilities, and revise the IHR. The creation of UNAIDS and attempts to revitalize WHO and the IHR highlight how badly global health politics, diplomacy, governance, and law had neglected the threat of infectious diseases for decades.

Thus began diplomatic activities to achieve a WHO better equipped to help countries address infectious disease problems. These activities included improving WHO's operational capacities, building global surveillance and response networks, and providing WHO with more governance and legal authority to lead global efforts against infectious disease threats. The fruits of this diplomacy became clear in the leadership role WHO played in the successful global response to the outbreak of severe acute respiratory syndrome (SARS) in 2003.[16] This success provided a catalyst for a radical transformation of the IHR in 2005, which incorporated into binding international law governance approaches WHO developed and applied during the SARS outbreak.[17]

---

the International Health Regulations (2005)." WHO, Report of the Ebola Interim Assessment Panel 5 (July 2015), available at http://who.int/csr/resources/publications/ebola/report-by-panel.pdf.

[12] UN Mission for Ebola Emergency Response (UNMEER), available at http://ebolaresponse.un.org/un-mission-ebola-emergency-response-unmeer.

[13] UN Security Council, Resolution 2177 (2014), S/RES/2177 (2014) (Sept. 18, 2014).

[14] Joint UN Programme on HIV/AIDS, UNAIDS: The First Ten Years (2008).

[15] Committee on Emerging Microbial Threats to Health, Emerging Infections: Microbial Threats to Health in the United States (1992), 132–133.

[16] David P. Fidler, SARS, Governance, and the Globalization of Disease (2004).

[17] David P. Fidler, *From International Sanitary Conventions to global health security: the new International Health Regulations*, 4(2) Chinese Journal of International Law 325–392 (2005).

However, less than a decade after the revised IHR was adopted, the Ebola outbreak exposed a WHO unable to handle a serious infectious disease event[18] and dismal compliance with the IHR by WHO member states.[19] The governance mechanisms and international law purpose-built for infectious disease threats appeared more fiction than fact. The weaknesses of WHO and the IHR laid bare by Ebola prompted much attention on possible governance and legal reforms (see later in this chapter), but the trajectory from the SARS zenith to the Ebola nadir involves the failure of diplomacy in global health contexts within WHO and beyond to sustain the governance and legal changes made. This failure points to the lack of political and foreign policy support for these changes. Without political commitment to sustain sufficient diplomatic attention and activities, governance and law suffered when the Ebola crisis hit.

Thus, the failure of global health diplomacy began before Ebola appeared in West Africa. Analyses of the outbreak frequently lamented that WHO and its member states did nothing with recommendations made by the IHR Review Committee after its evaluation of WHO's performance and the IHR's role in addressing the influenza A (H1N1) pandemic of 2009.[20] These recommendations sought action to strengthen WHO's surveillance and response capacities and improve the IHR's contributions to global health security.[21] Pursuing these suggestions would have required diplomatic activities in WHO on governance and legal issues, but neither the organization's leadership nor its member states were interested in undertaking such activities.

Even worse, WHO cut its budget and staffing for infectious disease surveillance and response in managing financial problems it confronted after the global recession of 2008–2010.[22] Faced with constrained funds, WHO de-emphasized infectious diseases and moved to give more attention and resources to other global health issues, such as noncommunicable diseases. These decisions reflected choices to realign global health diplomacy, governance, and law in ways that revealed different priorities for the organization's future activities.

The neglect of the Review Committee's recommendations and paring back political and financial support for WHO's surveillance and response capabilities suggest that diplomacy between SARS and Ebola had not transformed global health politics, governance, and law on infectious diseases. Instead, this period shows diplomatic activities responding to changes in political interests within WHO and its

---

[18] Adam Kamradt-Scott, *WHO's to blame? The World Health Organization and the 2014 Ebola outbreak in West Africa*, 37(3) Third World Quarterly 401-418 (2016).

[19] Adam Kamradt-Scott, Achieving Global Health Security: The Implementation of International Health Regulations (Geneva Centre for Security Policy Strategic Security Analysis No. 1) (Jan. 2016)

[20] WHO, Report of the Review Committee on the Functioning of the International Health Regulations (2005) and on Pandemic Influenza A (H1N1) 2009, WHO Doc. A/64 (May 5, 2011).

[21] *Id.* at 11–21.

[22] Sheri Fink, *Cuts at W.H.O. hurt response to Ebola crisis*, New York Times A1 (Sept. 4, 2014).

member states that undermined the governance and legal steps taken before and after SARS to shore up global health security against infectious diseases. Further, outside WHO, we find few diplomatic initiatives that proved useful in the Ebola crisis. The most notable effort was the US launch of the Global Health Security Agenda (GHSA) in February 2014, only 1 month before reports began to emerge about Ebola in West Africa.[23]

The global response to Ebola involved decisions and actions far removed from the strategies centered on global health security developed from the mid-1990s onward. Those strategies prioritized a strong, capable WHO, not the need for the UN to create emergency missions to address disease-triggered humanitarian crises. Those strategies emphasized the importance of public health capacities to handle microbial threats, not the need to deploy national military forces and health personnel to disease-stricken countries.[24] Those strategies empowered WHO officials to lead global efforts against pathogenic incidents, not the need to compensate for a leadership failure at WHO during a dangerous outbreak; required attention to rebuilding health capabilities in poor, conflict-scarred nations, not the need to prevent a disease outbreak from pushing such countries to the brink of political and social chaos; and depended on countries following the IHR before and during serious disease events, not the need to address noncompliance on a disconcerting scale.

These observations do not diminish the remarkable mobilization of political, health, humanitarian, and military resources during the Ebola crisis. The diplomacy necessary for this response was unprecedented and contributed to bringing the outbreak under control. However, these diplomatic efforts were ad hoc, crisis-driven, and unsustainable beyond the immediate emergency. The desperate straits in which Guinea, Liberia, and Sierra Leone found themselves motivated large-scale health and humanitarian responses by leading states and the UN, but this tragic context also signaled the complete failure of the intended strategy to receive sufficient political support and diplomatic attention within and outside WHO over many years.

The Ebola expeditionary campaign cannot serve as strategic guidance for global health diplomacy in the future. Reviews of the crisis agree that reforms are required within and beyond WHO to ensure that the emergency effort mounted against Ebola never has to be undertaken again.[25] No matter how necessary it was, health

---

[23] US Department of Health and Human Services, Global Health Security Agenda Launch (Feb. 13, 2014), available at http://www.globalhealth.gov/global-health-topics/global-health-security/ghsagenda-launch.html.

[24] Adam Kamradt-Scott, Sophie Harman, Clare Wenham, and Frank SmithIII, *Civil-military cooperation in Ebola and beyond*, 387 Lancet 104–105 (2016).

[25] WHO, *supra* note 11; Suerie Moon et al., *Will Ebola change the game? Ten essential reforms before the next pandemic. The report of the Harvard-LSHTM Independent Panel on the Global Response to Ebola*, 386 Lancet 2204–2221 (Nov. 28, 2015); Commission on a Global Health Risk Framework for the Future, The Neglected Dimension of Global Security: A Framework to Counter Infectious Disease Crises (2016); and UN Secretary-General's High-Level Panel on the Global Response to

experts do not believe the diplomacy that produced the global Ebola response has transformed global health politics, governance, or law. In fact, no one in global health ever wants to engage in this kind of desperation diplomacy in addressing future infectious disease events.

Little evidence can be found from before and during the Ebola outbreak that global health diplomacy on serious infectious disease threats within WHO and under the IHR produced transformative outcomes that advanced the normative cause of human health. Rather, diplomacy tracks the waxing and waning of political interests by states in global health security against infectious diseases. By the time Ebola emerged in West Africa, diplomacy reflected political neglect of infectious diseases in governance regimes and international law, even in the face of authoritative recommendations that WHO's weaknesses and problems with the IHR must be addressed. Further, diplomatic activities in WHO reduced the importance of infectious diseases in favor of increasing attention on other global health problems. Poor implementation of the IHR around the world exposed a gap between the rhetoric about the IHR's importance to global health security and the reality of how little states considered the IHR a political and diplomatic priority.

This neglect of diplomacy on infectious diseases is even more depressing because, historically, infectious diseases have been the most important global health issue for states in their foreign policy calculations, their conduct of health diplomacy, and their willingness to support governance regimes and international law in global health.[26] Addressing dangers posed by the cross-border spread of infectious diseases has been a core function of international health organizations since the beginning of the 20th century.[27] The revised IHR forms part of the use of international law for infectious disease surveillance and control that originated in the latter half of the 19th century.[28] Yet, by the time the world confronted the Ebola outbreak, states had weakened WHO's capacity to fulfill the core governance function of responding to serious infectious disease events and had failed to implement the applicable international law.

In sum, it is hard to exaggerate the disaster the Ebola crisis represents for global health diplomacy. The governance strategies and international law built through diplomacy prior to the outbreak proved feeble and ultimately irrelevant to the actions that brought the crisis under control. The diplomatic activities that

---

Health Crises, Protecting Humanity From Future Health Crises (Jan. 25, 2016), available at http://www.un.org/News/dh/infocus/HLP/2016-02-05_Final_Report_Global_Response_to_Health_Crises.pdf.

[26] David P. Fidler, International Law and Infectious Diseases (1999).

[27] Allyn L. Taylor, *Global health law*, in Ilona Kickbusch, Graham Lister, Michaela Todd, and Nick Drager (eds.) Global Health Diplomacy: Concepts, Issues, Actors, Instruments, Fora, and Cases 39 (2013).

[28] Fidler, *supra* note 26, at 21–57.

delivered the emergency health and humanitarian responses are not templates for future endeavors but something to avoid at almost all costs. Given this wreckage, the excitement the concept of global health diplomacy generated before Ebola now seems painfully quaint.

Global Health Diplomacy After Ebola

As already noted, reviews of what went wrong during the Ebola crisis have generated many recommendations for changes in global health governance and international law concerning infectious disease threats. Each proposal is a call for diplomatic activity to make the reform a reality. For many reasons, post-Ebola reform agendas do not dwell on diplomatic challenges the suggested reforms would create, let alone analyze the disaster the Ebola outbreak represents for global health diplomacy. However, given what happened before and during Ebola, some attention should be paid to the diplomatic implications of post-Ebola reform efforts.

To be successful, reforms must garner sufficient support from states and non-state actors that generates diplomatic efforts to translate these political interests into governance strategies and/or legal rules and to sustain them over time. Initial attempts at change demonstrated the difficulties these requirements create. Even after Ebola exposed the need for additional WHO funding, member states decided against increasing assessed contributions at the May 2015 meeting of the World Health Assembly,[29] approving instead an emergency contingency fund resourced by voluntary contributions[30]—but then they created more responsibilities for the organization in moving to develop WHO's emergency response capabilities.[31] This pattern of rejecting increased assessed contributions, mandating more responsibilities, and accepting voluntary funding for "vertical" programs has been repeated at WHO for decades,[32] suggesting that, despite how horrific it was, the Ebola outbreak was not a "game changer" for member states. Similarly, despite comprehensive criticism of the organization, its staff, and the director-general, member states showed little interest in holding anyone accountable for the mistakes and poor leadership.

---

[29] WHO, *supra* note 11, at 16.

[30] WHO, About the Contingency Fund for Emergencies, available at http://www.who.int/about/who_reform/emergency-capacities/contingency-fund/en/.

[31] WHO, First Report of the Advisory Group on Reform of WHO's Work in Outbreaks and Emergencies (Nov. 15, 2015), available at http://www.who.int/about/who_reform/emergency-capacities/first-report-advisory-group.pdf?ua=1.

[32] Charles Clift, What's the World Health Organization For? Final Report From the Centre on Global Health Security Working Group on Health Governance (May 2014), available at https://www.chathamhouse.org/sites/files/chathamhouse/field/field_document/20140521WHOHealthGovernanceClift.pdf.

Nor have states demonstrated serious interest in moving certain diplomatic and governance functions outside WHO, preferring instead to try to improve WHO without actually reforming how the organization operates. The Ebola outbreak created momentum for the US-supported GHSA, which expanded as the crisis deepened,[33] but indications that G7 countries were ready to accept greater global health leadership faded as the focus returned to fixing WHO. Plans to develop emergency response capabilities within WHO have progressed, but this project is proceeding with no additional assessed contributions to fund these capabilities and without changes to what many believe is WHO's dysfunctional governance structure. It is not clear how adding new capabilities to an already resource-starved organization, which remains essentially unchanged after the Ebola catastrophe, constitutes promising and sustainable reform.

What has happened in WHO in the aftermath of Ebola suggests political appetite for transformative change is lacking in member states, which makes it difficult to see how global health diplomacy will midwife significant reforms in governance or international law. This context does not bode well for proposals from review bodies that contemplate major changes in different areas of global health. Each proposed reform would require diplomatic negotiations to translate into collective action, and the places where such negotiations would have to happen under various proposals include WHO, the UN General Assembly, the UN Security Council, the World Bank, the International Monetary Fund, the World Trade Organization, and regional organizations. The number, diversity, and scope of proposals mean that much diplomacy would be needed just to sort out which reforms should become priorities.[34] Reports issued by review bodies do not provide much illumination on the critical need for political priority setting or on explaining how, diplomatically, priority reform efforts should unfold.

Reform proposals also raise questions about how review bodies framed the need for significant political commitment and diplomatic action to produce change. The dominant framing concept remains "security," as highlighted by the title of the report from the Commission on a Global Health Risk Framework for the Future—*The Neglected Dimension of Global Security: A Framework to Counter Infectious Disease Crises*.[35] However, infectious diseases have not been a neglected aspect of global

---

[33] White House, Fact Sheet: Global Health Security Agenda—Getting Ahead of the Curve on Epidemic Threats (Sept. 26, 2014), available at https://www.whitehouse.gov/the-press-office/2014/09/26/fact-sheet-global-health-security-agenda-getting-ahead-curve-epidemic-th.

[34] For example, the UN Secretary-General's High-Level Panel on the Global Response to Health Crises made 27 recommendations (many with multiple components) that encompassed proposals aimed at the national, regional, and international levels across a vast range of issues—from achieving better IHR implementation to fulfilling the Sustainable Development Goals. UN Secretary-General's High-Level Panel on the Global Response to Health Crises, Protecting Humanity from Future Health Crises, *supra* note 25.

[35] Commission on a Global Health Risk Framework for the Future, The Neglected Dimension of Global Security: A Framework to Counter Infectious Disease Crises, *supra* note 25.

security. Efforts to frame infectious disease threats as national, international, and human security threats began 20 years before the Ebola crisis. This outbreak suggests these efforts did not produce effective governance regimes, establish meaningful legal rules, or sustain diplomatic activities seeking these ends.

What transpired before and during the Ebola outbreak indicates states did not act as if framing infectious diseases as security threats was politically persuasive or diplomatically convincing. This framing did not generate sustained commitment or impact within WHO or under the IHR. Recall how, in the aftermath of an influenza pandemic—the most feared infectious disease threat in security terms—WHO and its member states ignored recommendations to shore up governance and legal aspects of global health security, cut budget and staff for infectious disease activities, and pivoted toward health issues not considered threats to security.

Further, WHO's ineffectiveness during the Ebola outbreak and the significant noncompliance with the IHR the outbreak exposed provide evidence that political and diplomatic commitment to global health security has been superficial. Continuing to frame infectious diseases as threats to security without grappling with why this approach produced such poor returns when Ebola hit avoids hard questions. The concept of global health security broke away from thinking about health in humanitarian and human rights terms, and this move sought to elevate health in foreign policy and international politics. The exposure of this shift as more rhetorical than transformational leaves global health vulnerable to the marginalization that characterized this policy area before it became associated with national and global security. Simply repeating the security mantra after Ebola will not be enough to sustain the kinds of diplomatic endeavors that reform proposals claim are critical.

Conclusion

Microbial crises have historically been inflection points for international cooperation on health. Diplomatic activity on infectious diseases developed in the latter half of the 19th century in response to frightening epidemics in Europe. The turn toward global health security occurred when HIV/AIDS and emerging and re-emerging infectious diseases presented clear and present dangers around the world. The SARS outbreak produced changes in international law on infectious diseases unlike anything previously seen. The proliferation of reform ideas in the wake of Ebola contains the hope that this devastating event will stimulate another wave of transformational political decisions and diplomatic breakthroughs in global health.

Although this history records dramatic changes, the political conditions needed for transformational global health diplomacy do not appear to be emerging from the Ebola crisis. The crisis exposed the depth of the failure of global health diplomacy undertaken before and during the outbreak, and this failure reflects the lack of sustained political commitment to achieving global health security through governance centered on WHO and international law enshrined in the IHR. This tragedy has punctured notions that global health diplomacy could reshape international politics to privilege the protection of human health from pathogenic harm. The Ebola disaster highlights how global health diplomacy remains dependent on, and subordinate to, the political calculations of states, which do not converge harmoniously on health issues, even on infectious diseases framed as threats to national and global security.[36]

Many reform proposals have been formulated and disseminated, and prospects for their translation into political interests, diplomatic negotiations, and governance activities decrease as more time passes after the Ebola outbreak. Another—but very different—infectious disease crisis that appeared in late 2015 and early 2016 also adversely affects taking advantage of this narrowing window of opportunity. This crisis involves the "explosive" spread of the mosquito-borne Zika virus[37] and unnerving correlations between the spread of Zika and increased cases of microcephaly in newborn infants and neurological disorders, perhaps including Guillain-Barré syndrome.[38] The WHO Director-General declared the spread of Zika and clusters of microcephaly associated with it a public health emergency of international concern under the IHR in early February 2016.[39]

This new global health crisis could divert political attention, diplomatic efforts, and financial resources away from the post-Ebola reform agenda. Responding to the Zika challenge involves little overlap with reform agendas proposed to address problems associated with the Ebola outbreak. The emergency response capacities being developed at WHO in the wake of Ebola are not particularly helpful for countries that must control the mosquitoes that transmit the Zika virus,[40] guide populations—especially pregnant women—to protect themselves against Zika infection,[41] and

---

[36] Harley Feldbaum and Joshua Michaud, *Health diplomacy and the enduring relevance of foreign policy interests*, PLOS Medicine (Apr. 20, 2010), available at http://journals.plos.org/plosmedicine/article?id=10.1371/journal.pmed.1000226.

[37] Sabrina Tavernise, *Zika virus "spreading explosively" in Americas, W.H.O. says*, New York Times A1 (Jan. 29, 2016).

[38] WHO, Zika Virus Fact Sheet (Feb. 2016), available at http://www.who.int/mediacentre/factsheets/zika/en/; Eric J. Rubin, Michael F. Green, and Lindsey R. Baden, *Zika virus and microcephaly*, 374 New England Journal of Medicine 984–985 (Feb. 10, 2016), available at http://www.nejm.org/doi/full/10.1056/NEJMe1601862.

[39] WHO, WHO Director-General Summarizes the Outcome of the Emergency Committee Regarding Clusters of Microcephaly and Guillain-Barré Syndrome (Feb. 1, 2016), available at http://www.who.int/mediacentre/news/statements/2016/emergency-committee-zika-microcephaly/en/.

[40] US Centers for Disease Control and Prevention, Surveillance and Control of Aedes Aegypoti and Aedes Albopictus in the United States, available at http://www.cdc.gov/chikungunya/resources/vector-control.html.

[41] US Centers for Disease Control and Prevention, Question and Answers: Zika Virus Infection (Zika) and Pregnancy, available at http://www.cdc.gov/zika/pregnancy/question-answers.html.

manage domestic political problems that unusual increases in microcephaly cases generate in affected countries, such as controversies over abortion.[42]

The post-Ebola reform effort must navigate enough difficult shoals without being blown off course by the political and diplomatic fallout of a new infectious disease emergency. As Ebola-related reform and Zika-response activities unfold concurrently, major changes in global health potentially loom on the horizon. The United States—the most important country in global health politics—will elect a new president in 2016, and whether the next presidential administration will make global health a foreign policy priority remains an open question. In addition, WHO chooses a new Director-General in 2017, and the damage the Ebola outbreak did to WHO will weigh heavily in this process. How these leadership changes might affect global health diplomacy is, at the moment, anyone's guess. But the prospects of significant shifts in US foreign policy and WHO governance might induce political caution in global health and leave much unfinished business for the next corps of diplomats to triage as best they can. After Ebola and in the midst of Zika, how the global management of infectious disease threats recovers politically and advances diplomatically is disturbingly unclear.

References

Clift, Charles. What's the World Health Organization For? Final Report From the Centre on Global Health Security Working Group on Health Governance (May 2014). Available at https://www.chathamhouse.org/sites/files/chathamhouse/field/field_document/20140521WHOHealthGovernanceClift.pdf.

Commission on a Global Health Risk Framework for the Future. The Neglected Dimension of Global Security: A Framework to Counter Infectious Disease Crises (2015).

Committee on Emerging Microbial Threats to Health. Emerging Infections: Microbial Threats to Health in the United States (1992).

Cooper, Andrew, Jorge Heine, and Ramesh Thakur. *Introduction: the challenges of 21st-century diplomacy.* In Andrew F. Cooper, Jorge Heine, and Ramesh Thakur (eds.) Oxford Handbook of Modern Diplomacy 1-31 (2013).

Davies, Sara E., Adam Kamradt-Scott, and Simon Rushton. Disease Diplomacy: International Norms and Global Health Security (2015).

Feldbaum, Harley, and Joshua Michaud. *Health diplomacy and the enduring relevance of foreign policy interests.* PLOS Medicine (Apr. 20, 2010).

Fidler, David. *From International Sanitary Conventions to global health security: the new International Health Regulations.* 4(2) Chinese Journal of International Law 325-392 (2005).

---

[42] Dom Phillips, Nick Miroff, and Julia Symmes Cobb, *Zika prompts urgent debate about abortion in Latin America*, Washington Post (Feb. 8, 2016), available at https://www.washingtonpost.com/world/the_americas/zika-prompts-urgent-debate-about-abortion-in-latin-america/2016/02/07/b4f3a718-cc6b-11e5-b9ab-26591104bb19_story.html; Sheilah Kaplan, "Abortion Politics Threatens to Derail Zika Funding in Congress," STAT (Feb. 10, 2016), available at http://www.statnews.com/2016/02/10/zika-hearing-congress-abortion/.

———. *Health diplomacy*. In Andrew F. Cooper, Jorge Heine, and Ramesh Thakur (eds.) Oxford Handbook of Modern Diplomacy 691-707 (2013).
———. International Law and Infectious Diseases (1999).
———. SARS, Governance, and the Globalization of Disease (2004).
Fink, Sheri, *Cuts at W.H.O. hurt response to Ebola crisis*. New York Times A1 (Sept. 4, 2014).
Garrett, Laurie. *The Zika virus isn't just an epidemic, it's here to stay*. Foreign Policy (Jan. 28, 2016). Available at http://foreignpolicy.com/2016/01/28/the-zika-virus-isnt-just-an-epidemic-its-here-to-stay-world-health-organization/.
Gostin, Lawrence O. Global Health Law (2014).
Heymann, David. *The true scope of health security*. 385 Lancet 1884–1887 (2015).
Joint UN Programme on HIV/AIDS. UNAIDS: The First Ten Years (2008).
Kamradt-Scott, Adam. Achieving Global Health Security: The Implementation of International Health Regulations (Geneva Centre for Security Policy Strategic Security Analysis No. 1) (Jan. 2016). Available at www.gcsp.ch/download/5089/12320.
———. *WHO's to blame? The World Health Organization and the 2014 Ebola outbreak in West Africa*. 37(3) Third World Quarterly 401–418 (2016).
Kamradt-Scott, Adam, Sophie Harman, Clare Wenham, and Frank SmithIII. *Civil-military cooperation in Ebola and beyond*. 387 Lancet 104–105 (2016).
Kaplan, Sheilah. *Abortion politics threatens to derail Zika funding in Congress*. STAT (Feb. 10, 2016). Available at http://www.statnews.com/2016/02/10/zika-hearing-congress-abortion/.
Lee, Kelley, and Adam Kamradt-Scott, *The multiple meanings of global health governance: a call for conceptual clarity*. Globalization and Health (2014). Available at https://globalizationand-health.biomedcentral.com/articles/10.1186/1744-8603-10-28.
Lee, Kelley, and Richard Smith, *What is "global health diplomacy?" A conceptual review*. 5(1) Global Health Governance (2011). Available at http://www.ghd-net.org/sites/default/files/Lee-and-Smith_What-is-Global-Health-Diplomacy_Fall-2011_0.pdf.
Moon, Suerie, et al. *Will Ebola change the game? Ten essential reforms before the next pandemic. The report of the Harvard-LSHTM Independent Panel on the Global Response to Ebola*. 386 Lancet 2204–2221 (Nov. 28, 2015).
Phillips, Dom, Nick Miroff, and Julia Symmes Cobb. *Zika prompts urgent debate about abortion in Latin America*. Washington Post (Feb. 8, 2016).
Rubin, Eric, Michael F. Green, and Lindsey R. Baden. *Zika virus and microcephaly*. 374 New England Journal of Medicine 984–985 (Feb. 10, 2016). Available at http://www.nejm.org/doi/full/10.1056/NEJMe1601862#t=article.
Tavernise, Sabrina. *Zika virus "spreading explosively" in Americas, W.H.O. says*. New York Times A1 (Jan. 29, 2016).
Taylor, Allyn. *Global health law*. In Ilona Kickbusch, Graham Lister, Michaela Todd, and Nick Drager (eds.) Global Health Diplomacy: Concepts, Issues, Actors, Instruments, Fora, and Cases 37-54 (2013).
US Centers for Disease Control and Prevention. Question and Answers: Zika Virus Infection (Zika) and Pregnancy. Available at http://www.cdc.gov/zika/pregnancy/question-answers.html.
———. Surveillance and Control of Aedes Aegypoti and Aedes Albopictus in the United States. Available at http://www.cdc.gov/chikungunya/resources/vector-control.html.
US Department of Health and Human Services. Global Health Security Agenda Launch (Feb. 13, 2014). Available at http://www.globalhealth.gov/global-health-topics/global-health-security/ghsagenda-launch.html.
UN Mission for Ebola Emergency Response (UNMEER). Available at http://ebolaresponse.un.org/un-mission-ebola-emergency-response-unmeer.
UN Secretary-General High-Level Panel on Global Response to Health Crises (2016). Available at http://www.un.org/News/dh/infocus/HLP/2016-02-05_Final_Report_Global_Response_to_Health_Crises.pdf.
UN Security Council. Resolution 2177 (2014), S/RES/2177 (2014) (Sept. 18, 2014).

White House. Fact Sheet: Global Health Security Agenda—Getting Ahead of the Curve on Epidemic Threats (Sept. 26, 2014). Available at https://www.whitehouse.gov/the-press-office/2014/09/26/fact-sheet-global-health-security-agenda-getting-ahead-curve-epidemic-th.

WHO. About the Contingency Fund for Emergencies. Available at http://www.who.int/about/who_reform/emergency-capacities/contingency-fund/en/.

———. First Report of the Advisory Group on Reform of WHO's Work in Outbreaks and Emergencies (Nov. 15, 2015). Available at http://www.who.int/about/who_reform/emergency-capacities/first-report-advisory-group.pdf?ua=1.

———. Report of the Ebola Interim Assessment Panel 5 (July 2015). Available at http://who.int/csr/resources/publications/ebola/report-by-panel.pdf.

———. Report of the Review Committee on the Functioning of the International Health Regulations (2005) and on Pandemic Influenza A (H1N1) 2009, WHO Doc. A/64 (May 5, 2011).

———. WHO Director-General Summarizes the Outcome of the Emergency Committee Regarding Clusters of Microcephaly and Guillain-Barré Syndrome (Feb. 1, 2016). Available at http://www.who.int/mediacentre/news/statements/2016/emergency-committee-zika-microcephaly/en/.

———. Zika Virus Fact Sheet (Feb. 2016). Available at http://www.who.int/mediacentre/factsheets/zika/en/.

8

The Future of Global Financing for Infectious Diseases

JENNIFER KATES AND ADAM WEXLER

The beginning of the 20th century saw rising global attention to the devastating toll that infectious diseases, particularly HIV, were imposing on the world's poor. Most notably, this included the creation of the Global Fund to Fight AIDS, Tuberculosis and Malaria (Global Fund) in 2002 and the launch of the US President's Emergency Plan for AIDS Relief (PEPFAR) in 2003, among others. Indeed, since 2002, official development assistance for health in low- and middle-income countries has increased fivefold, with assistance channeled to infectious diseases specifically representing between 33% and 59% of overall health funding.[1] While the global commitment to funding the fight against infectious diseases remains strong, there are some signs that this commitment is coming under strain, particularly in the wake of the global economic crisis that began in 2008, and there is an ongoing need to assess whether funding will sufficiently meet global need.

This chapter reviews global funding for infectious diseases by donors (both governments and multilateral organizations) based on analysis of data available through the Organization for Economic Cooperation and Development (OECD) Development Assistance Committee (DAC) Database and Creditor Reporting System (CRS).[2] This review covers trends in overall official development assistance

---

[1] Analysis of data obtained via online query of the OECD Development Assistance Committee (DAC) Database and Creditor Reporting System (CRS) (Mar 3, 2015).

[2] Official development assistance (ODA) is defined as government aid designed to promote the economic development and welfare of developing countries. Loans and credits for military purposes are excluded. Aid may be provided bilaterally, from donor to recipient, or channeled through a multilateral development agency such as the United Nations or the World Bank. Aid includes grants, "soft" loans, and the provision of technical assistance. Soft loans are those in which the grant element is at least 25% of the total. The OECD maintains a list of developing countries and territories; only aid to these countries counts as ODA. The list is periodically updated and currently contains more than 150

(ODA) for health as well as for infectious diseases specifically and as a share of health ODA. It also examines the roles played by each donor, with particular focus on the US government. In addition to OECD data, it uses data from the US federal Office of Management and Budget, Agency Congressional Budget Justifications, congressional appropriations bills, and the US Foreign Assistance Dashboard for known funding provided through the US Department of State, US Agency for International Development, Centers for Disease Control and Prevention, National Institutes of Health, and US Department of Defense. Finally, this chapter provides glimpses into future financing prospects and issues surrounding global funding for infectious diseases. All analyses were conducted by the Henry J. Kaiser Family Foundation.

Donor Funding for Health and Infectious Diseases

The Revolution in Donor Funding for Health and Infectious Diseases

There has been a revolution in funding for health and infectious diseases. That revolution began around the turn of the millennium, when the amount of funding for health and infectious diseases increased as a result of several interrelated initiatives. The 1980s and early 1990s witnessed the emergence of new infectious diseases like HIV, as well as the resurgence of other diseases like cholera.[3] These threats tended to impose their heaviest health and economic burdens on low- and middle-income countries, particularly those in sub-Saharan Africa. Between 2000 and 2005, major domestic and international funding mechanisms were established, including the Global Fund, the Gavi Alliance, PEPFAR, and the US President's Malaria Initiative (PMI).

As shown in Figure 8.1, health ODA rose from just US$4.4 billion in 2002 to US$22.8 billion in 2013 (the latest year of available data at the time of this analysis), a more than fivefold increase. In addition, despite the financial crisis experienced by global markets starting in 2008, ODA for health continued to increase, at least through 2013. Moreover, ODA for health has grown as a share of overall ODA, rising from 9.1% in 2002 to 14.3% in 2013, suggesting that donors have placed an increasing priority on health within their overall development portfolios (Figure 8.2).[4]

The United States is the largest donor to health ODA, accounting for approximately a third of funding in 2013 (33.5%). The second-largest donor to health was the Global Fund (17.6%), followed by the United Kingdom (8.9%) and Gavi (6.3%). These data indicate that despite their youth, international funding

countries or territories with per capita incomes below US$12,276 in 2010. Data on ODA flows are provided by the 29 OECD members of the Development Assistance Committee (DAC).

[3] Rebecca Katz and Julie Fischer, *The revised International Health Regulations: a framework for global pandemic response*, 3 Global Health Governance, 1, 2 (2010).

[4] Overall ODA totals do not include debt relief transactions.

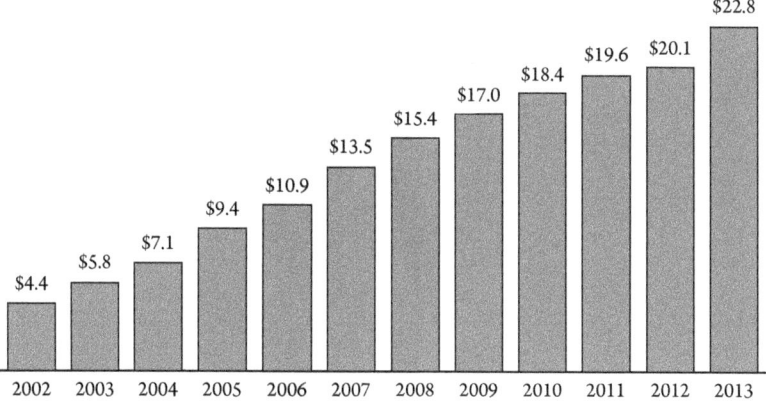

Figure 8.1 ODA for Health, 2002–2013.

organizations like the Global Fund and Gavi have quickly grown to become some of the most important providers of development assistance in the effort to control and eradicate infectious diseases (and, importantly, the United States is the top donor to the Global Fund[5] and one of the top donors to Gavi) (Figure 8.3).[6]

Much of the growth in health ODA has been driven by funding to combat infectious diseases (IDs), including funding for HIV, STD control, tuberculosis, malaria, and other IDs. In 2002, just as new initiatives targeting infectious diseases were beginning to be launched, funding for IDs constituted 32.5% of health ODA. By 2006, funding for IDs had grown to represent more than half (52.4%) of health

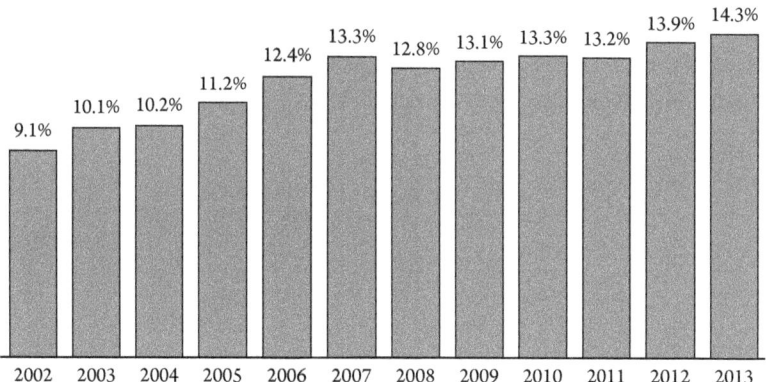

Figure 8.2 ODA for health as a share of total ODA, 2002–2013.

---

[5] The Global Fund, Financials, available at http://www.theglobalfund.org/en/financials/.
[6] The Henry J. Kaiser Family Foundation, The U.S. & Gavi, the Vaccine Alliance, available at http://kff.org/global-health-policy/fact-sheet/the-u-s-and-the-gavi-alliance/.

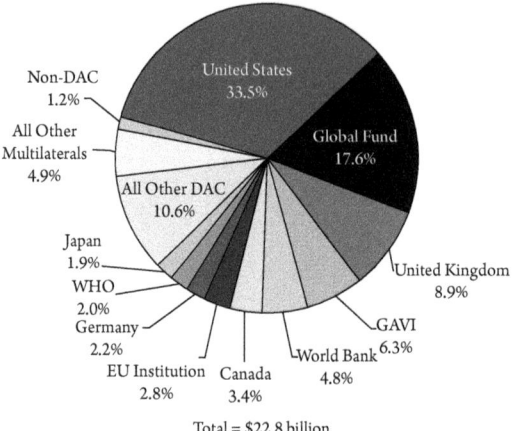

Figure 8.3 ODA for health by donor, 2013.

ODA and reached almost 60% in 2010, though it has since declined as a share of health ODA (Figure 8.4).

Funding for IDs totaled $1.4 billion in 2002, dedicated primarily to HIV and also other infectious diseases. By 2013, that assistance had reached $12.5 billion and was directed toward a broader range of infectious diseases, including tuberculosis and malaria. HIV remains the largest target of ODA for IDs (Figure 8.5).

As with health ODA overall, the United States is the largest donor to IDs, representing 47.6% of ID funding in 2013, followed by the Global Fund at 31.9%. While the United States and the Global Fund provided just over half of total health ODA in 2013, they accounted for more than three quarters (79.5%) of all health ODA for IDs. The United States is clearly fundamental to the global effort to support health generally and fight infectious disease specifically. As such, overall donor funding for such efforts is significantly influenced by changes in U.S. development assistance priorities.

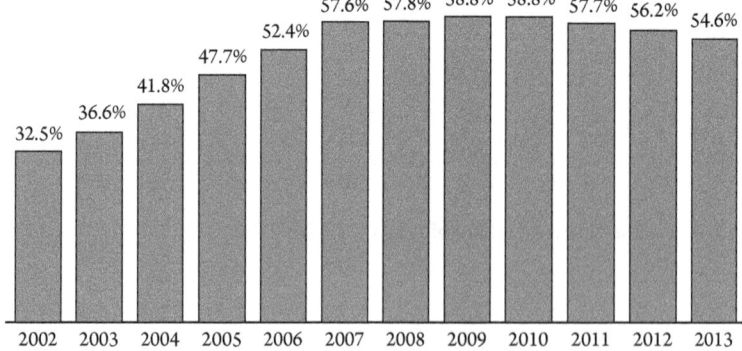

Figure 8.4 ODA for infectious diseases as share of health ODA, 2002–2013.

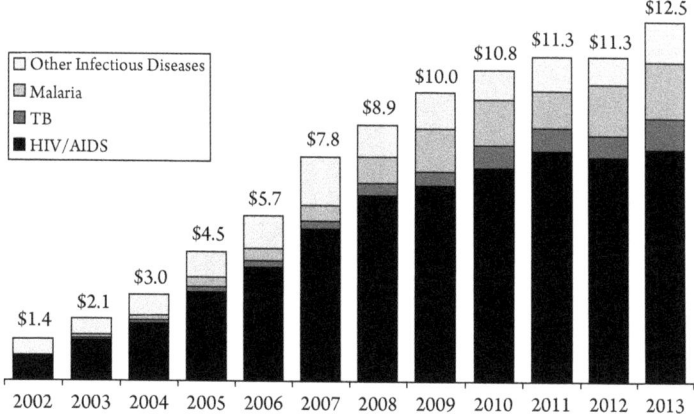

Figure 8.5 ODA for infectious diseases by type of infectious disease, 2002–2013.

Trends in U.S. Funding Priorities for Health and Infectious Disease

US funding for global health has increased over time, and, as shown earlier, the United States, through multiple agencies, is the largest single donor to health overall, and for infectious diseases specifically, in the world. In 2006, US funding for global health totaled $5.3 billion.[7] US funding for global health rose steadily, hitting $10.0 billion in 2010. Funding has remained relatively flat since then and has even fallen in some years and was $10.1 billion in 2015 (Figure 8.6).[8]

Similarly, the United States' contribution toward infectious disease efforts as a share of its global health funding climbed and peaked in tandem with the trend toward health assistance generally. Funding for infectious diseases within the US global health portfolio has represented approximately 80% of health funding over this period.

US funding for HIV, through PEPFAR, has received the highest proportion of assistance for all infectious diseases since 2006 (between 60% and 73% over the period), followed by the Global Fund (ranging between 12% and 20%). Funding for malaria, through the PMI, has ranged from 6% to 11%. The smallest shares have been allocated to neglected tropical diseases (NTDs) and funding for the Pandemic Influenza and Other Emerging Threats program, although the latter has recently

---

[7] Kaiser Family Foundation Analysis derived from www.foreignassistance.gov (last visited Mar. 3, 2015), Office of Management and Budget data, Agency Congressional Budget Justifications, and congressional appropriations bills.

[8] *Id.*; Consolidated and Further Appropriations Act, Pub. L. 113-235 (2015), available at https://www.congress.gov/113/plaws/publ235/PLAW-113publ235.pdf.

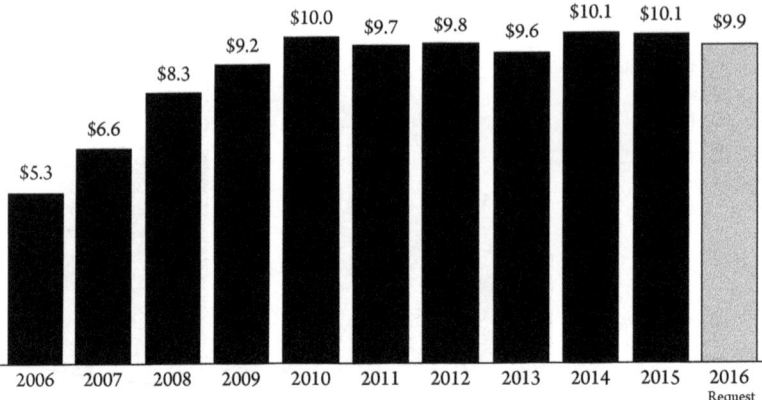

Figure 8.6 US global health spending, FY 2006–2016.

seen a shift with the US response to the West African Ebola epidemic of 2014 that included a significant $5.4 billion emergency funding in 2015 (Figure 8.7).[9] This funding from the United States is considered "supplemental" to the regular US budget for health. It is estimated that of the $5.4 billion, approximately $3.7 billion, or more than two thirds (69%), was designated for international efforts.[10] Still, this funding is largely considered a one-time boost, and it remains unclear how funding for infectious disease programs will fare over the next several years.

Conclusion

Since 2000, official development assistance for health has consistently risen as a share of overall ODA. Major increases are largely due to the creation of large, new initiatives, most notably PEPFAR and the Global Fund. The United States is consistently the largest donor to health ODA, and its role is even larger with respect to funding for infectious diseases. As of 2006, the majority of health ODA from all donors has been channeled to infectious diseases. However, because of the increasing attention given to noncommunicable diseases globally and continued strains on donor budgets, it is not clear that assistance to fight infectious disease will remain as robust in the near to medium term.

While critical for the global fight against infectious disease, these data also show that what the United States decides to do with respect to its development assistance

---

[9] Jennifer Kates, Josh Michaud, Adam Wexler, and Allison Valentine, The U.S. Response to Ebola: Status of the FY2015 Emergency Ebola Appropriation (Dec. 11, 2015), available at http://kff.org/global-health-policy/issue-brief/the-u-s-response-to-ebola-status-of-the-fy2015-emergency-ebola-appropriation/.

[10] *Id.*

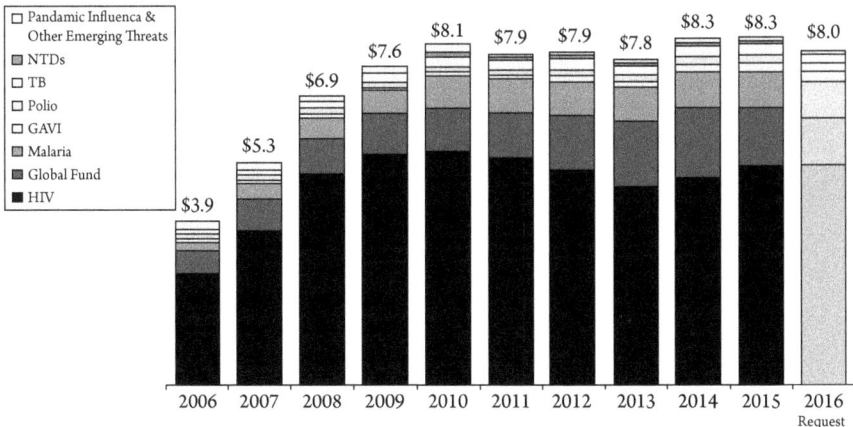

Figure 8.7 US global health funding by type of infectious disease, FY 2006–2016.

priorities has an outsized effect on the aggregate numbers. Since 2010, the United States' funding for infectious diseases has generally been stable, and it is likely to remain so at best. To the extent these trends reflected a general global responsiveness to the Millennium Development Goal (MDG) agenda, the future of funding for infectious disease management efforts is uncertain. While the 2000 MDGs emphasized control of infectious disease as a principal goal, the post-2015 Sustainable Development Goals (SDG) agenda is more expansive but less health specific. Infectious disease control is in fact one subgoal of health, which is, in turn, 1 of 17 broader goals.[11]

Infectious diseases continue to impose a heavy economic and health burden on the world's poor. The establishment of major international financing mechanisms and the willingness of wealthy countries, especially the United States, to address that burden is one of the great development gains made since 2000. However, as the outbreak of Ebola in three of the world's poorest countries has shown, there is still a tremendous amount of work to be done. Reducing the burden imposed by infectious disease will require the same willingness as during the last 15 years, if not more.

References

House Resolution 83 Consolidated and Further Continuing Appropriations Act, 2015 (113th Congress 2013–2014).
Katz, R., and Fischer, J. *The revised International Health Regulations: a framework for global pandemic response*, 3 Global Health Governance, 1, 2 (2010).
United Nations Economic and Social Council. The Millennium Development Goals and post- 2015 Development Agenda. Available at http://www.un.org/en/ecosoc/about/mdg.shtml.

---

[11] United Nations Economic and Social Council, the Millennium Development Goals and post-2015 Development Agenda, available at http://www.un.org/en/ecosoc/about/mdg.shtml.

9

International Public-Private Partnerships as Part of the Solution to Infectious Disease Threats

Operational, Legal, and Governance Considerations

KEVIN A. KLOCK

While global health law as a conceptual and academic field is relatively new, efforts to coordinate international measures against the outbreak and spread of disease are more than a century old. Between 1851 and 1892, predominantly European nations met intermittently in an effort to establish a list of internationally actionable diseases and the appropriate methods by which their spread might be limited.[1] Between 1893 and 1938, states convened additional conventions, steadily expanding the list of diseases deemed appropriate for cooperation and control.[2] Countries in the Americas formed the Pan American Health Organization in 1902 to "improve health and quality of life."[3] In 1946, the World Health Organization (WHO) was established to create a competent international body that could coordinate multilateral action.[4] Other treaty-based regimes emerged to deal with health issues ranging from opium and alcohol consumption to occupational safety and cross-boundary pollution.[5] In short, the history of global health law is, for the most part, a story

---

[1] Norman Howard-Jones, The scientific background of the International Sanitary Conferences 1851–1938 (1975), available at http://whqlibdoc.who.int/publications/1975/14549_eng.pdf.

[2] David P. Fidler, *The globalization of public health: the first 100 years of international health diplomacy*, 79 Bulletin of the World Health Organization 842, 843 (2001).

[3] Pan American Health Organization, available at www.paho.org.

[4] Constitution of the World Health Organization, Preamble, available at http://www.who.int/governance/eb/who_constitution_en.pdf.

[5] Jennifer Ruger, *Normative foundations of global health law*, 96 Geo. L.J. 423, 426 (2008).

of traditionally conceived sovereign states bargaining and coordinating to address common international challenges even as they coped with the collective-action problems inherent in those kinds of negotiations.[6] However, the maturation and proliferation of for-profit corporations and nonprofit organizations over the course of the 20th century offered alternative approaches to international public health challenges.

This chapter analyzes how the traditional state-centered model of cooperation has evolved to include actors not traditionally recognized under international law in order to raise global health outcomes. The international public-private partnerships behind this evolution have mobilized advantages offered by state and private actors while overcoming many of their relative disadvantages. After first examining the operational structures and legal formalities that characterize public-private partnerships, the chapter assesses common attributes of public and private entities and how these attributes may run in tension with one another. The chapter then turns to three public-private partnerships prominent in the global health field: the Global Fund to Fight AIDS, Tuberculosis and Malaria (Global Fund); the Global Alliance for Improved Nutrition (GAIN); and Gavi, the Vaccine Alliance (Gavi). The chapter analyzes the structure of those partnerships; identifies the attributes drawn from public and private sector financing; governance (including representatives on decision-making bodies); agenda setting; operational models; and, how each achieved successes in public health projects that would have been more difficult or impossible for any entity alone. The choices these partnerships make on these structural features affect their legitimacy as both international actors and effective global health organizations.

Public and Private Actors and Public-Private Partnerships Defined

It remains the case that the principal actor recognized under international law is the sovereign state. When a state possesses a permanent population, a defined territory, a functioning government, and an ability to enter into relations with other states, it is generally recognized as obtaining international personality.[7] The sovereign state must also have a functioning government with "the power, ability, and means to maintain the political organization of [its citizenry] with the assistance of the law, and to regulate and protect the rights of the members."[8]

---

[6] Kevin Klock, *The soft law alternative to the WHO's treaty powers*, 44 Geo. J. Int'l Law 828 (2013).
[7] Montevideo Convention on Rights and Duties of States (1933) art. 1.
[8] Thomas Grant, *Defining statehood: the Montevideo Convention and its discontents*, 37 Colum. J. Transnat'l L. 403, 409 (1999) (citing Fiore, P., International Law Codified and Its Legal Sanction or the Legal Organization of the Society of States 106).

Sovereign states may, in turn, create international organizations (IGOs) through treaty to coordinate efforts to solve common problems. Because their membership is predominantly composed of states, IGOs frequently possess international personality akin to state actors. For example, under the US International Organizations Immunities Act (IOIA) of 1945, recognized IGOs are given certain privileges and immunities under US law otherwise extended only to sovereigns.[9] IGOs are, in essence, unions of actors that already enjoy established international legal status.

Corporations, by contrast, are the creation of national or subnational governments that extend to fictional legal entities separate legal personality, limited liability, transferable ownership interests, centralized management (almost universally under a board structure), and shared ownership by capital contributors.[10] By granting such protections, the corporate form has emerged as "one of the most successful inventions in history, as evidenced by its widespread adoption and survival as a primary vehicle of capitalism."[11] Both its adoption and its influence were widespread. As early as the 1970s, corporations such as General Electric and Pfizer were said to make "daily business decisions which have more impact than those of most sovereign governments."[12]

A variation on the for-profit corporation is the nonprofit corporation. Nonprofit corporations share features of legal personality, limited liability, and board governance while capital contributors do not own the corporation, and interests in a nonprofit generally are not transferable. Income generated by nonprofit firms cannot inure to the benefit of those providing capital. Instead, they must convince donors to donate with no possibility of financial return. Nonprofit corporations work for public benefit purposes that may be narrow or broad in scope, support individuals or organizations, or serve specific functions. Prominent nonprofit corporations provide assistance monitoring (thereby helping to enforce) human rights, scrutinize government policies for fiscal responsibility, and, of course, facilitate access to healthcare, including essential medicines and vaccines. The most prominent among them share the same level of influence as large for-profit corporations. For instance, Médecins Sans Frontières is credited with mobilizing the global response to the Ebola outbreak in West Africa,[13] while traditional sovereign-state mechanisms like the International Health Regulations failed to work as anticipated.[14]

---

[9] 22 U.S.C. 288 "International organization" defined; authority of president.

[10] Reinier Kraakman et al. (eds.), The Anatomy of Corporate Law 5 (2009).

[11] Henry N. Butler, *The contractual theory of the corporation*, 11 Geo. Mason U. L. Rev. 99 (1989).

[12] Richard Barnet and Ronald E. Muller, Global Reach 15 (1974).

[13] Médecins Sans Frontières, Ebola: Pushed to the Limit and Beyond (2015), available at http://www.msf.org/article/ebola-pushed-limit-and-beyond.

[14] Lawrence Gostin and Eric Friedman, *Ebola: a crisis in global health leadership*, 384 Lancet 1323–1325 (2014).

Public-private partnerships "straddle the conventional divide between state and non-state actors. They often involve partners from government, business, and civil society [and] typically entail some joint decision-making and sharing of responsibilities, opportunities, and risks."[15] Successful partnerships mix each sector's methods for approaching problems and exploit their relative capabilities and constraints in managing them. They also create platforms for sharing information and technology.[16]

Despite their advantages, the legal personality of international public-private partnerships often presents complex problems with respect to financing, governance, and accountability. Even when sovereign governments are participants, public-private partnerships are rarely recognized as having international personality akin to states and IGOs. Alternatively, a partnership may opt for a corporate form organized under national or subnational law, but doing so raises difficult questions surrounding a national government's obligations and immunities when participating in an essentially contractually formed joint venture. So-called alliances between actors with separate legal personality often prevent public-private partnerships from serving as reliable contracting parties or earning confidence from stakeholders.[17]

The Swiss government was the first to reconcile these concerns when it crafted the Federal Act on the Privileges, Immunities and Facilities and the Financial Subsidies granted by Switzerland as a Host State (Host State Act). This statute extends to Swiss foundations that possess certain characteristics the same immunity from suit enjoyed by treaty-based international organizations.[18] Global Fund, GAIN, and Gavi each incorporated as Swiss foundations and benefit from the active participation of sovereign members. Unlike the Host State Act, the US IOIA does not extend to public-private partnerships, even when the United States itself is a member. As public-private partnerships multiply in number and force, legal accommodations like those in Switzerland may be necessary to provide the flexibility required to fulfill partnership objectives and design the kinds of governance arrangements needed to pursue their missions at scale.[19] For now, despite their

---

[15] Inge Kaul, *Exploring the policy space between markets and states: global public-private partnerships*, in The New Public Finance: Responding to Global Challenges 91 (2006).

[16] World Bank Group, Potential Benefits of Public Private Partnerships (2015), available at http://ppp.worldbank.org/public-private-partnership/overview/ppp-objectives.

[17] Anna Triponel, *A Global Fund to Fight AIDS, Tuberculosis and Malaria: a new legal and conceptual framework for providing international development aid*, 35 N.C.J. Int'l L. & Com. Reg. 173, 183 (2009).

[18] List of the Organizations With Which Switzerland Has Concluded an Agreement on Privileges, Immunities and Facilities (2015), available at https://www.eda.admin.ch/content/dam/eda/de/documents/aussenpolitik/voelkerrecht/20150909-DV-liste-abkommen-org_DE_FR_EN.pdf.

[19] Davinia Aziz, *Global public-private partnerships in international law*, 2 Asian Journal of International Law 339 (2012); Lisa Clarke, *Responsibility of international organizations under international law for the acts of global health public-private partnerships*, 12(1) Chicago Journal of International Law 55–84 (2011).

ascent in the global public health field, national and international law struggle with the appropriate legal approach.[20]

Public and Private Sector Governance

According to the World Bank:

> Conceptually, governance can be defined as the rule of the rulers, typically within a given set of rules. One might conclude that governance is the *process*—by which authority is conferred on rulers, by which they make the rules, and by which those rules are enforced and modified. Thus, understanding governance requires an identification of both the rulers and the rules, as well as the various processes by which they are selected, defined, and linked together and with the society generally.[21]

Governance therefore concerns *authority* for directing an enterprise, as well as the process by which that authority is exercised. A governance system must include a mechanism for disbursing and apportioning authority to particular members. Authority is established and distributed differently within private and public organizations, and there are nearly limitless possibilities for creating the hybrids at work in public-private partnerships.

Public Sector Governance Practices

IGOs generally borrow their governance practices from democratic legislative systems in which subgroups of the general population choose representatives to decide. For example, WHO's supreme governing authority is vested in the World Health Assembly (WHA).[22] Each WHO member state is authorized to appoint a limited number of delegates.[23] The concept of representation is key to public sector governance. The WHO Constitution provides that the WHA "shall be composed of delegates *representing* Members."[24]

---

[20] Inge Kaul, *Exploring the policy space between markets and states: global public-private partnerships*, in The New Public Finance: Responding to Global Challenges 92 (2006).

[21] The World Bank, What Is Governance?, available at http://web.worldbank.org/WBSITE/EXTERNAL/COUNTRIES/MENAEXT/EXTMNAREGTOPGOVERNANCE/0,,contentMDK:20513159~pagePK:34004173~piPK:34003707~theSitePK:497024,00.html (emphasis in original).

[22] WHO Const. Art. 18.

[23] WHO Const. Art. 11.

[24] WHO Const. Art. 18 (emphasis added).

One of the main mechanisms public institutions have to hold representatives accountable to the public is to manage their governance operations transparently. For example, responsible national parliaments engage in public debate and open voting to allow constituents, and the public at large, to hold parliamentarians accountable for their policy positions. IGOs engage in similar methods. The WHA and WHO's other decision-making bodies publish their agendas, resolutions, calendars, and other pertinent information for public inspection.[25] Many state and multilateral aid agencies are evaluated on the transparency of their operations.[26]

Private Sector Governance Practices

For-profit corporations (and related limited liability entities) also maintain rules that structure authority and decision-making. General corporation or company statutes, formation documents (in the United States, "articles of incorporation" or "articles of organization"), and bylaws distribute authority between those who contribute capital (the shareholders), those who oversee the corporation's affairs (the board of directors),[27] and the executives who manage the corporation on a day-to-day basis (the officers).[28] The latter two constituencies are not representatives in the sense that public sector representatives generally are understood to be; indeed, the nature of their selection and accountability is a complex and controversial question in corporate law.[29] However, for imprudent or disloyal decisions, they may be held personally accountable, a sanction most public authorities do not face.[30] They may also make poor business decisions that carry reputational or financial consequences even without legal liability.

---

[25] World Health Organization, Governing Body Documentation, available at http://apps.who.int/gb/gov/.

[26] Aid Transparency Index, available at http://ati.publishwhatyoufund.org/index-2014/results/.

[27] Wayne O. Hanewicz, *Director primacy, omnicare, and the function of corporate law*, 71 Tenn. L. Rev. 511–512 (2004).

[28] Robert Monks and Nell Minow, Corporate Governance (2011).

[29] Stephen M. Bainbridge, *Director primacy: the means and ends of corporate governance*, 97 Nw. U. L. Rev. 547, 605 (2003).

[30] The duty of care requires each director to become informed about issues on which he or she will make decisions, provide oversight, and "act with the care that an ordinarily prudent person would reasonably exercise in a like position and under similar circumstances." A.L.I., *Principles of the Law of Nonprofit Organizations*, § 315. The duty of loyalty requires that a director "act in a manner that he or she reasonably believes to be in the best interests of the charity, in light of its stated purposes." A.L.I., *Principles of the Law of Nonprofit Organizations*, § 310(a)–(b). These duties are incorporated into the law of many corporate governance systems throughout the world. See, e.g., Brazilian Institute of Corporate Governance, Code of Best Practice of Corporate Governance 22 (4th ed. 2009); Rebecca Lee, *Fiduciary duty without equity: "fiduciary duties" of directors under the Revised Company Law of the PRC*, 47 Va. J. Int'l. L. 897, 902 (2007).

One structural feature of board design aimed at the aforementioned problems is the inclusion of "independent" directors.[31] In 1975, Melvin Eisenberg observed that though American corporate law tasks boards with "managing," they could not do so in any meaningful sense given time and informational constraints.[32] He proposed a monitoring board that would make the most critical corporate decisions,[33] but argued that directors on the board must be "independent of those who are monitored" in order to perform meaningful oversight.[34] While definitions vary, the essential purpose of independence is having "only one non-trivial connection to the corporation—that of his or her directorship."[35]

The independence principle has gained traction globally. For example, the OECD Principles of Corporate Governance provide that "national principles, and in some cases laws, lay down specific duties for board members who can be regarded as independent and recommend that a significant part, in some instances a majority, of the board should be independent."[36] In the United States, independence is a relevant principle in assessing the legality of certain board judgments,[37] and it is required by the rules of stock exchanges.[38] The United Kingdom's Corporate Governance Code calls for an "appropriate combination of executive and non-executive directors (and, in particular, independent non-executive directors)."[39] Japanese companies are increasingly adding outside directors,[40] and African companies are being encouraged to do so as well.[41] The literature supporting participation of independent directors suggests that they are more likely to optimize risk oversight practices and challenge "unwise, unethical, or illegal behavior."[42]

---

[31] Jeffrey N. Gordon, *The rise of independent directors in the United States, 1950–2005: of shareholder value and stock market prices*, 59 Stan. L. Rev. 1465, 1468 (2007).

[32] See Melvin Aron Eisenberg, *Legal models of management structure in the modern corporation: officers, directors and accountants*, 63 Calif. L. Rev. 375, 141–144, 403–404 (1975).

[33] Melvin A. Eisenberg, The Structure of the Corporation, 156–168 (1976).

[34] *Id.* at 171.

[35] AFL-CIO, Exercising Authority, Restoring Accountability, 11 (2003).

[36] See G20/OECD Principles of Corporate Governance 40 (2015).

[37] See *China Auto. Sys.*, 2013 WL 4672059, at *6.

[38] See N.Y. Stock Exch., Inc., Listed Company Manual § 303A.01 (2009), available at http://nysemanual.nyse.com/lcm/sections/lcm-sections/chp_1_4/default.asp; NASDAQ Stock Market, Inc., Marketplace Rules, R. 5605(b)(1) (2014), available at http://nasdaq.cchwallstreet.com/NASDAQ/.

[39] UK Corporate Governance Code 10 (Sept. 2014), available at https://www.frc.org.uk/Our-Work/Publications/Corporate-Governance/UK-Corporate-Governance-Code-2014.pdf.

[40] Kazuaki Nagata, *New rules are pushing Japanese corporations to tap more outside directors*, Japan Times (Apr. 27, 2015), available at http://www.japantimes.co.jp/news/2015/04/27/reference/new-rules-pushing-japanese-corporations-tap-outside-directors/#.VsNQUfkrK71.

[41] Peter Were, *Add outside directors to add value to your company's board*, Business Daily (July 26, 2015), available at http://www.businessdailyafrica.com/Hire-outside-directors-to-add-value-to-your-company-s-board/-/539444/2809864/-/item/1/-/280uh8z/-/index.html.

[42] Nat'l Ass'n of Corp. Dirs., Report of the NACD Blue Ribbon Commission on Risk Oversight 17 (2002).

Even so, shareholders may still reject board decisions. When this occurs, they rarely have the opportunity to revisit specific actions and must rely on indirect pressures like selling their securities (if there is a ready market for them), suing the directors for breach of a legal duty, or exercising the relatively circumscribed authority allocated to them by law, articles of incorporation, or bylaws.[43]

In the nonprofit context, the board's allegiance is to the organization's charitable mission.[44] With no promise for a return on capital, nonprofit directors, officers, and agents must convince donors to give their money for the benefit of the mission. Donors rarely possess formal authority to control the selection and conduct of board members, although they may and often do use the promise of future gifts to influence governance generally and relevant board decisions specifically. As with for-profit corporations, independence has been viewed as an approach to solving certain accountability problems.[45]

Challenges in Negotiating Public-Private Partnership Governance

Table 9.1 provides a graphic representation of both the structure and the rhetoric surrounding public and private governance alternatives.[46] The matrix shows both how many hybrid forms of financing, governance, and legal status may be available to public-private partnership planners and also how values embedded in the norms of each may present challenges. For example, a public sector representative may counsel toward transparency of meeting minutes, decision-making processes, and agendas, while a private sector perspective may discourage doing so as a means to preserve efficiency, integrity, and candor in the decision-making process.

How Certain Global Health Partnerships Mobilize and Combine Public and Private Resources

The three international public-private partnerships featured in the following discussion borrow principles and structural features from both the public and the private sphere to achieve their missions. While their missions are distinct, they

---

[43] Robert B. Thompson, *Preemption and federalism in corporate governance*, 62 Law & Contemp. Probs. 215 (1999).

[44] John Carver, Creating a Mission That Makes a Difference 3 (1997).

[45] The United States Internal Revenue Service Form 990 *Return of Organization Exempt from Income Tax*, for example, requests nonprofit firms to identify the number "of independent voting members of the governing body" 1 (2014).

[46] Kevin A. Klock, *A house in order: a view inside charitable organizations*, speech to the O'Neill Colloquium, Georgetown Univ. Law Center, Washington (Sept. 17, 2014).

Table 9.1 **Finance and Governance Features of Public and Private Entities**

	Public: Governments	Public: IGOs	Private: Commercial Firms	Private: Nonprofits
Governed by	Parliament	Government assembly	Board of directors	Board of trustees
Elected by	Citizens	Fellow governments	Shareholders	Members/board
Governance buzzword	Accountability	Transparency	Independence	All of these ←
Governance outlet	Elections	Direct government representation	Sell securities, sue for breach of duty, shareholder vote	Sue for breach of duty, funding squeeze, tax status recission
Relevant law	National constitution, Montevideo Convention	International law (treaty, custom)	Domestic corporate and tax law, internal bylaws	Domestic corporate and securities law, internal bylaws
Capital/revenue generation	Taxes and bonds	Government treasuries (some private donor financing)	Profits and securities	Donor financing, excess oncome, securities

demonstrate the many ways in which public-private partnerships may address public health challenges.

The Global Fund

The Global Fund was created in 2002 as a partnership between governments, civil society, and affected communities to raise resources to address the disease burden imposed by AIDS, tuberculosis, and malaria.[47] The Global Fund, which is the main multilateral funder in global health, "channels 82 percent of the international financing for TB, 50 percent for malaria, and 21 percent of the international financing against AIDS" while also funding "health systems strengthening, as inadequate health systems are one of the main obstacles to scaling up interventions to secure better health outcomes for HIV, TB and malaria."[48] Through 2013, the Global Fund approved funding of more than US$29 billion, that has been used to support

---

[47] Triponel, *supra* note 17.
[48] The Global Fund, available at http://www.theglobalfund.org/en/about/diseases/.

more than 1,000 programs in over 150 countries.[49] In the battle against AIDS/HIV, 6.1 million people are now on antiretroviral therapy provided for by the Global Fund.[50] A total of 11.2 million cases of tuberculosis have been tested, diagnosed, and treated.[51] To fight the devastating effects of malaria, 360 million nets have been distributed to at-risk areas.[52]

Because the Global Fund is an international financing institution, it does not have a classic member state governance structure like some other international organizations. The Global Fund accepts donations and pledges from a wide variety of nations and from private foundations and private individuals. The Global Fund created a Partnership Forum, in which participation is open to stakeholders that actively support the fund's objectives. These stakeholders may include "representatives of donors, multilateral development cooperation agencies, developed and developing countries, civil society, nongovernmental and community-based organizations, technical and research agencies, and the private sector."[53]

The Global Fund is managed by a 28-member board composed of 20 voting members and 8 nonvoting members.[54] The board is separated into several groups of representatives. There are seven representatives from developing countries, including one from each WHO region and one additional representative from Africa.[55] Eight representatives come from donors, and five representatives come from civil society and the private sector. As specified in the Global Fund bylaws, the latter five are further separated into "one representative of a nongovernmental organization from a developing country, one representative of a nongovernmental organization from a developed country, one representative of the private sector, one representative of a private foundation, and one representative of a nongovernmental organization who is a person living with HIV/AIDS, or from a community living with tuberculosis or malaria."[56] The eight nonvoting members consist of the board chair, the board vice-chair, one representative from WHO, one representative from the Joint United Nations Programme on HIV/AIDS (UNAIDS), one representative from the partners constituency, one representative from the trustee of the Global Fund, one Swiss citizen with his or her domicile in Switzerland authorized to act on behalf of the Global Fund to the extent required by Swiss law, and the executive director of the Global Fund.[57] Each group decides on the process for selecting

---

[49] The Global Fund, available at http://www.theglobalfund.org/en/about/fundingspending/.
[50] *Id.*
[51] *Id.*
[52] *Id.*
[53] The Global Fund By-laws Art. 6.1, available at http://www.theglobalfund.org/documents/core/bylaws/Core_GlobalFund_Bylaws_en/ (last visited Apr. 5, 2014).
[54] *Id.* at Art. 7.1.
[55] *Id.*
[56] *Id.*
[57] *Id.*

its board representation, complying with the minimum standards established by the existing board. The members are considered to act as a representative of their constituencies.[58]

These internal governance features—both the constituencies and the rules under which the Global Fund operates—lean toward public sector representation and management. For example, the Global Fund has constituencies only; there are no unaffiliated board members. The board chair and vice-chair are selected by the board members for 2-year terms and play advocacy, partnership, and fundraising roles in addition to chairing board meetings.[59]

Financially, the Global Fund accepts donations from sovereign donors as well as private foundations and individuals. One prominent private sector initiative is the Product Red program, which allows commercial firms to demonstrate good corporate citizenship while raising finance for the Global Fund's mission. Companies such as Apple, Coca-Cola, and Starbucks can create "(PRODUCT)RED" branded items in return for remitting some of the revenue from sales of those items to the Global Fund.[60]

In addition, the Corporate Champions Program recruits companies with multinational footprints to make financial contributions to Global Fund–supported programs in countries where they operate and to lend their management skills and business infrastructure to develop and implement national strategies to combat AIDS, tuberculosis, and malaria. For instance, Chevron provides finance through the Global Fund to projects in seven countries in Africa and Asia. The company's support to these recipients focuses on capacity development initiatives, joint advocacy and communications campaigns, and other local projects. In addition, Chevron encourages staff members in these countries to share their skills with local program managers to assist them in improving grant reach and performance. In December 2013, BHP Billiton Sustainable Communities contributed US$10 million to support malaria efforts in Mozambique for the period 2014–2016, to reach universal malaria prevention coverage by 2014, and to maintain those levels every year with additional interventions.[61]

In addition, in 2009, Coca-Cola began sharing its supply chain management strategies with a Global Fund public sector partner, the Medical Stores Department of Tanzania. Together with the Bill and Melinda Gates Foundation and Accenture

---

[58] The Global Fund, *Private Sector and Non-government Partners*, available at http://www.theglobalfund.org/en/partners/privatesector/.

[59] *Id.* at Art. 7.3.

[60] The Global Fund, Project Red, available at http://www.theglobalfund.org/en/news/2012-12-01_(RED)_reaches_record_milestone_USD200_million_raised_to_fight_AIDS_in_Africa/.

[61] Devex Impact, BHP Billiton Sustainable Communities: Global Fund Corporate Champion Partner Funding Grants in Mozambique, available at https://www.devex.com/impact/partnerships/bhp-billiton-sustainable-communities-global-fund-corporate-champion-partner-funding-grants-in-mozambique-466.

Development Partnerships, they launched Project Last Mile, which is designed to improve pharmaceutical and medical supplies distribution in Tanzania.[62]

Global Alliance for Improved Nutrition

The mission of the Global Alliance for Improved Nutrition is to improve the health of the 3 billion people in the world who are considered malnourished.[63] As with other public-private partnerships, GAIN was founded after multiple stakeholders, especially major international organizations like the Food and Agricultural Organization, agreed that "no single sector was capable of singlehandedly doing what was going to be needed" to address malnutrition.[64] In particular, they concluded that the private sector must have a greater role.[65] While, unlike the Global Fund, GAIN is not directly committed to the fight against infectious disease, its objective of addressing nutrition deficiencies in at-risk populations is linked to basic health and susceptibility to infectious disease.

GAIN's governance structure reflects the close relationship it maintains between its mission and its stakeholders. While the Global Fund, like Gavi, works with governments, international organization partners, nongovernmental organizations, and for-profit firms, GAIN works with far more of the latter—more than 600 corporations or other business entities.[66] GAIN is managed by a 12-member board of directors who serve in their individual capacities.[67] While board members are drawn from both high-income and low-income countries, and from diverse institutions, the board manages GAIN through committees familiar to the for-profit corporate sector: finance and audit, board program, and nominations. GAIN is also least reliant on public sector donation. Only 51% of GAIN's activities are funded through public sector sources, with substantial private resources contributed by the Bill and Melinda Gates Foundation.

GAIN's principal contributions are through existing market mechanisms. For example, because GAIN operates a premix facility for added micronutrients, purchasers of fortification powders who would buy the product even without GAIN may do so with an assurance of quality and affordable price based on the facility's ability to purchase in large quantities. Similarly, GAIN supplies sachets of

---

[62] The Global Fund, Private and NGO Partners, available at http://www.theglobalfund.org/en/partners/privatesector/cocacola/

[63] http://www.gainhealth.org/about/.

[64] Kent Buse and Gill Walt, *Global public-private partnerships: part 1—a new development in health?*, 78 Bull World Health Organ 548–561 (2000).

[65] Fay Hanleybrown, John Kania, and Mark Kramer, *Channeling change, making collective impact work*, Stanford Social Innovation Review (Jan. 26, 2012), available at http://ssir.org/articles/entry/channeling_change_making_collective_impact_work.

[66] Id.

[67] GAIN, Transparency, available at http://www.gainhealth.org/about/our-policies/.

micronutrient powders to public health systems, also at affordable prices leveraged by its bulk purchasing power. A program to develop nutrient-enriched yogurt in Ecuador serves as a good example of a GAIN initiative that utilized the combined strengths of the public and private sectors.[68] GAIN secured the assistance of a traditional IGO, the International Finance Corporation, to provide capital to an Ecuadorian company, Reybanpac, to produce and market Lenutrit, a fortified yogurt-based complementary food supplement. This "partnership approach demonstrates how nutrition expertise can be combined with investment capital and business expertise to reduce business-related risks and to encourage the development of affordable, nutritious products."[69] In China, South Africa, and Kenya, for example, micronutrient deficiencies dropped between 11% and 30% among those who consumed GAIN's fortified products. During that time, GAIN has also raised $322 million in new financial commitments from its partners and leveraged many times more from its private sector and government partners.[70]

GAIN also works with government partners to craft national nutrition strategies.[71] It maintains an official relationship with WHO and works with World Food Program country offices to implement its in-country programs.[72] Civil society organizations have partnered with GAIN on the design and delivery of the 1000 Days Partnership, which aims to increase business investment in the nutritious foods needed between the start of pregnancy and a child's second birthday.[73]

Gavi, the Vaccine Alliance

Gavi was established in 2000 to expand the use and supply of existing and new vaccines in developing countries.[74] While previous childhood immunization initiatives were successful during their early stages, a lack of sustained international attention led to their decline.[75] Through the combined and coordinated efforts of governments and the private sector, including pharmaceutical companies and private charities, Gavi has established a public-private partnership that has vertically integrated the production, finance, and delivery of vaccines to developing country populations.

Gavi's board composition plays a major role in ensuring voices from the public and private sector are considered.[76] Ten governments—five sovereign donors

---

[68] http://www.gainhealth.org/knowledge-centre/project/innovative-finance-lns-ecuador/.
[69] http://www.gainhealth.org/knowledge-centre/project/innovative-finance-lns-ecuador/.
[70] Ibid.
[71] GAIN, About, available at http://www.gainhealth.org/about/alliances/#government.
[72] Id.
[73] GAIN, 1,000 Days, Our Mission, available at http://www.thousanddays.org.
[74] Clarke, *supra* note 19, at 55, 59.
[75] Id. at 57.
[76] Gavi, Governance, available at http://www.gavi.org/about/governance/gavi-board/composition/.

and five recipient countries—maintain voting seats, as do three IGOs (WHO, UNICEF, and the World Bank). The private sector is also well represented: executives from vaccine manufacturers in developing and industrialized countries possess two seats, as do representatives from civil society and the Gates Foundation. The other 10 seats—1 for research and technical health institutes and 9 for independent members—can be apportioned to persons with public and/or private sector experience based on the partnership's needs from time to time.

Gavi's revenue model also incorporates public and private sector features, with governments, corporations, foundations, and private individuals making direct financial contributions to Gavi.[77] Roughly a quarter of Gavi's funding comes from foundations, corporations, and individuals, many of whom are located in the United States. The remainder of Gavi's funding is from governments committed to its mission.[78] As of December 2013, the United States has donated more than $532.8 million to the GAVI Alliance, representing 7.3% of all Gavi donations.[79] The Gavi Matching Fund is a partnership between the government of the United Kingdom and the Bill and Melinda Gates Foundation to match contributions from corporations, foundations, and their customers, members, employees, and business partners. The International Finance Facility for Immunisation (IFFIm) allows Gavi to take longer-term pledges made by participating governments and sell debt instruments ("vaccine bonds") based on those pledges to investors to make cash resources available for immediate use.

Gavi also shapes global vaccine markets, which requires deep engagement with procurement agencies such as UNICEF and private sector manufacturers. As a condition of participation, manufacturers must guarantee vaccine prices over certain periods in addition to the price advantages Gavi obtains through large purchases made through UNICEF. For example, Biological E, an Indian manufacturer, is offering a 5-year price commitment to Gavi-graduated (moved off Gavi support) countries for its pentavalent vaccine. Pfizer has agreed to reduce the price per dose of its four-dose, multidose vial presentation pneumococcal vaccine to US$3.10 for all Gavi-eligible and Gavi-graduated countries until the end of 2025. Not only does Gavi procure vaccines at low rates but the prices of Gavi-covered vaccines on the open market generally have declined over the course of its activities. The co-financing aspect of Gavi's mission is not intended to be a principal source of revenue and instead operates to familiarize and normalize the inclusion of immunization as part of national healthcare plans.

Gavi also draws on public sector strengths, including the technical expertise of the Center for Disease Control and Prevention (CDC) and WHO, the purchasing power of UNICEF, financial advice from the World Bank, and the priorities

---

[77] Gavi, Donor Profiles, available at http://www.gavialliance.org/funding/donor-profiles/.
[78] *Id.*
[79] *Id.*

of low-income countries in designing national immunization programs. Technical standards developed by WHO's Department of Immunizations, Vaccines and Biologicals are used to ensure the quality and safety of vaccines and provide technical guidance to Gavi. UNICEF procures vaccines and safe injection materials for Gavi. Both WHO and UNICEF play essential roles in their in-country offices through their support of countries' applications, implementation, and monitoring of Gavi's immunization programs. Other public sector partners include national governments, bilateral development agencies (e.g., USAID and the UK Department for International Development), and technical and research agencies such as the CDC.[80] Partners may be involved in several aspects of the immunization process by (1) developing Gavi's policies and programs, (2) facilitating delivery and administration of vaccines, and (3) providing the governance of Gavi.[81]

Private sector partners play logistical roles as well as funding roles at Gavi. In January 2015, Gavi entered a 3-year partnership with the International Federation of Pharmaceutical Wholesalers (IFPW), a global association of pharmaceutical wholesalers focused on the storage and delivery of medicines, which will bolster regional supply chain training centers in Benin and Rwanda, serving multiple countries in Africa. The IFPW will provide a package of support, including US$1.5 million in cash and member expertise to ensure that students in Gavi-supported countries receive the training needed to become effective supply chain managers.[82] Gavi is also working with UPS and its Global Healthcare Logistics Strategy Group to assist Gavi in developing and implementing an executive training and mentorship program to enhance the capability of local supply chains.[83]

With access to mobile phones rapidly growing in the developing world, a significant opportunity exists for mobile technology to help healthcare providers increase the take-up of vaccinations. Gavi has partnered with Vodafone to facilitate the use of cell phones to alert mothers to the availability of vaccinations by text message, enabling health workers to access health records and schedule appointments through their phones and helping health facilities in remote locations monitor stocks to ensure that vaccinations are available when mothers and children arrive.[84]

---

[80] A. Saul, *Vaccines for neglected diseases* 248 (Rino Rappuoli and Fabio Bagnoli eds., 2011).

[81] Gavi, GAVI's Partnership Model, available at http://www.gavialliance.org/about/gavis-partnership-model/.

[82] Gavi, New Private Sector Partners Bring Technical Expertise and Innovative Finance to Help Save Children's Lives, available at http://www.gavi.org/Library/News/Press-releases/2015/New-private-sector-partners-bring-technical-expertise-and-innovative-finance-to-help-save-children-s-lives/.

[83] *Id.*

[84] Gavi, GAVI Partners With Vodafone to Bolster the Supply Chain in Africa, available at http://www.gavi.org/library/news/gavi-features/2012/gavi-partners-with-vodafone-to-bolster-the-supply-chain-in-africa/.

How Global Health Partnerships Balance Public and Private Sector Governance Elements

The governing bodies of the Global Fund, GAIN, and Gavi all include members with skills and experiences from the public and private sectors. Yet the three partnerships maintain diverse arrangements, with the Global Fund having the most public-oriented approach, GAIN having a structure that is most similar to private sector entities, and Gavi having a structure somewhere in between.

The Global Fund

The Global Fund's governance structure favors the practices of its public sector stakeholders. As noted earlier, sovereigns constitute 75% of the board's voting members. All members of the board are considered to act in a representative capacity.[85] Three members—the chair, vice-chair, and Swiss citizen—possess the characteristics typically associated with independent governance, but they lack voting rights.

This orientation has yielded outcomes one might expect of a traditional IGO while limiting some of the comparative advantages of a private enterprise. For example, a 2014 review of the Global Fund's governance by its inspector general found that partnership engagement was quite high.[86] This is unsurprising, since, as with traditional IGOs, each of the main stakeholders has a seat at the decision-making table. Further, by possessing privileges and immunities under Swiss law,[87] the Global Fund may conduct its decision-making and operations transparently, with limited concern for legal liability. It publishes its board's meeting agendas and minutes on a public website.[88] The organization achieves a high ranking on the Aid Transparency Index.[89]

However, the same inspector general report found that the board needed to spend more time evaluating performance, pay more attention to risk, and improve management oversight.[90] In fact, the report found that in "contrast to many private

---

[85] The Global Fund, Private Sector and Non-government Partners, http://www.theglobalfund.org/en/partners/privatesector/.

[86] Office of the Inspector General of the Global Fund to Fight AIDS, Tuberculosis and Malaria, Governance Review 10 (2014), available at http://www.theglobalfund.org/documents/oig/reports/OIG_GF-OIG-14-008_Report_en/.

[87] List of the Organizations With Which Switzerland Has Concluded an Agreement on Privileges, Immunities and Facilities 4 (2015), available at https://www.eda.admin.ch/content/dam/eda/de/documents/aussenpolitik/voelkerrecht/20150909-DV-liste-abkommen-org_DE_FR_EN.pdf.

[88] The Global Fund, Board Decisions, available at http://www.theglobalfund.org/en/board/decisions/.

[89] Aid Transparency Index, available at http://ati.publishwhatyoufund.org/index-2014/results/.

[90] Office of the Inspector General of the Global Fund to Fight AIDS, Tuberculosis and Malaria, Governance Review 10 (2014), available at http://www.theglobalfund.org/documents/oig/reports/OIG_GF-OIG-14-008_Report_en/.

sector organizations which have fewer conflicts of interest yet more robust management and control of those conflicts, the Global Fund has many conflicts and little control."[91] As noted earlier, a board without independent directors may be relatively less likely to address these areas well.

Global Alliance for Improved Nutrition

At the other end of the spectrum, GAIN's arrangements most closely resemble a corporate governance model. Its governing documents contemplate appointing up to 13 board members who must "not represent any particular interest" in deliberations or decision-making.[92] Those affiliated with donor governments or other related organizations, while not conforming to the common private sector definitions of independence, are nevertheless charged to "not see themselves as representing the interest of another organization."[93] Of the three partnerships reviewed in this chapter, GAIN maintains the smallest board, a feature more prominent in the corporate and nonprofit spheres.[94]

GAIN's governance arrangements may therefore result in outcomes that contrast with those of the Global Fund. For example, GAIN's board performs regular risk oversight by identifying major threats and recording them on a register that is regularly reviewed and discussed by its Finance and Audit Committee and Operations Committee.[95] Further, despite being entitled to privileges and immunities under the Swiss Host State Act,[96] GAIN's directors have agreed to be subject to the traditional duties of care and loyalty.[97]

On the other hand, GAIN appears to be the least transparent of the three partnerships reviewed here as regards the decision-making processes of its board. Though it makes its governing documents and board member names available to

---

[91] Office of the Inspector General of the Global Fund to Fight AIDS, Tuberculosis and Malaria, Governance Review 24 (2014), available at http://www.theglobalfund.org/documents/oig/reports/OIG_GF-OIG-14-008_Report_en/.

[92] GAIN statutes Article 8.1.

[93] Id.

[94] The average corporate board in the United States in 2014 had 11.2 members. Joann S. Lublin, *Smaller boards get bigger returns*, Wall Street Journal (Aug. 26, 2014). The average nonprofit board in the United States in 2013 had 15.3 members. Nat'l Ass'n of Corp. Dirs., 2013–2014 NACD Nonprofit Governance Survey 5 (2014).

[95] Global Alliance for Improved Nutrition, GAIN Annual Financial Report 2015, 16.

[96] List of the Organizations With Which Switzerland Has Concluded an Agreement on Privileges, Immunities and Facilities 4 (2015), available at https://www.eda.admin.ch/content/dam/eda/de/documents/aussenpolitik/voelkerrecht/20150909-DV-liste-abkommen-org_DE_FR_EN.pdf.

[97] Global Alliance for Improved Nutrition, GAIN Conflict of Interest Policy for Board Members 2 (2008), available at http://www.gainhealth.org/wp-content/uploads/2014/10/conflict_of_interest.pdf.

the public (which is typical for private sector entities),[98] it does not publish the agenda of its meetings and places only a summary of its minutes on the organization's website.[99]

Gavi, the Vaccine Alliance

Gavi has adopted public and private features in closer balance, a result likely tied to its evolution. It was conceived as a time-limited multistakeholder project and so initially had no organizational form. Instead, partners met in semiannual "board meetings" to set, coordinate, and monitor the partnership's programmatic activities. To house the project's finances and give it some contractual capability, a Washington State charity named the Global Fund for Children's Vaccines (and later called the Vaccine Fund and the GAVI Fund) was formed.[100] As a nonprofit corporation, the fund was governed by a board of directors who possessed traditional fiduciary duties.

For a number of years, the two boards worked together to fulfill a joint immunization mandate. The partnership board used a parliamentary/international institution governance style, which emphasized representation, transparency, and consensus. The Global Fund board used a private charity/corporate governance style that emphasized independence and fiduciary control. When in 2006 the boards took decisions at odds with one another, they decided the dual governance system was no longer tenable and negotiated a new set of arrangements.

The governance structure Gavi uses today is a product of its dual-system history. Eighteen members of the board represent constituencies, and nine directors fit the traditional definition of independence. Gavi possesses privileges and immunities under Swiss law,[101] but unlike GAIN, the board members have not chosen to make themselves subject to Swiss fiduciary duties. Nevertheless the board members are aware of what the duties of care and loyalty entail and make it their intention to exceed those expectations.[102]

As to outcomes, Gavi has been recognized as being among the most transparent aid agencies in the world.[103] From a governance standpoint, Gavi publishes the agendas of its board and committee meetings along with non–commercially sensitive meeting minutes.[104] Gavi also possesses a strong risk program, which includes

---

[98] GAIN, Governance, available at http://www.gainhealth.org/organization/governance/.

[99] GAIN, Board Decisions, available at http://www.gainhealth.org/wp-content/uploads/2014/05/26th-Board-of-Directors-meeting.pdf

[100] http://www.gavi.org/funding/financial-reports/.

[101] List of the Organizations With Which Switzerland Has Concluded an Agreement on Privileges, Immunities and Facilities 4 (2015), available at https://www.eda.admin.ch/content/dam/eda/de/documents/aussenpolitik/voelkerrecht/20150909-DV-liste-abkommen-org_DE_FR_EN.pdf.

[102] Dagfinn Høybråten, *Presentation to the Gavi Board Retreat on the Role of Board Members* (Mar. 24 2015).

[103] Aid Transparency Index, supra note 122.

[104] Gavi, Gavi, the Vaccine Alliance Board, available at http://www.gavi.org/about/governance/gavi-board/.

a results framework,[105] risk appetite statement,[106] and overall risk policy.[107] The partnership conducts regular assessments of organizational achievement[108] and the board's performance.[109]

However, there is often disagreement over what a board member's role entails.[110] Predictably, the governance expectations of individual board members tend to be linked to whether they serve in a representative or an independent capacity. Given that the last board self-evaluation highlighted board member turnover as a concern,[111] there will remain a process of re-education of new members on how the balance of public sector and corporate governance practices is maintained. In that respect, while a properly managed balance can yield the best outcomes, it may be the least stable given its hybrid mixture of governance principles.

Conclusion

In all three examples analyzed in this chapter, public-private partnerships emerged because existing international mechanisms plateaued in their impact, although for reasons not systematically studied here. Novel forms of shared decision-making and operations are giving public and private actors a space within which to build innovative, implementable solutions. In other words, in the broader context of public goods, public-private partnerships have played a pivotal role that government and corporate actors could not play alone. While it is too early to tell definitively, these partnerships have succeeded in placing public health matters at the top of the development agenda.

Public-private partnerships, at least for the time being, enjoy evidence to support their desirability and proliferation. Given that they create opportunities for consensus-building and resource mobilization, the most important issue for managers and future founders is to determine the appropriate governing and operating principles that will lay the foundation for the best results.

---

[105] Gavi, Gavi Risk Policy Results Framework, available at http://www.gavi.org/Library/GAVI-documents/Policies/Risk-policy-results-framework/.

[106] Gavi, Gavi Risk Appetite Statement, available at http://www.gavi.org/Library/GAVI-documents/Policies/Risk-appetite-statement/.

[107] Gavi, Gavi's Risk Policy, available at http://www.gavi.org/Library/GAVI-documents/Policies/Risk-policy/.

[108] Gavi, Results: Evaluations, available at http://www.gavi.org/results/evaluations/.

[109] Minutes of the Gavi Alliance Governance Committee Meeting, 24 March 2014, 1–3, available at http://www.gavi.org/About/Governance/GAVI-Board/Governance-committee/2014/Governance-Committee-Meeting,-24-March-2014,-Final-Minutes/.

[110] Minutes of the Gavi Alliance Governance Committee Meeting, 24 March 2014, 2, available at http://www.gavi.org/About/Governance/GAVI-Board/Governance-committee/2014/Governance-Committee-Meeting,-24-March-2014,-Final-Minutes/.

[111] Minutes of the Gavi Alliance Governance Committee Meeting, 24 March 2014, 1, available at http://www.gavi.org/About/Governance/GAVI-Board/Governance-committee/2014/Governance-Committee-Meeting,-24-March-2014,-Final-Minutes/.

References

Aziz, D. *Global public-private partnerships in international law*, 2 Asian Journal of International Law 339 (2012).

Barnet, R., and Ronald E. Muller. Global Reach (1974).

Buse, K., and G. Walt. *Global public-private partnerships: part 1—a new development in health?* 78 Bull World Health Organ 548–561 (2000).

Clarke, L. *Responsibility of international organizations under international law for the acts of global health public-private partnerships*. 12 Chicago Journal of International Law 55–84 (2011).

Devex Impact. BHP Billiton Sustainable Communities: Global Fund Corporate Champion Partner Funding Grants in Mozambique. Available at https://www.devex.com/impact/partnerships/bhp-billiton-sustainable-communities-global-fund-corporate-champion-partner-funding-grants-in-mozambique-466.

Fidler, D. *The globalization of public health: the first 100 years of international health diplomacy*. 79 Bulletin of the World Health Organization 842, 843 (2001).

GAIN. Donors. Available at http://www.gainhealth.org/organization/donors/.

———. 1,000 Days, Our Mission. Available at http://www.thousanddays.org.

———. Transparency. Available at http://www.gainhealth.org/about/our-policies/.

Gavi. Donor Profiles. Available at http://www.gavialliance.org/funding/donor-profiles/.

———. GAVI Partners With Vodafone to Bolster the Supply Chain in Africa. Available at http://www.gavi.org/library/news/gavi-features/2012/gavi-partners-with-vodafone-to-bolster-the-supply-chain-in-africa/.

———. GAVI's Partnership Model. Available at http://www.gavialliance.org/about/gavis-partnership-model/.

———. Gavi's Strategy. Available at http://www.gavi.org/about/strategy/ (last visited July 14, 2015).

———. Governing Gavi. Available at http://www.gavi.org/about/governance/.

———. How Gavi Is Funded. Available at http://www.gavi.org/funding/how-gavi-is-funded/.

———. New Private Sector Partners Bring Technical Expertise and Innovative Finance to Help Save Children's Lives. Available at http://www.gavi.org/Library/News/Press-releases/2015/New-private-sector-partners-bring-technical-expertise-and-innovative-finance-to-help-save-children-s-lives/.

Global Fund. About Diseases. Available at http://www.theglobalfund.org/en/about/diseases/.

———. About Funding. Available at http://www.theglobalfund.org/en/about/fundingspending/.

———. By-laws Art. 6.1. Available at http://www.theglobalfund.org/documents/core/bylaws/Core_GlobalFund_Bylaws_en/.

———. Private Sector and Non-government Partners. Available at http://www.theglobalfund.org/en/partners/privatesector/.

———. Results. Available at http://www.theglobalfund.org/en/about/results/.

Global Health Workforce Alliance. GAVI—The Global Alliance for Vaccines and Immunizations. Available at http://www.who.int/workforcealliance/members_partners/member_list/gavi/en/.

Hanleybrown, F., John Kania, and Mark Kramer. *Channeling change, making collective impact work*. Stanford Social Innovation Review (Jan. 26, 2012).

Howard-Jones, N. The Scientific Background of the International Sanitary Conferences, 1851–1938 (1975).

Kaul, I. *Exploring the policy space between markets and states: global public-private partnerships*. In The New Public Finance: Responding to Global Challenges 91 (2006).

Klock, K. *The soft law alternative to the WHO's treaty powers*. 44 Geo. J. Int'l Law 828–829 (2013).

Montevideo Convention on the Rights and Duties of States. Available at http://www.cfr.org/sovereignty/montevideo-convention-rights-duties-states/p15897.

OECD. From Lessons to Principles for the Use of Public-Private Partnerships. Available at http://www.oecd.org/gov/budgeting/48144872.pdf.

Ruger, J. P. *Normative foundations of global health law*. 96 Georgetown Law Journal 423, 426 (2008).

Saul, A. *Vaccines for neglected diseases* 248 (Rino Rappuoli and Fabio Bagnoli eds., 2011).

Triponel, A. *Global Fund to Fight Aids, Tuberculosis and Malaria: A new legal and conceptual framework for providing international development aid*. 35 North Carolina Journal of International Law and Commercial Regulation 173 (2009).

10

Global Vaccine Access as a Critical Intervention to Fight Infectious Disease, Antibiotic Resistance, and Poverty

SETH BERKLEY

Worldwide, more than 30 vaccine doses are delivered every second through routine immunization programs. This number has increased dramatically as more vaccines are developed for the largest killers of children, and the global community acknowledges that vaccines, as a fundamental medical intervention, positively affect more lives than any other. Vaccine delivery has become the base of the primary healthcare delivery system and a principal mechanism by which global health outcomes have been improved precisely because they protect against common infectious diseases that disproportionately burden the lives and well-being of children, in particular those living in the world's poorest countries. As noted at the UNICEF World Summit for Children 1990, "Preventable childhood diseases . . . against which there are effective vaccines . . . are currently responsible for the great majority of the world's 14 million deaths of children under five years and disability of millions more every year."[1] Since then, the annual number of child deaths has fallen to just under 6 million, but far too many children still die unnecessarily.

The purpose of this chapter is to broaden the scope through which the social impact of vaccines is viewed—a scope traditionally focused on infectious disease—to include the full range of public health threats vaccines combat, the substantial contribution vaccines play in alleviating the most severe forms of poverty around the world, and the role of routine immunization programs as the foundation of national primary healthcare and public health systems. Viewed through this widened lens, it becomes clear that funding and effecting global access to vaccines

---

[1] UNICEF, Plan of Action for Implementing the World Declaration on the Survival, Protection and Development of Children in the 1990s (1990), available at http://www.unicef.org/wsc/plan.htm.

should be at the highest priority for low-, middle-, and high-income countries alike. The chapter further outlines specific development, delivery, and financing mechanisms that may facilitate the achievement of access to new and underused vaccines for children living in the world's poorest countries.

Background

Vaccines have, of course, served as an important medical intervention for hundreds of years, and in some forms even longer. Ancient physicians ground dried scabs from smallpox victims and used the resulting powder to immunize healthy people. In 1796, Edward Jenner observed that exposure to cowpox provided protection against smallpox, a breakthrough credited with giving birth to the field of immunology.[2] After Jenner's discovery, which built on earlier experiments by Dorset farmer Benjamin Jesty, nearly 80 years passed before Louis Pasteur's work on cholera, anthrax, and rabies led to methods for inactivating whole bacteria, which could then be used as vaccines. This also paved the way for the discovery of bacterial toxins, the production of antitoxins, and the realization that immune serum contained antibodies that neutralized toxins or bacterial replication.[3] In the middle part of the 20th century, improvement of those methods and discovery of others led to a rapid increase in the number of vaccines, from 10 to a point where today we have nearly 60 vaccines, capable of protecting against approximately 30 diseases. While advances in medical technology assure that this number will continue to increase in the future, the question that remains is: How do we get these vaccines, with their vast potential to save lives, to all the people that need them?

In the 1960s and 1970s, vaccine coverage in low-income countries was often less than 5%. As a result, in 1974, the World Health Organization (WHO) initiated the Expanded Program on Immunization (EPI) with the objective of vaccinating children throughout the world against six diseases: diphtheria, tetanus, pertussis (whooping cough), measles, poliomyelitis, and tuberculosis. In 1977, the Pan-American Health Organization (PAHO) formed its Revolving Fund, which allows participant countries to pool their resources to procure high-quality vaccines, syringes, and related supplies for their populations at relatively low prices.[4] Around the same time, James Grant used his leadership of the United Nations Children's Fund (UNICEF) to press for universal childhood immunization as one of the pillars

---

[2] Stanley A. Plotkin and Susan L. Plotkin, *The development of vaccines: how the past led to the future*, 9 Nature Reviews Microbiology 889–893 (2011), available at http://www.nature.com/nrmicro/journal/v9/n12/full/nrmicro2668.html.

[3] *Id.*

[4] World Health Organization, Pan American Health Organization Revolving Fund, available at http://www.who.int/immunization/newsroom/PAHO_Revolving_Fun_FINAL.pdf.

of low-cost, high-impact interventions that could drastically reduce child mortality.[5] In 1984, Dr. William Foege, former director of the Centers for Disease Control and Prevention (CDC) and two of his former CDC colleagues, Carol Walters and Bill Watson, founded the Task Force for Child Survival, which adopted immunization and vaccines as one of its core strategies to improve child wellness and survival worldwide. As a result of all these efforts, immunization rates in the poorest countries rose steadily during the 1980s. By 1990, UNICEF was able to declare "universal childhood immunisation," with global rates rising to close to 80%. Rates in the poorest countries still remained lower, with around 60% of children in the 73 poorest countries, which later became eligible for Gavi support, receiving three doses of a combination vaccine that protects against diphtheria, tetanus, and pertussis (DTP3—traditionally used as the primary measure of immunization coverage), up from less than 30% in 1980.

In 1990, the Declaration of Manhattan, the founding document of the Children's Vaccine Initiative, was adopted at the World Summit for Children.[6] Its target was to achieve universal immunization, defined as approximately 80% coverage. However, DTP3 coverage in the poorest countries actually fell in the early 1990s and continued to stagnate for the rest of the decade.

Gavi and the Global Mobilization of Resources for Immunization

Gavi was launched in 2000 to help reinvigorate immunization efforts. Its objective was twofold: to catalyze renewed momentum in vaccine coverage in developing countries (as measured by DTP3 coverage growth) and to accelerate introductions of new and powerful vaccines that were becoming available in high-income countries but were not yet being introduced in the poorest countries. The creation of Gavi, made possible through the priority given to vaccines by the Bill and Melinda Gates Foundation, facilitated the use of breakthrough technologies to expand access to new vaccines, as well as traditional immunizations that may have been delayed for decades without Gavi support. For example, between Gavi's inception and 2014, DTP3 coverage in Gavi-supported countries rose from 60% to 81%.[7] This change had a direct impact on disease burden: between 1980 and 2014, cases of diphtheria declined by 92%, pertussis by 91%, and tetanus by 90%.[8] At the same time, Gavi supported

[5] Jim Grant, UNICEF Visionary (Richard Jolly ed.), available at http://www.unicef.org/about/history/files/Jim_Grant_unicef_visionary.pdf.

[6] Paul F. Basch, Vaccines and World Health: Science Policy and Practice 188 (1994).

[7] *Id.* Based on data officially reported to WHO and UNICEF by current member states. Note: includes DTP-containing vaccines, such as pentavalent vaccine.

[8] Christopher J. L. Murray et al., *Disability-adjusted life years (DALYs) for 291 diseases and injuries in 21 regions, 1990–2010: a systematic analysis for the Global Burden of Disease Study 2010*, 380(9859)

countries to introduce powerful new vaccines, including those against pneumococcal, rotavirus, and *Haemophilus influenzae* type b (Hib) that protect against pneumonia and diarrhea, two of the leading causes of child mortality. Gavi also supported countries to introduce two vaccines that protect against cancer—hepatitis B vaccine, which protects against liver cancer, and human papillomavirus (HPV) vaccine, which protects against cervical cancer. Today, every Gavi-supported country has introduced hepatitis B and Hib vaccines, and the majority have also introduced rotavirus and pneumococcal vaccines only a decade after these latter vaccines were first licensed (by contrast, there was a delay of 11 years between the first high-income country introducing Hib and its first introduction in a low-income country).

In this same period, the global population has increased by 60%. Beyond the direct health impact against specific diseases, vaccines provide long-term socioeconomic benefits: vaccinated children remain healthy, which contributes to better cognitive development and therefore better use of educational resources. Keeping people healthy also lowers societal healthcare costs, while reductions in child mortality contributes to smaller families. Fewer cases of illness also help protect families from out-of-pocket healthcare expenses, which they may not be able to afford and can tip them into poverty, and prevent parents from having to take time off from work to care for their sick children. In all these ways, vaccines help create a healthier workforce population and contribute significantly to economic growth. In fact, every dollar invested in childhood immunization saves US$16 in healthcare costs, lost wages, and lost productivity due to illness. Taking into account the full value people place on living longer, healthier lives, then that return on investment increases to US$44.[9] Gavi estimates that over the next 5 years alone, the vaccines it supports will generate economic benefits of at least US$80 to US$100 billion. The evidence is clear that vaccines work and that they are worth the kind of international, public-private investment Gavi represents.

Gavi as an institution is unique. It is a public-private partnership, organized not only to leverage what are regarded as the traditional strengths of the public and private sectors but also to bring together the entire field of public health and immunology around the objective of expanding access to vaccines for the world's poorest countries. Gavi's board includes representatives from all key stakeholders in the field of immunization: vaccine industry representatives from both industrialized and middle-income countries, civil society organizations, the Bill and Melinda Gates Foundation, research and technical health institutes, governments from both high-income and low-income countries, the World Bank, the World Health Organization, and UNICEF. A critical feature of Gavi's board is that one third of its members are

---

Lancet 2197–2223 (2012), available at http://www.thelancet.com/journals/lancet/article/PIIS0140-6736(12)61689-4/abstract.

[9] Sachiko Ozawa et al., *Return on investment from childhood immunization in low- and middle-income countries, 2011–2020*, 35(2) Health Affairs 199–207 (2016).

unaffiliated directors who bring an independent perspective to board discussions, more typical of a corporate board of directors than an international organization.

The Gavi model of expanding vaccine access is premised on co-financing and market shaping. The principal concept of its market shaping is that Gavi uses its scale—supporting countries that are home to 60% of the world's children—and predictable funding to reduce the price of vaccines that are normally prohibitively expensive at the price point at which they enter high-income markets. By creating stable markets for developing country vaccines, Gavi has also led to many new entrants, particularly from middle-income country manufacturers, and this is facilitating a more competitive and healthier vaccine market. Co-financing is an arrangement in which Gavi-eligible countries pay a share of the price of their Gavi-supported vaccines. For the poorest countries (those classified as "low income" by the World Bank), this is $0.20 a dose—typically a small proportion of the total price but important to help mobilize domestic resources for immunization and ensure these vaccines are included in the national budget. Once a country crosses the low-income threshold, its co-financing increases by 15% every year. This continues until the country's gross national income per capita reaches Gavi's eligibility threshold (currently $1,580), at which point it begins a process of transitioning away from Gavi support. Over the following 5 years, the country will gradually increase its share of the cost of Gavi-supported vaccines until Gavi support ends and the country becomes fully self-financing. Gavi is working with manufacturers to ensure that countries can continue to access prices similar to those paid by Gavi for at least 5 years after they transition out of Gavi support to ensure that the transition is financially sustainable.

As the following sections describe, there is good evidence that Gavi's model and its mission—to both promote health and build financial capacity—are succeeding.

Immunization Programs

Pneumococcal Bacteria

The pneumococcus bacterium is one of the most common causes of severe pneumonia as well as ear infections, sinus infections, meningitis (infection of the covering around the brain and spinal cord), and bacteremia (bloodstream infection). There are more than 80 serotypes of pneumococcal bacteria, and vaccines are aimed at reducing the public health burden of those types most likely to cause severe illness. The earliest pneumococcal conjugate vaccine targeted 7 of these bacteria (PCV7), and its use between 2001 and 2009 in the United States alone was determined to have prevented about 131,000 cases of invasive pneumococcal disease (IPD) in children younger than 5 years of age.[10] In the Kilifi District of Kenya, the

---

[10] Centers for Disease Control and Prevention, Pneumococcal Disease (2013), available at http://www.cdc.gov/vaccines/vpd-vac/pneumo/downloads/dis-pneumo-color.pdf.

introduction of PCV10 in 2011 has been associated with a radical decline in the number of cases of children under the age of 5 suffering from vaccine-specific serotypes of invasive pneumococcal disease: from 39 in 2011 to only 1 in 2014.[11] Kenya was one of the first Gavi-supported countries to introduce pneumococcal conjugate vaccine; the vaccine has now been introduced with Gavi support in more than 50 countries (approximately 70% of those that Gavi supports). Today, there is also a 13-valent vaccine that Gavi countries may use.

The public health benefits of increased access to vaccines are not limited to individual recipients or even to "herd immunity," the phrase used to describe the indirect protection from infectious disease created when a substantial percentage of a population has become immune to that infection. When the spread of the infection through the population is prevented, individuals who are not immune benefit from this protection. In the case of pneumococcal bacteria, vaccines have also suppressed the selection mechanisms that give rise to drug-resistant pathogens. South Africa's gold mining communities served as one of the earliest foci for public health research because prevalent pneumococcal bacteria caused severe pneumonia with a high fatality rate. Development of drug resistance among those bacteria was common, and it was an early site of research into the efficacy of polyvalent pneumococcal vaccines. With the introduction of PCV7 in 2009, incidence of penicillin-resistant, ceftriaxone-resistant, and multidrug-resistant pneumococcal cases declined significantly, and with the introduction of PCV13 in 2011, it declined even further.[12] The cumulative effect was likely caused by the vaccines diminishing the selective pressure for drug resistance.

Meningitis A

The impact of Gavi's work on meningitis A in Africa has been similarly far-reaching. Meningitis A is caused by a strain of *Neisseria meningitidis*, a bacterium that routinely results in meningitis, meningococcemia, and septicemia, and which particularly affects 26 countries in sub-Saharan Africa's "meningitis belt." The vaccine was developed by the Serum Institute of India with the specific objective of creating an affordable meningitis A–specific vaccine. Gavi provided the funding to procure the vaccine once it was licensed. From 2010 to 2014, Gavi-funded campaigns immunized more than 220 million children and young adults in 15 countries. On average, the campaigns reached more than 85% of those at risk of contracting the deadly disease. The impact has been immediate: there were no new cases of meningitis A in

---

[11] KEMRI-Wellcome Trust Research Programme, Pneumococcal vaccination of children in Kenya can provide 'herd protection' to unvaccinated population, (2014) available at http://kemri-wellcome.org/news/pneumococcal-vaccination-of-children-in-kenya-can-provide-herd-protection-to-unvaccinated-population/.

[12] Anne von Gottberg et al., *Effects of vaccination on invasive pneumococcal disease in South Africa*, 371 N Engl J Med 1889–1899 (2014).

vaccinated countries in 2014, and epidemics in the meningitis belt reached their lowest-ever recorded levels. Burkina Faso and Chad, for example, have reported significant reductions in meningitis A rates across the population thanks to high vaccination coverage.

Hepatitis B and Pentavalent Vaccine

Gavi's initial mandate was focused on hepatitis B vaccine. Chronic hepatitis B is a major cause of liver cancer, which may be prevented by immunization. When hepatitis B vaccine first became available in high-income countries in 1982, it was not accessible to developing countries largely because of its cost. More than a decade passed before the first developing country used the vaccine for routine immunization. Through Gavi support, by 2006, the proportion of low-income countries with hepatitis B in their routine immunization plans had overtaken that in high-income countries. In Gavi's first decade, an additional 267 million children were immunized with hepatitis B vaccines. As a result, an estimated 3 million future deaths from liver cancer and other hepatitis B–related infections were prevented. Hepatitis B vaccine is now available in every Gavi-supported country as part of the pentavalent five-in-one vaccine, which protects children against five diseases (diphtheria, tetanus, pertussis, hepatitis B, and Hib with South Sudan becoming the last Gavi country to introduce the vaccine, in 2014.

Human Papillomavirus Vaccine

Human papillomavirus causes virtually all cases of cervical cancer. Unlike in high-income countries, where a wide range of treatment options may be available, cervical cancer in low-income countries results in high mortality rates with associated burdens imposed by the loss of often young, otherwise healthy women. Historically, maternal deaths—the death of a woman while pregnant or within 42 days of termination of pregnancy—were the leading killer of women in developing countries.[13] Now, the number of deaths caused by cervical cancer is nearly the same as the number of maternal deaths.[14] In developing countries, cervical cancer is the leading

---

[13] World Health Organization, Trends in Maternal Mortality: 1990 to 2013 Estimates by WHO, UNICEF, UNFPA, The World Bank and the United Nations Population Division (2014), available at http://apps.who.int/iris/bitstream/10665/112682/2/9789241507226_eng.pdf?ua=1.

[14] Rafael Lozano et al., *Global and regional mortality from 235 causes of death for 20 age groups in 1990 and 2010: a systematic analysis for the Global Burden of Disease Study 2010* 380(9859) Lancet 2095–2128 (2012), available at http://www.thelancet.com/journals/lancet/article/PIIS0140-6736(12)61728-0/abstract; Institute for Health Metrics and Evaluation Maternal Health Infographics (2010) available at http://www.healthdata.org/maternal-health/infographics; Bernard W. Stewart and Christopher P. Wild, World Cancer Report 2014 (2014), International Agency for Research on Cancer, WHO, available at http://whocp3.codemantra.com/Marketing.aspx?ID=WCR2014&ISBN=9789283204299&sts=b#1.

cause of cancer death in women, and 91% of global estimated HPV-related cancer deaths are due to cervical cancer (HPV is also linked to head and neck cancer, as well as anal and penile cancer). Cervical cancer kills approximately 260,000 women each year, of whom 85% live in developing countries. Malawi, Mozambique, and Zambia, for example, suffer from high cervical cancer rates.[15] Since the first Gavi-supported HPV vaccine demonstration program in Kenya in 2013, more than 1 million girls have been vaccinated with Gavi support. In 2014, Gavi helped seven countries to initiate HPV vaccine demonstration programs—the first step toward national introductions—and several countries have now introduced the vaccine nationwide following the lead of Rwanda in 2011. Due to large-scale commitments, it is predicted that 30 million girls in 40 Gavi-supported countries will be vaccinated against HPV by 2020.[16]

Equitable Access to Vaccines

The collective result of these efforts has been the dramatic narrowing of the gap between rich and poor in the context of vaccine access. High-income and low-income countries have reached near parity in hepatitis B and Hib vaccine access, and the gap is closing for pneumococcal conjugate and other vaccines.[17] Despite this progress, less than 5% of children in Gavi-supported countries currently receive all 11 antigens universally recommended by WHO for infants. Thanks to Gavi-supported efforts, that coverage will increase to reach 50% of children by 2020. Indeed, in 2016–2020 alone, Gavi hopes to support the vaccination of an additional 300 million children, helping to avert 5 to 6 million deaths.[18]

Financial Sustainability

Global commitment to vaccine access has not just led to substantial gains in reducing child mortality and in narrowing gaps in health outcomes. Evidence is also

---

[15] World Health Organization, International Agency for Cancer Research, Cervical Cancer Estimated Incidence, Mortality and Prevalence Worldwide in 2012, available at http://globocan.iarc.fr/old/FactSheets/cancers/cervix-new.asp.

[16] Gavi, 2014 Strategic Demand Forecast (2014), available at http://www.Gavi.org/Library/Gavi-documents/Supply-procurement/Gavi-Strategic-Demand-Forecast-2014/.

[17] The International Vaccine Access Center (IVAC) VIMS database, available at http://www.jhsph.edu/research/centers-and-institutes/ivac/vims/.

[18] Preliminary Gavi projections based on WHO/UNICEF coverage estimates and Strategic Demand Forecast version 9; Gavi, Gavi Strategic Demand Forecasts 9 and 10 (2015); Gavi, Investing Together for a Healthy Future: the 2016-2020 Investment Opportunity, available at http://www.Gavi.org/Library/Publications/Publications-Gavi/The-2016-2020-Gavi-Alliance-Investment-Opportunity/.

growing that supports Gavi's development and resource mobilization model. That approach is defined by three features: co-financing, donor commitments, and shaping the market for vaccines. These features are, in turn, supported by innovative financing mechanisms that have helped attract additional donor support and contributed to Gavi's market shaping efforts.

Co-Financing

Gavi's co-financing model is based on sharing nominal costs per vaccine dose at year 1 of support and gradually moving toward self-sufficiency. China's experience with Gavi support provides an illustration of how this process is intended to work. China has historically suffered from relatively high rates of hepatitis B infection, a disease that also transmits at high rates from mother to newborn. Fifteen years ago, barely 40% of children in China's poorest areas were immunized against hepatitis B. Approximately 10% of China's population were chronic carriers of the disease, which at the time was responsible for hundreds of thousands of deaths every year due to liver cancer and cirrhosis. In 2002, Gavi, the government of China, and the China Center for Disease Control (CDC) started a partnership that lasted until December 2010 to combat the disease. The collaboration provided first-dose hepB vaccines at birth free of charge to more than 25 million newborns in the poorest and most remote provinces of western and central China. The Chinese government introduced the vaccine into its routine immunization program in 2005. Since the start of the project, the percentage of newborn children immunized with the first dose at birth has climbed from 64% to more than 90% in most areas. Less than 1% of children under age 5 are now chronic carriers of hepatitis B. China now entirely self-finances the program and has transitioned from being a recipient of Gavi support to becoming a Gavi donor. China is also now a provider of vaccines to Gavi, following the prequalification of a Chinese Japanese encephalitis vaccine by WHO in 2013.

Market Shaping

Because of its purchasing power and the nature of its mandate, Gavi is able to secure the lowest prices for vaccines in the world, often achieving 95% to 97% reductions in prices available in high-income markets.[19] Gavi procures rotavirus vaccine, for example, at a price of $2.50 per dose, whereas in high-income markets the price can be more than $100.00. Gavi's market-shaping efforts have also helped drive improvement in long-term market dynamics, including incentivizing the entry of new manufacturers into vaccine markets and securing continued reductions in

---

[19] UNICEF Supply Division, Working together for healthy vaccine markets available at http://www.gavi.org/progress-report/.

vaccine prices. The cost of fully immunizing a child with pentavalent, pneumococcal, and rotavirus vaccines has declined by 39% since 2010.[20] This is in large part due to a significant increase in the supply base for Gavi-supported vaccines, which increased from 5 suppliers in 2001 to 16 in 2015. Gavi has also used an advance market commitment to support its market-shaping efforts for pneumococcal vaccine, which helped mobilize additional donor support for vaccine procurement while incentivizing manufacturers to make sufficient supply available at affordable prices.

Donor Base

Gavi's model also relies on long-term donor funding commitments, which enable Gavi to approve multiyear support for countries and provide manufacturers with confidence on the viability of the Gavi market. At Gavi's replenishment in January 2015, 31 donors pledged an additional US$7.5 billion for the 2016–2020 period, a large majority of which was as part of a multiyear commitment for the entire period. These long-term pledges are complemented by innovative financing instruments, including the International Finance Facility for Immunisation (IFFIm). IFFIm allows long-term pledges made by governments to be converted into immediately available cash resources by selling "vaccine bonds" to investors and using government commitments to pay for those pledges over the period of the debt instruments. The World Bank acts as financial adviser and treasury manager to IFFIm.

Gavi also seeks to mobilize expertise and resources—both in kind and operational support—from the private sector. To help catalyze these partnerships, Gavi established the Gavi Matching Fund with US$ 130 million combined (UK£ 50 million and US$ 50 million, respectively) of support from the UK Department for International Development (DFID) and the Bill & Melinda Gates Foundation in order to match contributions from corporations, foundations, their customers, members, employees and business partners.

Conclusion

The benefits following the world's large-scale commitment to increasing access to vaccines has been extraordinary. Millions of deaths have been averted, diseases that have long plagued those in the poorest countries are in retreat, and there are identifiable improvements in workforces and economies as a result. Despite this success, much remains to be done. One in five children still do not receive even three doses of a DTP-containing vaccine while, as described earlier, less than 5% receive all 11

---

[20] *Id.*

vaccines recommended by WHO. Moreover, the Ebola crisis and now Zika are reminders that there are many deadly diseases for which vaccines are not yet available. Gavi's priority for the next 5 years will be to improve coverage and equity of immunization and to support countries that are getting wealthier by increasing their own domestic investment in immunization (including more than 20 that will transition out of Gavi support by 2020). Given the overwhelming return on investments in vaccines in terms of both human quality of life and economic growth, it is critical that immunization remain a global priority. While much work remains, the progress so far represents one of the tremendous public health achievements of this century.

References

Basch, P. Vaccines and World Health: Science Policy and Practice 188 (1994).
Centers for Disease Control and Prevention. Pneumococcal Disease. Available at http://www.cdc.gov/vaccines/vpd-vac/pneumo/downloads/dis-pneumo-color.pdf.
Gavi. 2014 Strategic Demand Forecast (2014). Available at http://www.Gavi.org/Library/Gavi-documents/Supply-procurement/Gavi-Strategic-Demand-Forecast-2014/.
———. Strategic Demand Forecast version 9; Gavi Strategic Demand Forecasts 9 and 10, Gavi The Vaccine Alliance (2015).
———. Investing together for a healthy future: the 2016–2020 investment opportunity. *Gavi The Vaccine Alliance*. Available at http://www.Gavi.org/Library/Publications/Publications-Gavi/The-2016-2020-Gavi-Alliance-Investment-Opportunity/.
Institute for Health Metrics and Evaluation Maternal Health Infographics (2010) available at http://www.healthdata.org/maternal-health/infographics International Vaccine Access Center (IVAC) VIMS database. Data as of Dec. 31, 2014 available at http://www.jhsph.edu/research/centers-and-institutes/ivac/view-hub/
Jolly, R. (ed.) Jim Grant, UNICEF Visionary. Available at http://www.unicef.org/about/history/files/Jim_Grant_unicef_visionary.pdf.
KEMRI-Wellcome Trust Research Programme, Pneumococcal vaccination of children in Kenya can provide 'herd protection' to unvaccinated population, (2014) available at http://kemri-wellcome.org/news/pneumococcal-vaccination-of-children-in-kenya-can-provide-herd-protection-to-unvaccinated-population
Murray, C. J., et al. *Disability-adjusted life years (DALYs) for 291 diseases and injuries in 21 regions, 1990–2010: a systematic analysis for the Global Burden of Disease Study 2010* 380(9859) Lancet 2197–2223 (2012).
Plotkin, S. A., and S. L. Plotkin. *The development of vaccines: how the past led to the future.* 9 Nature Reviews Microbiology 889–893(2011).
KEMRI-Wellcome Trust Research Programme, Kilifi, Kenya.
Stewart, Bernard, and Christopher P. Wild. (2014). World Cancer Report 2014. International Agency for Research on Cancer, WHO. Available at http://whocp3.codemantra.com/Marketing.aspx?ID=WCR2014&ISBN=9789283204299&sts=b#1.
UNICEF. Plan of Action for Implementing the World Declaration on the Survival, Protection and Development of Children in the 1990s. Available at http://www.unicef.org/wsc/plan.htm.
von Gottberg, A., et al. *Effects of vaccination on invasive pneumococcal disease in South Africa.* 371 N Engl J Med 1889–1899 (2014).
WHO-UNICEF. Estimates of DTP3 Coverage. Available at http://apps.who.int/immunization_monitoring/globalsummary/timeseries/tswucoveragedtp3.html.

World Health Organization. Pan American Health Organization Revolving Fund. Available at http://www.who.int/immunization/newsroom/PAHO_Revolving_Fun_FINAL.pdf.

———. Trends in Maternal Mortality: 1990 to 2013 Estimates by WHO, UNICEF, UNFPA, The World Bank and the United Nations Population Division (2014). Available at http://apps.who.int/iris/bitstream/10665/112682/2/9789241507226_eng.pdf?ua=1.

World Health Organization, International Agency for Cancer Research. Cervical Cancer Estimated Incidence, Mortality and Prevalence Worldwide in 2012. Available at http://globocan.iarc.fr/old/FactSheets/cancers/cervix-new.asp.

PART III

ETHICAL AND HUMAN RIGHTS OBLIGATIONS IN PUBLIC HEALTH EMERGENCIES

11

Bridging the Gap Between Biomedical Innovation and Access to Treatments to Fight Infectious Disease

VERONICA MILLER

The outbreak of Ebola virus disease in West Africa exposed multiple weaknesses in the global system for detecting, preventing, and responding to infectious disease threats, some of which had been fully understood and some of which had been known to the global public health community for some time. Until the West African epidemic, Ebola did not appear to pose a major threat to public health.[1] The irregular outbreaks that did occur were quickly contained using orthodox approaches.[2] The ability of the disease to spread the way it did and the poor performance of formal global mechanisms that had existed since 2005 were unanticipated. Ebola represented a neglected tropical disease in which few private actors had invested any research and development resources, largely because the likely market appeared minuscule. That was an old story. US and Canadian governments had, years before, made national security–related investments in Ebola research.[3] That research had yielded a few experimental drug and vaccine candidates, although all were early in the development pathway, and regulatory review was distant.[4]

When the Ebola epidemic exploded, critics pointed to the nascent state of Ebola diagnostics, therapeutics, and candidate vaccines as demonstrating precisely why

---

[1] Suerie Moon et al., *Will Ebola change the game? Ten essential reforms before the next pandemic. The report of the Harvard-LSHTM Independent Panel on the Global Response to Ebola*, 386 (10009), Lancet 2204–2221 (Nov. 28, 2015).

[2] CDC, Outbreaks Chronology: Ebola Virus Disease, available at http://www.cdc.gov/vhf/ebola/outbreaks/history/chronology.html.

[3] Frank L. Smith, *We have military research to thank for Ebola vaccines*, Mediacom (Aug. 28, 2014), available at https://medium.com/war-is-boring/we-have-military-research-to-thank-for-ebola-vaccines-565897c3f1bc#.so7cq0hcx.

[4] Thomas Hoenen and Heinz Feldmann, *Ebola virus in West Africa, and the use of experimental therapies or vaccines*, 12 BMC Biol. 80 (2014).

the system for biomedical innovation was broken.[5] Although reported to have a case fatality rate above 65%, with no available therapeutics or vaccines, Ebola was neglected because of how many people it affected and where.[6]

The threat of global transmission of Ebola accelerated governmental, philanthropic, and private industry interest and pushed the few promising diagnostic, therapeutic, and vaccine candidates toward regulatory evaluation of safety and efficacy.[7] The US Congress provided emergency supplemental funding, which facilitated these efforts, and large pharmaceutical firms acquired, licensed, or developed vaccine candidates and formed partnerships with national and international health authorities. The US Department of Health and Human Services (HHS) declared that it would provide liability protection for activities related to three specific Ebola vaccine candidates.[8]

The purpose of this chapter is to analyze the gap between biomedical innovation and access to treatment that has characterized much of the debate surrounding the Ebola response as well as other infectious diseases. While that gap generally consists of three parts—discovery, regulatory review, and health system integration—this chapter focuses on the latter while indicating how aspects of the former, such as clinical trial design and regulatory collaboration, may work for expanding access. Using the planning and implementation histories for treatments of two other viral diseases, HIV and hepatitis C, the chapter explores achievements, challenges, and lessons learned regarding how biomedical innovation may be efficiently and fairly translated into treatment access around the world.

From Biomedical Innovation to Treatment Access

For biomedical innovation to reach the widest number of patients, medical products must pass through three phases. The first is from discovery (bench) to clinical

[5] *How many Ebola patients have been treated outside of Africa?*, New York Times (Jan. 26, 2015), available at http://www.nytimes.com/interactive/2014/07/31/world/africa/ebola-virus-outbreak-qa.html?; WHO Ebola Response Team, *Ebola virus disease in West Africa—the first 9 Months of the epidemic and forward projections*, 371 N Engl J Med 1481–1495 (2014).

[6] A. Lefebvre et al., *Case fatality rates of Ebola virus diseases: a meta-analysis of World Health Organization data*, 44(9) Med Mal Infect. 412–416 (2014); J. Millman, *Why the drug industry hasn't come up with an Ebola cure*, Washington Post (Aug. 13, 2014), available at https://www.washingtonpost.com/news/wonk/wp/2014/08/13/why-the-drug-industry-hasnt-come-up-with-an-ebola-cure/.

[7] World Health Organization, Ethical Considerations for Use of Unregistered Interventions for Ebola Virus Disease (Aug. 11, 2014), available at http://apps.who.int/iris/bitstream/10665/130997/1/WHO_HIS_KER_GHE_14.1_eng.pdf.

[8] Alexander Gaffney, *US government immunizes future manufacturers of Ebola vaccines from legal liability*, 1 Regulatory Affairs Professionals Society (2014), available at http://www.raps.org/Regulatory-Focus/News/2014/12/09/20947/US-Government-Immunizes-Future-Manufacturers-of-Ebola-Vaccines-from-Legal-Liability/.

trial; the second is from clinical trial to demonstration of efficacy and regulatory approval; and the third is implementation. This chapter will focus on the latter phase.

Premarketing Clinical Research

It is well known that the number of new drug applications and newly approved drugs has, over a fairly long time horizon, plateaued or declined. Without delving too far into the heated debate over whether drug development is too costly or regulatory opacity and inefficiency (clinical trial design and endpoints) is to blame, there are promising cooperative models in the precompetitive space that have shown that reducing time to approval is possible. The Forum for Collaborative HIV Research, for example, has created a "safe space" for regulators, researchers, and firms to analyze existing data and identify important aspects of drug development such as biomarkers, practical aspects of drug delivery, and details of regulatory review. The forum reduces the costs of drug development by minimizing the number of competitive spaces innovators must target.[9] The HCV Drug Development Advisory group similarly brings together representatives from the US and European regulatory agencies, academia, patient advocates, and industry to clarify barriers to drug development and access. The Ebola crisis has prompted calls for an internationally organized and funded entity to focus on research and development on neglected diseases that portend global public health risks.[10]

Regulatory Mechanisms to Accelerate Approval

Although the main purpose of the clinical research phase is to bring a product to market, important groundwork to support—or not—global access is laid during the clinical research and development period. Clinical research programs before approval and postmarketing commitments determine what and how much is known about how a new intervention affects different patient subgroups (e.g., men vs. women; HCV genotype 1 vs. HCV genotype 4 infected patients) with respect to efficacy and safety over the short and long term. Well-planned clinical trials offer the opportunity for determining correlates of clinical outcomes that inform dosing and delivery options and may reduce trial duration.

---

[9] Veronica Miller, *The forum for collaborative HIV research: a model for an integrated and inclusive approach to clinical research and drug development*, 86(3) Clinical Pharmacology and Therapeutics 332–335 (2009).

[10] Monica Balasegaram et al., *A global biomedical R&D fund and mechanism for innovations of public health importance* 12(5) PLoS Medicine (2015); Stanley A. Plotkin, Adel Mahmoud, and Jeremy Farrar, *Establishing a global vaccine development fund*, 373 N Engl J Med 297–300 (July 23, 2015).

There are many possible variations of adaptive design, but the basic concept is to rapidly incorporate results (clinical, biomarker, imaging) during the study to inform the design, favor winning products, reject failures, match responses and enrollment to specific biomarker/drug mates, and select doses. A good example is monitoring and potentially halting a study if futility or clear benefit is seen based on interim analysis. This requires appropriate statistical approaches and corrections for what are essentially multiple analyses. Adaptive design "incorporates prospectively planned opportunities for modification of one or more specified aspects of the study design and integrates hypotheses based on analysis of accumulating data while the study is ongoing."[11] For example, for accelerated approval pathways, the US Food and Drug Administration approved antiretroviral drugs for HIV based on favorable changes in CD4 T-lymphocyte counts and/or plasma HIV RNA, but it required clinical endpoint trials for traditional approval. The disadvantage of requiring clinical endpoint studies for AIDS was that participants had to remain on randomized study regimens until the occurrences of a clinical endpoint, such as an opportunistic infection or death. Compared with an endpoint of disease progression, plasma HIV RNA, an analysis of how many copies of the virus are present in the blood, had practical advantages such as routine use in clinical practice and ease of measurement. Given these practical advantages, the use of plasma HIV RNA for purposes of drug approval was adopted even for traditional approvals similar to the way in which blood pressure and cholesterol measurements have been used for the approval of antihypertensive and hypolipidemic drugs.[12] Similar innovations have been used to test drug resistance.[13]

Regulatory Approval and Postmarketing Regulatory Oversight

In most instances, sponsors negotiate approval of their medical product with each national regulatory authority. This in itself is an onerous process, and additional requirements imposed by national regulatory authorities that lack the capacity of agencies in higher-resource countries often cause disparities in access to medicines. In some cases, individual country agencies, such as Mexico's health authority, COFEPRIS, accept approval certifications from designated foreign regulatory authorities like the US Food and Drug Administration (FDA) or European Medicines Agency (EMA). The World Health Organization (WHO)

---

[11] Brian Alexander and Patrick Wen, *Biomarker-based adaptive trials for patients with glioblastoma—lessons from I-SPY2*, 15(8) Neuro-Oncology 972–978 (2013).

[12] Jeffrey Murray et al., *The use of plasma HIV RNA as a study endpoint in efficacy trials of antiretroviral drugs*, 13(7) AIDS 797–804 (1999).

[13] Victor DeGruttola et al., *The relation between baseline HIV drug resistance and response to antiretroviral therapy: re-analysis of retrospective and prospective studies using a standardized data analysis plan*, A5(1) Antiviral Therapy 41–48 (2000).

also provides a prequalification service for medicines, pharmaceutical quality control laboratories, and active pharmaceutical ingredients and conducts considerable advocacy for medicines of guaranteed quality. Expansion of laws that authorize WHO prequalification to substitute for national registration is one of the frequent recommendations made for facilitating medicines in emergency contexts.

In Europe, new drugs are approved through national regulatory authorities or through the centralized EMA process in which individual country regulatory agencies participate. However, individual country health technology assessments play a significant role in establishing access. Not uncommonly, European country-level health technology assessment review and approval request additional data (i.e., additional clinical studies) to satisfy idiosyncratic information requirements. These additional pathways add substantial cost to the approval process.

The requirement for regional regulatory review and approval is not without benefits. Populations vary with respect to genetics, environmental factors that may influence outcome (e.g., common co-infections), as well as customs regarding the use of health technologies; thus locally generated data provide unique value and should facilitate regional/local registration. Ironically, the notion that "we don't know if this will work for our women because it wasn't tested in our women" (South Africa) may compete with "we won't allow you to use our women as guinea pigs" (Cambodia). As with other aspects of registration, national regulatory authorities are not of equal capacity, and resource constraints in low- and middle-income countries often erect structural barriers to access to new (and sometimes old) medical interventions.

Experts from major global regulatory agencies have called for more cross-stakeholder and cross-jurisdictional engagement and collaboration to increase efficiencies in regulatory approval and health technology assessment approvals.[14] In addition to formal international harmonization processes, mechanisms such as the Forum for Collaborative HIV Research provide opportunities for informal discussions between agencies in the presence of scientific experts from all stakeholder groups, a process that helps reduce misunderstanding and increase attention to regulatory requirements.[15]

In short, global access requires global registration. The process toward global registration requires significant additional resources and commitment from sponsors. The global public health community has not been as engaged as needed in working to reduce the bureaucracies and other barriers in local and regional registration; these barriers contribute to disparities and inequities in access.

---

[14] L. G. Baird et al., *Accelerated access to innovative medicines for patients in need*, 96(5) Clinical Pharmacology and Therapeutics, 559–571 (2014).

[15] Miller, *supra* note 9.

Emergency Pathways

Regulatory agencies such as the US FDA and the EMA maintain specific regulatory processes for responses to public health emergencies that may be expanded and adapted based on the experience with Ebola. A diversity of mechanisms accelerate access to drugs in areas of unmet clinical need.[16] For example, the accelerated access pathway described here shortens clinical development time by basing the approval on not fully validated surrogate markers that are reasonably likely to predict a clinical endpoint. Sponsors commit to evaluate the effects on their drug on clinical outcome for full approval. In the priority review pathway, review time is shortened to 6 months. The Food and Drug Administration Safety and Innovation Act of 2012 provided the "breakthrough therapy designation," which expedites development time through intensive discussions between the FDA and the sponsor and high-level organizational commitment, including senior staff involvement. Other pathways, such as staggered approval, special medical use, and limited population antibacterial drugs (for severe infections and an unmet medical need) are ways to expand specialized approval pathways and reduce the time and expense of drug and therapeutic development. The EMA announced the initiation of staggered approval, or "adaptive licensing," pilot projects in 2014. Under that regime, drugs to treat an unmet clinical need for a serious condition (e.g., multi-drug-resistant bacteria) are approved based on a limited set of data, with broader approval once sufficient data are gathered through monitoring utilization and clinical experience. Finally, the possibility of approval under exceptional circumstances exists in Europe for medicines for which there are urgent public health needs, based on noncomprehensive nonclinical and clinical data where there is little likelihood that such data will be collected. Under this scenario, benefit-risk profiles are reviewed on an annual basis. Of note, these changes and adaptations came about because of strong advocacy, in the first instance, by the HIV-affected community calling for more efficient review and approval processes for antiretrovirals to help stem what had become an alarming and frightening pandemic.

Implementation and Access

Once a drug, diagnostic, or vaccine is approved, health services, systems, and policies shape access to the approved biomedical intervention. The rapid support and collaboration behind Ebola vaccines may be, and should be, applied in nonemergency contexts with interventions that have passed vigorous regulatory review. One Ebola vaccine candidate, rVSV-ZEBOV, was deployed through a consortium of healthcare delivery entities, financing organizations, and sovereign governments, including the Guinean government, Merck, the Canadian government, the

---

[16] Baird et al., *supra* note 14.

Norwegian government, Médecins Sans Frontiéres, the London School of Hygiene and Tropical Medicine, the Wellcome Trust, and WHO. [17] The vaccine, which consists of a livestock virus that has been genetically engineered to express the Ebola surface glycoprotein,[18] was given to more than 3,500 people via a strategy known as "ring vaccination", encircling patients with Ebola or those exposed to Ebola by vaccinating their contacts[19] to study the safety and efficacy of the vaccine.[20] The results suggested (although they did not prove) that the vaccine provided substantial protection.[21]

Lessons learned from past responses and again with Ebola reinforced the need for coordination across many disciplines, not just the biomedical sciences, in order to break discipline-based silos. Insights from natural sciences, public health, and clinical medicine need to be integrated into aid, health systems support, and emergency preparedness planning. There are disease-specific models that show commitment matters, such as the eradication of smallpox and (nearly) polio. Even under ideal circumstances, success will be modified by structural and sociobehavioral barriers. Again using Ebola as an example, we saw that social structures, living environments, and human behavior have significant impact on the course of an epidemic.

HIV: Advocacy, Innovation, and Access

In many respects, the global experience with HIV/AIDS provides important, positive lessons for bridging the gap between biomedical innovation and patient access to life-saving medicines. Legislators and regulators developed accelerated approval pathways (with HIV/AIDS drugs principally in mind) based on surrogate endpoints rather than traditional clinical criteria, substantial resources for drug development and access were committed by public and private coffers at the national and international levels, and health systems strengthening took on a core role as part of the response to the HIV/AIDS epidemic.

Rigorous science and biomedical innovation have provided the tools to end the HIV pandemic.[22] But HIV began as an emergency, requiring emergency responses. Not everyone agreed on the nature or scope of the emergency: Surgeon General C. Everett Koop fought a battle within the Reagan White House for destigmatization,

---

[17] Gavi, Encouraging trial results offer significant hope for rapid availability of Ebola vaccine to end current outbreak (2015), available at http://www.gavi.org/contact/.

[18] Declan Butler, Ewen Callaway, and Erika Check Hayden, *How Ebola-vaccine success could reshape clinical-trial policy*, 524 Nature 13–14 (2015).

[19] Gavi, *supra* note 17.

[20] *Id.*

[21] *Id.*

[22] Anthony Fauci and Hilary Marston, *Ending the HIV-AIDS pandemic—follow the science*, 373(23) New England Journal of Medicine, 2197–2199 (2015).

open access to information, and tailored public health policies.[23] Funding for research flowed slowly. Even after life-saving, efficacious treatments became available, globally, the epidemic exploded with disproportionate effect in sub-Saharan Africa. As recently as 2001, leaders of US agencies argued that deploying expensive treatments there would waste resources and spawn drug-resistant viral strains.[24]

From the beginning, advocacy was tied to biomedical and public health research. Scientists and public health researchers established that less virus load in the body led to less transmission; that individuals on treatment with suppressed virus replication do not transmit HIV to their sexual partners;[25] and that antiretrovirals, if present in sufficient quantity at the point of entry (vaginal or rectal tissue, blood), may prevent HIV acquisition. These principles were first demonstrated through prevention of mother-to-child transmission as far back as 1994.[26] It took until 2011 to convince policymakers that the benefit of antiretrovirals (whose mechanism of action is to inhibit virus replication and spread from cell to cell) is similarly evident in adults.

Now, HIV-infected individuals may live for a nearly normal lifespan, although inflammation based on co-morbidities continues to take a toll. Although drug innovation was driven by the private sector, significant public funding was made available to develop clinical trial networks for treatment of adults and children, behavioral and biomedical preventative interventions, and vaccine studies. Publicly funded observational cohorts have made substantial contributions in the form of hypothesis testing, detection and confirmation of toxicity signals, and best practices for treatment implementation. For example, IeDEA is an international research consortium established in 2005 by the National Institute of Allergy and Infectious Diseases to provide a resource for globally diverse HIV/AIDS data. Sites in various regions throughout the world collaborate to collect and define key variables, harmonize data, and implement methodologies to pool data to address priority research questions. IeDEA collects HIV/AIDS data from seven international regional data centers, including four in Africa and one each in the Asia/Pacific region, the Central/South America/Caribbean region, and North America. This type of data and resource pooling allows researchers to address unique and evolving research questions that individual cohorts are unable to answer. The principal clinical guidelines panel setting the standard

---

[23] C. Everett Koop, *The early days of AIDS as I remember them*, 13(2) Ann Forum Collab HIV Res. 1–10 (2011).

[24] Celia W. Dugger, *Clinton makes up for lost time in battling AIDS*, New York Times (Aug. 29, 2006), available at http://www.nytimes.com/2006/08/29/health/29clinton.html?pagewanted=all&_r=0.

[25] Myron S. Cohen et al. *Prevention of HIV-1 infection with early antiretroviral therapy* 365(6) New England Journal of Medicine, 493–505 (2011); Nancy Padian et al., *HIV prevention transformed: the new prevention research agenda*, 378(9787) Lancet 269–278 2011).

[26] K. Luzuriaga and L. M. Mofenson, *Challenges in the elimination of pediatric HIV-1 infection*. 374(8) New England Journal of Medicine 761–770 (2016).

of care for the United States and adapted by other groups around the world is funded and managed by HHS, setting a novel precedent for "living document"–based guidelines—allowing rapid turnaround to incorporate new data as they become available.

The availability of antiretroviral drugs at affordable prices around the world illustrates the willpower and commitment behind the efforts. As the emergency response evolved, it quickly became apparent that the cost of drugs, even with tiered pricing, was prohibitive and that existing manufacturing capacity would not keep up with the demand. The leadership of HHS worked in concert with the FDA's Division of Antiviral Products to generate guidance and offer technical support for non-US generic manufacturers to prepare dossiers for submission to and review by the FDA for generic drug products to be distributed outside of the United States.[27] Since the implementation of this program, more than 150 generic drug products have been approved and have been or are in use around the world, including several fixed-dose combination products for infants and children.[28] This unique achievement has not been repeated for any other disease.

Nor is biomedical research limited to postinfection pharmaceutical regimens. There is robust funding for studies examining pre-exposure prophylaxis (PrEP), an oral pharmaceutical regimen that prevents infection for those at high risk; microbicides that can be applied inside the vagina or rectum to protect against sexually transmitted infections; and vaginal rings that deliver slow-release chemicals that inhibit viral replication. Some of the most important findings include the sexual behaviors and practices of vulnerable groups like young women.

The best evidence that these policies acting in concert may close the gap between innovation and access is found in the relative outcomes in high-income and low-income countries. For example, Botswana is close to reaching the 90-90-90 target for testing, treatment, and viral suppression, ahead of the United States and most European countries.[29] In Kenya, "almost nine out of ten HIV positive people who know their status and are eligible for ART are receiving treatment."[30]

These achievements would not have been possible without the *concerted* commitment from and engagement of donor countries (US PEPFAR and Global Fund) working with and through countries; strong and persistent advocacy at regional, national, and international levels; and the personal engagement of political leaders.

---

[27] Andrea Quinones-Rivera, *The untold story of how high quality and low-cost drugs were incorporated into PEPFAR*, 13 Ann Forum Collab HIV Res, 1–8 (2013).

[28] Quinones-Rivera, *supra* note 27; CB Holmes et al., *Id.*

[29] Christine Lubinski, CROI 2016: Botswana Within Reach of UNAIDS 90-90-90 (Feb. 29, 2016), available at http://sciencespeaksblog.org/2016/02/29/croi-2016-botswana-within-reach-of-unaids-90-90-90/.

[30] Katy Migiro, *Kenya Making "huge progress" in fight against HIV/AIDS* (Sept. 10, 2013), available at http://news.trust.org//item/20130910131526-iak2j.

What started off as an emergency response has become a strategic, targeted, and implementation science–based program.[31] In fact, the HIV pandemic has contributed to implementation science more than any other disease.[32]

HCV: Private Sector–Led Innovation, Cost Barriers to Access, and Little Coordination

Hepatitis C is a serious liver disease that results from infection with the hepatitis C virus (HCV). People with hepatitis C often have no symptoms, may live with an infection for decades without feeling ill, or may be successfully treated with medications. Over time, chronic hepatitis C can cause serious health problems, including liver damage, cirrhosis, liver cancer, and even death.

Globally, the number of those affected has reached around 130 to 150 million infections and 350,000 to 500,000 deaths each year.[33] The disease disproportionately impacts the most vulnerable—low-income communities, injecting drug users, prisoners, and veterans are the populations most at risk.[34] For example, in the United States, injecting drug users are 150 times more likely than the general population to be infected with HCV.[35] China, Vietnam, India, Pakistan, Georgia, and Egypt have the highest prevalence of hepatitis C. These six countries represent 41% of global population, 62% of global burden of hepatitis B virus, and 39% of global burden of hepatitis C.

The remarkable story of antiretroviral development (more than 30 drugs and drug combinations in six drug classes developed within 30 years) is rivaled only by the "arch of a medical triumph" of HCV direct-acting antiviral development. More than 95% of chronically infected HCV patients with pan-genotypic all-oral regimens are curable in as short a time as 6 to 8 weeks. As with antiretrovirals, regulatory flexibility played a role in the development of breakthrough treatments. Regulatory policies allowing the use of historical controls instead of the then current standard of care (48 weeks of injectable pegylated interferon and ribavirin) and shortening the sustained viral response time from 24

---

[31] Wafaa Al-Sadr et al., *Scale-up of HIV treatment through PEPFAR: a historic public health achievement*, 60 Suppl 3 Journal of Acquired Immune Deficiency Syndromes S96–S104 (2012); Eric Goosby et al., *Raising the bar: PEPFAR and new paradigms for global health*, 60 Suppl 3 Journal of Acquired Immune Deficiency Syndromes, S158–S162 (2012).

[32] Nancy Padian et al., *Implementation science for the US President's Emergency Plan for AIDS Relief (PEPFAR)*, 56(3) Journal of Acquired Immune Deficiency Syndromes, 199–203 (2011).

[33] WHO, Hepatitis C, available at http://www.who.int/mediacentre/factsheets/fs164/en/.

[34] CDC, Hepatitis C FAQs for the Public, available at http://www.cdc.gov/hepatitis/C/cFAQ.htm#overview.

[35] California Healthcare Institute in collaboration with Boston Consulting Group, Innovation in Hepatitis C Treatment: New Opportunities for Action (July 2014).

weeks to 12 weeks based on emerging data greatly increased the efficiency of drug development.[36]

Three new antivirals for hepatitis C have been developed in the past few years. These medicines, called direct antiviral agents (DAA), are more effective, safer, and better tolerated than the older therapies. Although the production cost of DAAs is low, the initial prices are very high and are likely to make access to these drugs difficult even in high-income countries.

The first of these agents is Sovaldi (or sofosbuvir). Sovaldi, which is a one-pill-per-day regimen, as part of a combination therapy, time limited at 12 weeks, has been shown to work for genotypes 1, 2, 3, and 4 in just 12 or 24 weeks, depending on the patient's genotype. The second therapy is a combination treatment—Harvoni, or a combination of ledipasvir and sofosbuvir. This medicine may be used only for genotype 1. No other combination treatment is needed for Harvoni. The duration of treatment varies depending on the patient's cirrhotic condition, treatment experience, and viral load. In clinical studies, 96% to 99% of patients who had no prior treatment were cured with just 12 weeks of therapy. The third new treatment is Viekira Pak, which is composed of two different tablets: ombitasvir, paritaprevir, and ritonavir tablets, and dasabuvir tablets.

Despite advocacy efforts, HHS has not established a treatment guidelines panel following the HIV model. Instead, professional societies collaborate in the development and generation of treatment guidelines, with less uniformity and, implicitly, less relevance. Treatment guidelines provided by professional societies raise concerns about Pharmaceutical companies' influence influence on the process.

In contrast to HIV, there are no NIH-funded networks for treatment and prevention for HCV, and publicly funded cohort collaborations are limited. Cohorts such as HCV TARGET were initiated and are maintained with industry funding. Funding and resources (e.g., staffing at the CDC and WHO) for HCV programs are minuscule when compared with those for HIV. HCV lacks a dedicated PEPFAR, Global Fund, and the commitment of political leadership.

Global HCV eradication is in fact more straightforward than HIV eradication: there is a known cure that poses no unique difficulty for established health systems. The contrast between domestic and global access to HCV versus HIV treatments is attributable to lack of commitment, engagement of donor nations and organizations, and lack of effective advocacy. The HCV-affected community is marginalized and stigmatized as the HIV community was in its early years.

These factors have influenced the commitment to affordable access both by pharmaceutical developers and by purchasing governments. The market price for a course of treatment for these drugs ranges between $83,000 and $153,000 per

---

[36] C. Hutchison et al., *Accelerating drug development through collaboration: the Hepatitis C Drug Development Advisory Group*, 96(2) Clinical Pharmacology and Therapeutics, 162–165 (2014).

patient. In the United States, the wholesale price of Harvoni is $1,125 per pill. Although most insurers negotiate lower bulk prices with pharmaceutical firms, treating hepatitis C patients with these new drugs is incredibly costly.

The high costs of the DAA drugs have posed real barriers to treatment. The US CDC recommends that all infected persons should receive treatment. However, many insurers have imposed limitations—some require that a patient already have mild to moderate liver scarring before receiving DAA treatment; others require that HCV patients with alcohol or substance abuse problems show sustained sobriety for a period of time before qualifying for treatment. In November 2015, the Centers for Medicare and Medicaid Services (CMS) issued a formal letter to states that instructed them to remove these and any other "unreasonable" limitations to DAA drug treatment for the HCV patients insured under Medicaid.[37]

Globally, cost poses an even greater challenge to access. The firms that developed HCV treatments earn nearly all their profits from sales in the United States and Europe, because those countries are able to pay the high prices demanded. Pharmaceutical firms do offer tiered pricing, but still at rates that make widespread access unlikely especially in the six countries that need the treatments most. For example in Egypt, 9 million people, or 10% of the population, are infected with hepatitis C. Gilead has offered to charge the Egyptian government just $14 per day per patient for Harvoni, and AbbVie is providing Viekira Pak for $13 a day. Despite these reduced prices, they are not standardized, and drug companies tend to negotiate drug prices on a country-by-country, drug-by-drug basis. Inclusion of the DAA drugs on WHO's Model List of Essential Medicines signals to governments, regulators, and drug companies that those medicines should be made available to poor countries at low prices.

Global access is evolving, but it is driven by the pharmaceutical sector rather than by public, bilateral and multilateral funding organizations. Building on the HIV experience, innovator and generics firms are collaborating on licensing and pricing arrangements. Gilead made news by licensing its medicines to India-based generic manufacturers. Overall, the approach is to work through tiered pricing and generic licensing in more than 130 countries according to the level of income: low-income, lower-middle-income, and high-income countries. In parallel, Gilead implemented and executed an aggressive drug registration program on a country-by-country basis. By 2015, Gilead had expanded licensing agreements to manufacturers in more countries and reached more than 165,000 HCV-infected patients with branded or licensed generic drugs. Their achievements in the HIV and HCV spaces are dependent on partnerships with other for-profit companies, public sector agencies, local and regional business partners, and not-for-profit

---

[37] Centers for Medicare and Medicaid Services, Assuring Medicaid Beneficiaries Access to HCV Drugs, available at https://www.medicaid.gov/Medicaid-CHIP-Program-Information/By-Topics/Benefits/Prescription-Drugs/Downloads/Rx-Releases/State-Releases/state-rel-172.pdf.

service providers. The unique arrangement with generic manufacturers offers control over the quality of the distributed medicines. Clearly, the visionary business strategy was in place from the time of marketing approval in the United States, and the program was directed and executed according to private sector expectations in terms of deliverables and outcomes, including antidiversion strategies. The result is slowly expanding access to proven treatments, no strategic long-range planning, and a lack of coordination across stakeholders; correspondingly, little work has been done on studying implementation models, including monitoring and evaluation across programs.

Conclusion

As the examples of HIV and HCV show, there are different models by which biomedical breakthroughs may be accelerated and made more widely available, from clinical trial design to the coalitions of donors and health planners that have made HIV access a relative success and HCV access relatively less so.

References

Baird LG, Banken R, Eichler HG, Kristensen FB, Lee DK, Lim JC, et al. *Accelerated access to innovative medicines for patients in need*. 96(5) Clinical Pharmacology and Therapeutics 559–571 (2014).

Balasegaram M et al., *A global biomedical R&D fund and mechanism for innovations of public health importance* 12(5) PLoS Medicine e1001831 (2015).

CDC. Outbreaks Chronology: Ebola Virus Disease. Available at http://www.cdc.gov/vhf/ebola/outbreaks/history/chronology.html.

Cohen MS, Chen YQ, McCauley M, Gamble T, Hosseinipour MC, Kumarasamy N, et al. *Prevention of HIV-1 infection with early antiretroviral therapy*. 365(6) New England Journal of Medicine 493–505 (2011).

DeGruttola V, Dix L, D'Aquila R, Holder D, Phillips A, Ait-Khaled M, et al. *The relation between baseline HIV drug resistance and response to antiretroviral therapy: re-analysis of retrospective and prospective studies using a standardized data analysis plan*. A5(1) Antiviral Therapy 41–48 (2000).

El-Sadr WM, Holmes CB, Mugyenyi P, Thirumurthy H, Ellerbrock T, Ferris R, et al. *Scale-up of HIV treatment through PEPFAR: a historic public health achievement*. 60 Suppl 3 Journal of Acquired Immune Deficiency Syndromes S96–S104 (2012).

Everett Koop C *The early days of AIDS as I remember them*, 13(2) Ann Forum Collab HIV Res. 1–10 (2011).

Fauci AS, Marston HD. *Ending the HIV-AIDS pandemic—follow the science*. 373(23) New England Journal of Medicine 2197–2199 (2015).

Gaffney, A. *US government immunizes future manufacturers of Ebola vaccines from legal liability*. 1 Regulatory Affairs Professionals Society (2014). Available at http://www.raps.org/Regulatory-Focus/News/2014/12/09/20947/US-Government-Immunizes-Future-Manufacturers-of-Ebola-Vaccines-from-Legal-Liability/.

Goosby E, Von Zinkernagel D, Holmes C, Haroz D, Walsh T. *Raising the bar: PEPFAR and new paradigms for global health*. 60 Suppl 3 Journal of Acquired Immune Deficiency Syndromes S158–S162 (2012).

Hoenen T, Feldmann H. *Ebola virus in West Africa, and the use of experimental therapies or vaccines.* 12 BMC Biol. 80 (2014).

Holmes CB, Coggin W, Jamieson D, Mihm H., Granich R, Savio P, et al. *Use of generic antiretroviral agents and cost savings in PEPFAR treatment programs,* 304(3) JAMA 313–320 (2010).

How many Ebola patients have been treated outside of Africa? New York Times (Jan 26, 2015). Available at http://www.nytimes.com/interactive/2014/07/31/world/africa/ebola-virus-outbreak-qa.html?

Hutchison C, Kwong A, Ray S, Struble K, Swan T, Miller V. *Accelerating drug development through collaboration: the Hepatitis C Drug Development Advisory Group.* 96(2) Clinical Pharmacology and Therapeutics 162–165 (2014).

Lefebvre A, et al. *Case fatality rates of Ebola virus diseases: a meta-analysis of World Health Organization data.* 44(9) Med Mal Infect. 412–416 (2014).

Luzuriaga K, Mofenson LM. *Challenges in the elimination of pediatric HIV-1 infection.* 374(8) New England Journal of Medicine 761–770 (2016).

Miller V. *The forum for collaborative HIV research: a model for an integrated and inclusive approach to clinical research and drug development.* 86(3) Clinical Pharmacology and Therapeutics 332–335 (2009).

Miller V, Grant RM. *Regulatory considerations for antiretroviral prophylaxis to prevent HIV acquisition.* 96(2) Clinical Pharmacology and Therapeutics 153–155 (2014).

Millman J. *Why the drug industry hasn't come up with an Ebola cure.* Washington Post (Aug. 13, 2014). Available at https://www.washingtonpost.com/news/wonk/wp/2014/08/13/why-the-drug-industry-hasnt-come-up-with-an-ebola-cure/.

Moon S, et al. *Will Ebola change the game? Ten essential reforms before the next pandemic. The report of the Harvard-LSHTM Independent Panel on the Global Response to Ebola.* 386 (10009) Lancet 2204–2221 (Nov. 28, 2015).

Murray JS, Elashoff MR, Iacono-Connors LC, Cvetkovich TA, Struble KA. *The use of plasma HIV RNA as a study endpoint in efficacy trials of antiretroviral drugs.* 13(7) AIDS 797–804 (1999).

Padian NS, Holmes CB, McCoy SI, Lyerla R, Bouey PD, Goosby EP. *Implementation science for the US President's Emergency Plan for AIDS Relief (PEPFAR).* 56(3) Journal of Acquired Immune Deficiency Syndromes 199–203 (2011).

Padian NS, McCoy SI, Karim SS, Hasen N, Kim J, Bartos M, et al. *HIV prevention transformed: the new prevention research agenda.* 378(9787) Lancet 269–278 (2011).

Plotkin SA, Mahmoud A and Farrar J. *Establishing a global vaccine development fund,* 373 N Engl J Med 297–300 (July 23, 2015).

Smith FL. *We have military research to thank for Ebola vaccines.* Mediacom. Available at https://medium.com/war-is-boring/we-have-military-research-to-thank-for-ebola-vaccines-565897c3f1bc#.yexv8p9vf.

WHO Ebola Response Team. *Ebola virus disease in West Africa—the first 9 months of the epidemic and forward projections.* 371 New England Journal of Medicine 1481–1495 (2014).

12

Ethical Challenges in the Development and Deployment of Medical Therapies and Vaccines in the Context of Public Health Emergencies

ANNICK ANTIERENS

Introduction

In late summer 2014, the Ebola epidemic in West Africa exploded,[1] involving primarily three countries but with cases managed in at least seven others[2] on three different continents. When incidence rates seemed to increase exponentially and statistical models were forecasting thousands of cases per week in the following months,[3] many questions were raised about why no medical countermeasures were available and how to fast-track research and development of promising experimental interventions. At that time, Ebola virus disease (EVD) was daily news, but until then it had been a neglected disease. Although reported to have a case fatality rate (CFR) above 65%,[4] with no available therapeutics or vaccines,[5] EVD was

---

[1] Centers for Disease Control and Prevention, Ebola Virus Disease Outbreak—West Africa, September 2014, 63(39) MMWR (Oct. 3, 2014), available at http://www.cdc.gov/mmwr/preview/mmwrhtml/mm6339a4.htm. G. Chowell and H. Nishiura, Transmission dynamics and control of Ebola virus disease (EVD): a review, 12 BMC Medicine 196 (2014).

[2] *How many Ebola patients have been treated outside of Africa?*, New York Times (Jan 26, 2015), available at http://www.nytimes.com/interactive/2014/07/31/world/africa/ebola-virus-outbreak-qa.html?.

[3] WHO Ebola Response Team, *Ebola virus disease in West Africa—the first 9 months of the epidemic and forward projections*, 371 N Engl J Med 1481–1495 (2014); G. Chowell and H. Nishiura, *Transmission dynamics and control of Ebola virus disease (EVD): a review*, 12 BMC Medicine 196 (2014).

[4] A. Lefebvre et al., *Case fatality rates of Ebola virus diseases: a meta-analysis of World Health Organization data*, 44(9) Med Mal Infect. 412–416 (2014).

[5] Thomas Hoenen and Heinz Feldmann, *Ebola virus in West Africa, and the use of experimental therapies or vaccines*, 12 BMC Biol. 80 (2014).

neglected because of the low number of cases and their origin. Since its discovery in 1976, 26 outbreaks had been reported with a total of 2,427 cases, most of them in Central African countries.[6] This disease profile does not generate much if any interest from the private sector to develop new products because the market is negligible. Market failures are seen for a whole category of neglected diseases in low-income countries.[7] In the case of EVD, at least some research and development had been initiated, mainly by the public sector, including military research,[8] most likely for preparedness against possible bioterrorism. But none of the products had been evaluated beyond preclinical research,[9] possibly because EVD presents only in outbreaks, most of them identified late, in remote settings and of short duration,[10] which does not make it conducive for the preparation and implementation of clinical trials.

With the recognition of the Ebola outbreak as a public health emergency of international concern by the World Health Organization (WHO) and the subsequently convened WHO ethics panel's conclusion that "it would be acceptable on ethical and evidential grounds to use as potential treatments or for prevention unregistered interventions, that have shown promising results in laboratory and animal models but have not yet been evaluated for safety and efficacy in humans," researchers, medical service providers, and pharmaceutical companies were called to engage in clinical field research on experimental Ebola products.[11] But implementation of clinical trials in the midst of an uncontrolled devastating outbreak in vulnerable resource-poor and trial-illiterate communities brought about specific ethical challenges.

Relevance of Unregistered Interventions

Tackling an Ebola-like epidemic requires a range of public health measures such as surveillance, contact tracing, health promotion, patient transport, and infection control and prevention covering, among others, home spraying and ensuring safe

---

[6] Centers for Disease Control and Prevention, Outbreaks Chronology: Ebola Virus Disease, available at http://www.cdc.gov/vhf/ebola/outbreaks/history/chronology.html.

[7] J. Millman, *Why the drug industry hasn't come up with an Ebola cure*, Washington Post (Aug. 13, 2014), available at https://www.washingtonpost.com/news/wonk/wp/2014/08/13/why-the-drug-industry-hasnt-come-up-with-an-ebola-cure/.

[8] Frank L. Smith, *We have military research to thank for Ebola vaccines*, Mediacom (Aug. 28, 2014), available at https://medium.com/war-is-boring/we-have-military-research-to-thank-for-ebola-vaccines-565897c3f1bc#.so7cq0hcx.

[9] Hoenen and Feldmann, *supra* note 5.

[10] CDC, *supra* note 6.

[11] World Health Organization, Ethical Considerations for Use of Unregistered Interventions for Ebola Virus Disease (Aug. 11, 2014), available at http://apps.who.int/iris/bitstream/10665/130997/1/WHO_HIS_KER_GHE_14.1_eng.pdf.

burials. When the epidemic curve is steeply rising, teams on the ground are rapidly overwhelmed and overstretched. It is therefore a legitimate opening question to ask whether medical professionals and scientists in emergency contexts should even undertake clinical trials, considering the additional burden doing so adds to processes and resources that could compromise patient care and community interventions. Moreover, in any given context, research and development yields only a limited number of products that will survive regulatory review.[12] Even if they are determined to be effective and subsequently licensed, therapeutics may not be the most efficient means to manage an epidemic. An alternative may be to focus on clinical research to improve supportive therapies instead of evaluating unregistered products. In the context of distrust, poor communication, and strained relations between communities and governments or international aid organizations that characterized the response to Ebola in its early days,[13] trials with experimental products, potentially perceived as experimentation, might fuel resistance to the work of health care and front-line workers.

On the other hand, drugs and vaccines for Ebola or other emerging infections with no endemic persistence can only be tested for efficacy in human studies during epidemics. Demonstrating their efficacy and safety in animal models has limitations because animals do not react to the infection in the same way as humans, considerable difference exists between animal models,[14] and the standardized procedures in preclinical studies do not correspond to the reality of human contamination, disease evolution, and access to treatment.[15] When CFR remains high, both caregivers and communities at risk are heavily affected. Caregivers have an increasing sense of powerlessness, despondency, and distress and are aware of the nonnegligible risks for their own life, which makes them willing and eager to be able to provide potentially effective therapies.[16] Communities legitimately mistrust health structures in which more than one out of two patients do not come out alive and, as a result, will rather seek help from traditional healers or hide in their homes.[17] The possibility of a higher chance of survival with life-saving therapeutics may encourage people

---

[12] PhRMA, 2015 Profile: Biopharmaceutical Research Industry, available at http://www.phrma.org/sites/default/files/pdf/2015_phrma_profile.pdf.

[13] Samuel Cohn and Ruth Kutalek, *Historical parallels, Ebola virus disease and cholera: understanding community distrust and social violence with epidemics*, PLoS Currents (Jan. 26, 2016), available at http://currents.plos.org/outbreaks/article/historical-parallels-ebola-virus-disease-and-cholera-understanding-community-distrust-and-social-violence-with-epidemics/.

[14] Victoria Wahl-Jensen et al., *Use of the Syrian hamster as a new model of Ebola virus disease and other viral hemorrhagic fevers*, 4 Viruses 3754–3784 (2012).

[15] *Ebola: a call to action*, 20(9) Nat Med. 967 (2014).

[16] Bonnie L. Hewlett, *Providing care and facing death: nursing during Ebola outbreaks in Central Africa*, 16 J Transcult Nurs. 289–297 (Oct. 2005).

[17] Cohn and Kutalek, *supra* note 13; P. Omidian et al., Medical Anthropology Study of the Ebola Virus Disease (EVD) Outbreak in Liberia/West Africa (2014), available at http://www.medbox.org/ebola/medical-anthropology-study-of-the-ebola-virus-disease-evd-outbreak-in-liberiawest-africa/

with suspected symptoms to present early and by doing so increase their survival chances and diminish transmission. Similar effects apply for vaccines, when community outreach activities would be accompanied by offering additional active protection for the people at risk. All these potential positive effects may counterbalance the increased workload and resources, of which part, if not all, could be absorbed by researchers provided they work collaboratively with the caregivers, patient care is not compromised, and coherence is maintained in operational strategies and links to the communities.

With respect to the decision to plan and commence clinical trials during public health emergencies, balancing these advantages and disadvantages requires an initial assessment of the resource and communication context in which the outbreak is underway, the epidemic profile of the disease, and preventive or therapeutic options. Factors that aid organizations and service providers must consider in this assessment include risks linked to patient safety, community misconceptions, possible security incidents and institutional risks (and therefore chose to decline trial participation), or ensuring there is no missed opportunity to evaluate experimental interventions that could benefit current and future patients (and therefore accepting trial involvement). This ethical dilemma is even more pronounced when there are only a few therapeutic centers that may be used as trials sites.

Choice of an Intervention

Whether for use in the frame of a clinical trial or in emergency access, any unregistered or experimental agent must have a plausible safety profile and promise a probable benefit to patients and/or targeted populations.[18] During the recent Ebola epidemic, more than 200 interventions were proposed to prevent or cure EVD, ranging from novel antiviral drugs and antibody products, to repurposed drugs with potential antiviral activity, host immunity stimulators, and anti-inflammatory activity modulators, to natural allopathic agents, multivitamins, ozone therapy, and silver nanoparticles.[19]

---

toolboxes/preview; *Ebola in West Africa: gaining community trust and confidence*, 383(9933) Lancet 1946 (June 7, 2014).

[18] H. Clifford Lane, Hilary Marston, and Anthony Fauci, *Conducting clinical trials in outbreak settings: Points to consider*, 13(1) Clin Trials 92–95 (Feb. 2016), available at http://www.ncbi.nlm.nih.gov/pubmed/26768564.

[19] Tia Ghose, *Nano silver? Nigeria's potential Ebola treatment unlikely to work*, Live Science (Aug. 15, 2014), available at http://www.livescience.com/47389-nigerian-experimental-ebola-drug.html; *Ebola—saving lives with natural allopathic medicine*, Dr Sircus.com (Aug. 4, 2014), available at http://drsircus.com/medicine/ebola-saving-lives-natural-allopathic-medicine/; Azizul Haque, Didier Hober, and Joel Blondiaux, *Addressing therapeutic options for Ebola virus infection in current and future outbreaks*, 59(10) Antimicrob Agents Chemother, 5892–5902 (Oct. 2015); Robert Rowen, *Ozone*

Although, in view of the very high mortality, it is tempting to give patients agents that have shown efficacy for other pathologies (e.g., in improving immunity or in reducing symptoms of sepsis), the justification for their use is debatable. As long as no data are available on their efficacy in the disease to be targeted, it will be challenging to choose an agent or the combination of several agents—as it will be difficult to determine individual effect—and questionable to impose on patients the burden of additional pharmaceuticals and on clinical staff of additional drug administration and monitoring. Furthermore, safety profiles of repurposed or off-label drugs should not be overestimated because data coming from use for different pathologies and symptomatologies (and in some case in different doses or regimen) may not effectively predict results in critically ill patients.

Candidate therapeutics or vaccines must first show good efficacy results in appropriate preclinical studies and safety data at least from phase I human studies.[20] But in the case of a disease with only epidemic occurrence where the potential research sites are few and epidemic dynamics unpredictable, additional criteria must be developed to identify priority agents. Selection criteria based on practical considerations in addition to therapeutic promise must be included: means of administration (oral or intramuscular route would be preferred to intravenous infusion), duration of treatment (shorter over longer), and the storage conditions (outside over cold chain). The potential quantities of a promising agent (even after scale-up) generated fierce debates about prioritizing agents that would be scarce even if found effective.[21] One therapeutic candidate, ZMapp, represented just this dilemma: even if proved effective, it was unclear how much of the drug might be produced even over a long time horizon.[22] Positive study outcomes are expected to enhance production scale-up, although only provided scarcity is not a result of slow production capacity, regulatory review, or market calculations. Critics of ZMapp's early administration of scarce doses to two Americans argued that in the prioritizing process of candidate agents, it would be more justified to test a largely available product, even if potentially less effective, to guarantee, in case of positive results, posttrial access to a maximum of patients in need. Additionally healthcare workers and international aid organizations might also consider the lack of posttrial access unethical and unfeasible because the research

---

therapy: a possible answer to Ebola?, available at http://articles.mercola.com/sites/articles/archive/2014/10/26/ozone-therapy-ebola.aspx.

[20] Lane, Marston, and Fauci, *supra* note 18.

[21] Steven Joffe, *Evaluating novel therapies during the Ebola epidemic*, 312(13) JAMA 1299–1300 (2014).

[22] Andrew Pollack, *Ebola drug could save a few lives, but whose?*, New York Times (Aug. 8, 2014), available at http://www.nytimes.com/2014/08/09/health/in-ebola-outbreak-who-should-get-experimental-drug.html.

could then be assimilated by patients and communities to scientific imperialism and exploitation.[23] This may negatively affect the possibility of new research on other potentially effective agents.

Scarcity of a promising intervention raises other questions such as to whom the product would be allocated and under what circumstances. Most people would agree that allocation should be fair and objective, and in the absence of evidence on modalities of efficacy, this could correspond to a first-come, first-served basis[24] or to the principle of a lottery.[25] Another point of view would be to prioritize healthcare workers because they take enormous risks for the benefit of others and will be needed to care for future patients, trace contacts, and participate in burial teams.[26] This might apply only to national staff because international personnel usually have access to a high-quality standard of care, giving them much higher survival chances.[27] Prioritizing the neediest or the most vulnerable may also be an option, provided it is feasible to identify them and there is a genuine expectation that the experimental treatment will benefit them.[28]

Arguably, use of scarce experimental interventions should be accompanied by rigorous data collection on safety and efficacy to ensure generation of robust results for ongoing or future epidemics.[29] While the randomized control trial (RCT) remains the preferred gold standard to demonstrate safety and efficacy, context and available treatment courses may not allow that the threshold of statistically needed sample size to be reached. Single-arm designs or emergency use with strong data collection, on the other hand, might not compromise the acquisition of knowledge while being much more acceptable for communities and caregivers.[30] Prioritization of unregistered novel agents to be evaluated in clinical trials should be based on objective criteria such as existing promising efficacy and safety data in previously conducted preclinical, animal and/or human studies, combined with availability of the product and guarantees for posttrial access if appropriate.

---

[23] P. Wilmshurst, *Scientific imperialism: if they won't benefit from the findings, poor people in the developing world shouldn't be used in research*, 314 BMJ 840–841 (1997).

[24] Morenike Folayan et al., *Compassionate use of experimental drugs in the Ebola outbreak*, 384(9957) Lancet 1843–1844 (2015).

[25] Mayeni Jones, *Ebola outbreak: informed consent must be central to experimental drug testing*, International Bar Association (Sept. 3, 2014), available at http://www.ibanet.org/Article/Detail.aspx?ArticleUid=920c89de-c0de-4bbf-8c76-4d65d95be993.

[26] Annette Rid and Ezekiel Emanuel, *Ethical considerations of experimental interventions in the Ebola outbreak*, 384(9957) Lancet 1896–1899 (2014).

[27] Lawrence Gostin, *Ethical allocation of drugs and vaccines in the West African Ebola epidemic*, 92(4) Millbank Quarterly 662–666 (2014).

[28] *Id.*

[29] Joffe, *supra* note 21; Rid and Emmanuel, *supra* note 26.

[30] Folayan et al., *supra* note 24.

Trial Designs

The choice of the trial design when evaluating new interventions in epidemic emergencies requires careful consideration. As noted earlier, the RCT is generally considered the most solid design to prove efficacy and safety of new therapeutics and vaccines.[31] The presence of a randomly allocated control group supports the certainty that the measured effects are due to the evaluated intervention as opposed to being caused by changes in context or pathogen, participants' profile, standard of care, caregivers' experience, or other factors.[32] Most researchers agree that the evaluation of a novel therapeutic agent against a deadly disease such as EVD would not involve a placebo (use of an inactive substance physically indistinguishable from the studied product) in the control group because the risks linked to the placebo administration for patients and health staff would not be acceptable. Observation bias can thus not be excluded. Therefore, in the absence of an existing approved alternative, a therapeutic RCT would imply randomly assigning confirmed patients to receiving standard of care and the novel agent or to receiving standard of care alone.

In the Ebola context, the choice of the design must necessarily be confronted to a series of questions. How feasible and ethical is conventional trial design in the context of a ravaging epidemic with a virus causing more than 50% mortality within 2 weeks of disease onset? How to ask clinical staff to consciously, although without being fully responsible, deny half of their patients a potentially life-saving treatment option? How to accept randomization when in some patient groups CFR was demonstrated to reach 80% or more? In an RCT, enrolled participants share benefits and risks, and randomization toward the control group might diminish the chances of benefit but also the risks. But what would be the ethical rationale in the Ebola context considering that catastrophically ill patients who run a fairly high risk of death would prefer to avoid the risks linked to an experimental treatment at the expense of taking their chances with it?[33] How do clinical trial designers ensure that patients have a meaningful choice when asked to choose between agreeing to participate in an RCT or refusing to participate and thereby forgoing an opportunity to access a potentially life-saving treatment? What is the autonomy of patients in this regard? There is little chance that in such context and circumstances patients would accept participation in an RCT out of altruism for the higher public good or the benefit of future patients; instead, they would be inclined to agree to be enrolled out of

---

[31] Gail Sullivan, *Getting off the "gold standard": randomized controlled trials and education research*, 3(3) Journal of Graduate Medical Education, 285–289 (2011).

[32] JM Kendall, *Designing a research project: randomised controlled trials and their principles*, 20 Emerg Med J 164–168 (2003).

[33] Udo Schuklenk and Christopher Lowry, *Terminal illness and access to phase 1 experimental agents, surgeries and devices: reviewing the ethical arguments*, 89(1) Br Med Bull 7–22 (2009).

despair.[34] How to ensure acceptability when patients present in family clusters and randomization is done within the families?

Feasibility is also linked to the perception and acceptance of communities. Full engagement with communities is known to be crucial but may not always prevent misconceptions and disagreements that may interrupt public health measures like surveillance and contact tracing and may cause security problems.

Is a concurrent control group really crucial? How relevant is a concurrent control group when the adequate sample size may not be obtained? How comparable is a concurrent control when randomization may not guarantee similar groups because of slow recruitment or different settings or unknown prognostic factors? In these circumstances, the concurrent control group may have an allocation bias and be less representative than a large historical control group. An important element to consider is the expected outcome of the evaluation of the novel therapeutic. In the case of an uncontrolled epidemic with high CFR, it is reasonable to target the rapid identification of therapeutic agents with high efficacy or to rapidly reject the ones that are futile or toxic. Determining whether a new agent reduces mortality by 1% or 2% is less relevant when CFR is above 50%. Alternative single-arm designs exist whereby results are analyzed each time a new 14-day outcome is received and clear stopping rules are established for determining when treatments are effective or ineffective. Changes in mortality rate would be seen faster, study results would be reached earlier, and more unnecessary deaths avoided compared with a classic RCT design.[35]

In vaccination trials, the stakes are different. If efficacy must be measured through incidence rates, then as epidemic dynamics and geographical spread become more difficult to predict, a concurrent control group would be necessary. Because potential participants are not ill, the informed consent procedure should be easier, more genuine, and less prone to be perceived as a coercive offer. The benefit of possible protection is less attractive than for treatment, while the risks linked to an experimental intervention are less acceptable. As with other therapeutics, different trial design alternatives are available. Selection of the most appropriate design should depend on the context, the CFRs, and the existing proven medical countermeasures. Public health measures should not be jeopardized, and patients and communities should be given as much autonomy as possible to choose to receive or not receive an experimental intervention.

Inclusions

In clinical research, some patient groups are traditionally excluded, such as pregnant and lactating women, children, and the elderly. Researchers and sponsors

---

[34] Sarah Edwards, RJ Lilford, and J Hewison, *The ethics of randomised controlled trials from the perspectives of patients, the public, and healthcare professionals*, 317(7167) BMJ 1209–1212 (1998).

[35] Ben Cooper et al., *Evaluating clinical trial designs for investigational treatments of Ebola virus disease*, 12(4) PLoS Med, available at http://journals.plos.org/plosmedicine/article?id=10.1371/journal.pmed.1001815.

justify these exclusions as precautions to diminish the risk-taking in fragile individuals who are more prone to suffer from toxic effects. Neglecting these patient groups in clinical trials may result either in product access denial because they are not included for indication of use or in harm due to potentially ill-adapted dose, regimen, or pharmacovigilance.[36]

In epidemic emergencies, where adequate medical countermeasures are nonexistent, where a lot of transmission occurs within families, and CFR is high especially in these same patient groups, the risk-benefit balance must be analyzed under less conventional criteria. Pregnant women are traditionally excluded because of potential teratogenic effect. In epidemics where CFR in pregnancy is very high as in EVD, the justification to deny pregnant women the chances to access potential therapeutics in order to avoid possible adverse events in the unborn child is questionable.[37] There is little chance a fetus will survive if the mother dies. When fetal survival rates are close to zero, endeavoring to save a condemned fetus at the expense of the mother's life contravenes fundamental canons of medical ethics. In EVD, for example, no positive outcome in pregnancy has ever been described; rather, all reported pregnancies in Ebola-infected women ended in spontaneous miscarriage, stillbirth, or neonatal death.[38]

Small children are generally excluded from clinical trials because of lack of safety data in phase I trials and their different metabolic and immunologic maturity, making it challenging to define the optimal dosage.[39] But in epidemic emergencies this should be contextualized against the CFR, which can be particularly high in young children; the nonexistence of therapeutic alternatives; the chances the tolerance profile would substantially differ from the adult one (and therefore reduce the need for specific phase I trial for children); and the possibility of using a pharmacokinetic model to define dosage regimen for children as was done for favipiravir in the EVD outbreak.[40] In these cases children should also be given access to potentially lifesaving treatment options.

When sponsors, trial insurance companies, or manufacturers fail to agree on inclusion of the previously mentioned groups, there is still the option to propose the therapeutic intervention in emergency access, provided a clear protocol has

---

[36] Government of Canada, Panel on Research, Fairness and Equity in Research Participation, available at http://www.pre.ethics.gc.ca/eng/policy-politique/initiatives/tcps2-eptc2/chapter4-chapitre4/.

[37] Kibadi Mupapa et al., *Ebola hemorrhagic fever and pregnancy*, 179(Suppl 1) J Infect Dis S11–S12 (1999).

[38] World Health Organization, Trends in Maternal Mortality: 1990 to 2013. Estimates by WHO, UNICEF, UNFPA, the World Bank, and the United Nations Population Division, available at http://apps.who.int/iris/bitstream/10665/112682/2/9789241507226_eng.pdf; Benjamin O. Black, Severine Caluwaerts, and Jay Achar, *Ebola virus disease and pregnancy*, 8(3) Obstet Med. 108–113 (2015).

[39] Government of Canada, *supra* note 36.

[40] Naïm Bouazza et al., *Favipiravir in children with Ebola*, 385 (9968) Lancet 603–604 (Feb. 2015).

been validated by the appropriate ethics committees. Patients with high mortality risk who are excluded from clinical trials, and in the absence of an acceptable alternative, should be given the autonomy of choice to access experimental treatments after full disclosure of potential benefits and risks. In reality, emergency access is not regulated in many countries. Additionally, trial sponsors should not use the existence of this option as a reason to shirk their responsibility by systematically excluding the most fragile patients and offloading the liability to clinicians and patients.

In research and development of vaccines, plans should be made to rapidly conduct phase I trials with groups of people comparable to the ones more at risk of being contaminated by the disease or more likely to die if they are infected.

Risks for severe adverse events seem less acceptable in preventive interventions like for eample vaccination, because the product is given to healthy individuals. But when trial partpation includes individuals that have had high-risk exposure to the deadly disease, the potential harm caused by the experimental preventive intervention should be balanced against the risk these participants are running of contracting the infection and subsequentialy of dying.

Informed Consent

Any proposition to provide an unregistered or experimental intervention to a patient should be preceded by voluntary informed consent. But how feasible and valid is the consent procedure for patients with a fast-acting life-threatening infection in the context of an epidemic emergency? How will care providers or investigators explain to critically ill patients how a novel agent works and what side effects can be expected? In that context, how to ensure potential trial participants grasp the concept of randomization and its consequences? In addition to all these barriers, face-concealing protective equipment worn by the consent takers, cross-cultural communication problems, and educational limitations hinder the possibility of patients' understanding and their ability to give meaningful consent.

Even in ideal circumstances of communication and discussion, it is difficult to ascertain whether patients, known to distrust the formal health system and modern medical practices, would feel confident that they would receive the best available treatment if they refused to participate in the proposed trial. For very ill patients or unaccompanied minors, proxy consent should be sought, but identifying the traditionally accepted family representation to give consent can be complex and time-consuming, if not impossible due to the difficulties involved in reaching them, given that they may have died or be ill themselves or may live in faraway areas. This reduces the chances for patients to access potentially effective treatment options in a timely manner. Community consent is another option, but it also may be difficult due to time constraints and the possibility that any given individual may not accept community consent on his or her behalf.

Meaningful informed consent is easier to obtain for vaccine trials because time is less an issue, and participants are healthy. Nevertheless, in some epidemic contexts, ethical challenges still arise. When facility-based isolation or quarantine of contacts of infected patients is imposed by health authorities, particularly if enforced by military personnel, then consent appears tainted by coercion. While voluntary informed consent is an ethical requirement for any trial involving experimental interventions, many factors influence the meaningfulness of any given consent. There is a need to reflect on how ethical judgments change in extreme circumstances and what models for adaptation that assure patient autonomy might be consulted.

Community Engagement

In many ethical research frameworks, active community engagement is considered essential to foster collaborative partnership with affected communities. Ideally, this collaboration includes building relationships between different stakeholders, discussing research objectives and therapeutic misconceptions with participating communities to counter misinterpretation, involving communities in decision-making around study design, studying implementation and benefit sharing, and spreading research literacy.[41]

But in epidemic emergencies, when it seems essential to minimize delays to commence clinical trials on preventive and therapeutic interventions, the time and resources required to ensure meaningful community engagement are scarce. If it has not been achieved earlier in the outbreak, time is needed to establish trust with communities, understand cultural practices and beliefs, refute misconceptions and rumors around a poorly understood disease, induce adapted behavioral changes, and build confidence in conventional health sector and international aid organizations, all preferably before engaging in discussions around the relevance, objectives, design, and expected outcome of clinical trials.[42] Depending on the context, defining the communities and ensuring valid community representation can be difficult when there is no sense of community belonging or when community leadership is a complex structure consisting of different key members. Partnership with national or local authorities is a key requirement for trial implementation but might not guarantee facilitating community engagement when they are mistrusted or even opposed by the targeted communities. A real tension exists between the urgency of proposing potential life-saving or life-protecting solutions and the ethical principle of ensuring communities' autonomy to participate in decisions around

---

[41] Morenike Folayan et al., *Stakeholders' engagement with Ebola therapy research in resource limited settings*, 15 BMC Inf. Dis. 242 (2015).

[42] Morenike Folayan et al., *Ethics, emergencies and Ebola clinical trials: the role of governments and communities in offshored research*, 22(Suppl 1) Pan African Medical Journal 10 (2015).

clinical research. Vaccine trials cannot be unlinked to valuable community engagement: Time constraints are less pressing Healthy individuals are enrolled, who are not always at risk of contracting the disease and have to present spontaneously for participation. Phase I and II trials can also be conducted in non-affected communities or countries, making it essential to ensure the buy-in of all stakeholders and in particular of the participating communities, Phase III trials usually require large recruitment numbers in affected and scared communities that need to fully understand and trust the principle of vaccination trials. Finally most vaccine trials will define communities or geographical location for recruitment which enables targeted community engagement.

For therapeutic trials, inclusion only concerns infected patients presenting at treatment centers. Targetting their communities of origin for valuable enagement before trial implementation is challenging when the epidemic's geographical spread is wide and unpredictable and ensuring that all the communities that could potentially be affected are being involved might not be feasible in time or require substantial amounts of resources, which could have been allocated to more "pressing" and impactful activities.

While pretrial meaningful community engagement might not be achievable, this should not be the case for any form of benefit sharing. Trial results, whether positive or negative, their interpretation, and the future plans for research and development of the investigational agent should be disclosed and discussed with the trial participants and the affected communities. Participating communities should receive fair access to the investigational agent, if proven safe and effective, or any other product resulting from the research. Additionally capacity building through partnership with national researchers and policymakers and straightening of national ethics committees and regulatory authorities should be ensured

Data Sharing and Use of Human Samples

For any deadly disease about which important knowledge gaps exist and no proven medical countermeasures are available, analysis of data and further research on human samples are crucial to understanding the pathogen, the disease it causes, and how to treat it. This principle applies to the development of therapeutics or vaccines. During epidemic emergencies, data and samples are collected, analyzed, and stored by many service providers, the vast majority for patient management or follow-up of transmission chains and contacts; therefore, with the exception of research, no consent is requested from the patient for the further use of his or her data and samples in studies or research. This raises important ethical questions. How acceptable would it be to use the routinely collected data and samples for research? Risks for patients and communities should be minimized. Data and samples should be anonymized, knowing this will not always be possible: some patients might still be identifiable after removal of their names and addresses. Consent could be sought retrospectively, although doing so may be unfeasible or undesirable because patients might have died or moved or may not be willing to be contacted. Community consent might be discussed but only provided community representation is acceptable for most of the patients. Survivors' organizations should be involved even if their governance is not necessarily validated by all survivors. Approval of national and international ethics review boards should be obtained. Involvement of national researchers and benefit sharing should be guaranteed.

International response teams should be prepared for the next outbreak and integrate the further use of routinely collected data and samples as part of the steps toward acquisition of knowledge and research and development. This means ethical questions should be answered and processes prepared to ensure adequate involvement of communities, national authorities, and ethics committees and consent of subjects from which data or samples will be collected.

Conclusion

All clinical research should comply to the greatest extent possible with the framework for ethical principles and benchmarks, particularly in developing countries. In public health emergencies and particularly when mortality rates are high and medical countermeasures limited, particular weight should be placed on equitable and fair access to experimental interventions, how to facilitate feasibility of community engagement and ensure patients' or participants' autonomy. While many analysts now focus on the integrity of the global system for detecting, preventing, and responding to infectious disease outbreaks as a result of failures accompanying the Ebola crisis, as many or more lessons may be learned about ethical obligations to patients, communities, providers, and researchers during public health emergencies.

References

Black BO, Caluwaerts S, Achar J. *Ebola virus disease and pregnancy*. 8(3) Obstet Med. 108–113 (2015).
Bouazza N, et al. *Favipiravir in children with Ebola*. 385 (9968) Lancet. 603–604 (Feb. 2015).
Centers for Disease Control and Prevention. 63(39) MMWR (Oct. 3, 2014). Available at http://www.cdc.gov/mmwr/preview/mmwrhtml/mm6339a4.htm.
Centers for Disease Control and Prevention. Outbreaks Chronology: Ebola Virus Disease. Available at http://www.cdc.gov/vhf/ebola/outbreaks/history/chronology.html.
Chowell G, Abdirizak F, Lee S, Lee J, Jung E, Nishiura H, et al. *Transmission dynamics and control of Ebola virus disease (EVD): a review*. 12 BMC Medicine 196 (2014).
Cohn S, Kutalek R. *Historical parallels, Ebola virus disease and cholera: understanding community distrust and social violence with epidemics*. PLoS Currents (Jan. 26, 2016). Available at

http://currents.plos.org/outbreaks/article/historical-parallels-ebola-virus-disease-and-cholera-understanding-community-distrust-and-social-violence-with-epidemics/.

Cooper BS, Boni MF, Pan-ngum W, Day NPJ, Horby PW, Olliaro P, et al. *Evaluating clinical trial designs for investigational treatments of Ebola virus disease.* 12(4) PLoS Med (2015).

Ebola: a call to action. 20(9) Nat Med. 967 (2014).

Ebola in West Africa: gaining community trust and confidence. 383(9933) Lancet 1946 (June 7, 2014).

Ebola—saving lives with natural allopathic medicine. DrSircus.com. (Aug. 4, 2014). Available at http://drsircus.com/medicine/ebola-saving-lives-natural-allopathic-medicine/.

Edwards SJL, Lilford RJ, Hewison J. *The ethics of randomised controlled trials from the perspectives of patients, the public, and healthcare professionals.* 317(7167) BMJ 1209–1212 (1998).

Folayan MO, Brown B, Haire B, Yakubu A, Peterson K, Tegli J. *Stakeholders' engagement with Ebola therapy research in resource limited settings.* 15 BMC Inf. Dis. 242 (2015).

Folayan, Brown B, Yakubu A, Peterson K, Haire B. *Compassionate use of experimental drugs in the Ebola outbreak.* 384(9957) Lancet 1843–1844 (2015).

Folayan MO, Peterson K, Kombe F. *Ethics, emergencies and Ebola clinical trials: the role of governments and communities in offshored research.* 22(Suppl 1) Pan African Medical Journal 10 (2015).

Ghose T. *Nano silver? Nigeria's potential Ebola treatment unlikely to work.* Live Science (Aug. 15, 2014). Available at http://www.livescience.com/47389-nigerian-experimental-ebola-drug.html.

Gostin LO. *Ethical allocation of drugs and vaccines in the West African Ebola epidemic.* 92(4) Millbank Quarterly 662–666 (2014).

Government of Canada, Panel on Research. Fairness and Equity in Research Participation. Available at http://www.pre.ethics.gc.ca/eng/policy-politique/initiatives/tcps2-eptc2/chapter4-chapitre4/.

Haque A, Hober D, Blondiaux J. *Addressing therapeutic options for Ebola virus infection in current and future outbreaks.* 59(10) Antimicrob Agents Chemother 5892–5902 (Oct. 2015).

Hewlett BL, Hewlett BS. *Providing care and facing death: nursing during Ebola outbreaks in central Africa.* 16 J Transcult Nurs 289–297 (Oct. 2005).

Hoenen T, Feldmann H. *Ebola virus in West Africa, and the use of experimental therapies or vaccines.* 12 BMC Biol. 80 (2014).

How many Ebola patients have been treated outside of Africa? New York Times (Jan. 26, 2015). Available at http://www.nytimes.com/interactive/2014/07/31/world/africa/ebola-virus-outbreak-qa.html?.

Joffe S. *Evaluating Novel Therapies During the Ebola Epidemic,* 312(13) JAMA 1299–1300 (2014).

Jones M. *Ebola outbreak: informed consent must be central to experimental drug testing.* International Bar Association (Sept. 3, 2014). Available at http://www.ibanet.org/Article/Detail.aspx?ArticleUid=920c89de-c0de-4bbf-8c76-4d65d95be993.

Kendal JM. *Designing a research project: randomised controlled trials and their principles.* 20 Emerg Med J 164–168 (2003).

Lane HC, Marston HD, Fauci AS. *Conducting clinical trials in outbreak settings: points to consider.* 13(1) Clin Trials 92–95 (Feb. 2016).

Lefebvre A, Fiet C, Belpois-Duchamp C, Tiv M, Astruc K, Aho Glélé LS. *Case fatality rates of Ebola virus diseases: a meta-analysis of World Health Organization data.* 44(9) Med Mal Infect. 412–416 (2014).

Millman J. *Why the drug industry hasn't come up with an Ebola cure.* Washington Post (Aug. 13, 2014).

Mupapa K, Mukundu W, Bwaka MA, et al. *Ebola hemorrhagic fever and pregnancy.* 179(Suppl 1) J Infect Dis S11–S12 (1999).

PhRMA. 2015 Profile: Biopharmaceutical Research Industry (2015). Available at http://www.phrma.org/sites/default/files/pdf/2015_phrma_profile.pdf.

Rid A, Emanuel EJ. *Ethical considerations of experimental interventions in the Ebola outbreak.* 384(9957) Lancet 1896–1899 (2014).

Rowen R. Ozone Therapy: A Possible Answer to Ebola? Available at http://articles.mercola.com/sites/articles/archive/2014/10/26/ozone-therapy-ebola.aspx.

Schuklenk U, Lowry C. *Terminal illness and access to phase 1 experimental agents, surgeries and devices: reviewing the ethical arguments.* 89(1) Br Med Bull 7–22 (2009).

Smith FL. *We have military research to thank for Ebola vaccines.* Mediacom. Available at https://medium.com/war-is-boring/we-have-military-research-to-thank-for-ebola-vaccines-565897c3f1bc#.yexv8p9vf.

Sullivan GM. *Getting off the "gold standard": randomized controlled trials and education research.* 3(3) Journal of Graduate Medical Education 285–289 (2011).

Wahl-Jensen V, Bollinger L, Safronetz D, de Kok-Mercado F, Scott DP, Ebihara H. *Use of the Syrian hamster as a new model of Ebola virus disease and other viral hemorrhagic fevers.* 4 Viruses 3754–3784 (2012).

WHO. Report of an Advisory Panel to WHO: Ethical Considerations for Use of Unregistered Interventions for Ebola Virus Disease (Aug. 11, 2014).

WHO Ebola Response Team. *Ebola virus disease in West Africa—the first 9 months of the epidemic and forward projections.* 371 N Engl J Med 1481–1495 (2014).

Wilmshurst P. *Scientific imperialism: if they won't benefit from the findings, poor people in the developing world shouldn't be used in research.* 314 BMJ 840–841 (1997).

World Health Organization. Trends in Maternal Mortality: 1990 to 2013. Estimates by WHO, UNICEF, UNFPA, The World Bank and the United Nations Population Division. Available at http://apps.who.int/iris/bitstream/10665/112682/2/9789241507226_eng.pdf.

13

Evidence, Strategies, and Challenges for Assuring Vaccine Availability, Efficacy, and Safety

SAAD B. OMER AND SAM F. HALABI

Vaccines are our most effective and cost-saving tools for disease prevention, preventing untold suffering and saving tens of thousands of lives and billions of dollars in treatment costs each year.[1] Routine immunization programs protect most of the world's children from a number of infectious diseases that previously claimed millions of lives. Safe and effective vaccines have been developed for dozens of infectious diseases, and promising candidates are under development for several of the most life-threatening infections, including Ebola virus disease, malaria, tuberculosis, and HIV/AIDS. Global support for vaccination programs has explained the significant progress made toward achieving Millennium Development Goal 4, with its aim of reducing childhood mortality by two thirds. In 2013, 6.3 million children under age 5 died, compared with 12.7 million in 1990. Between 1990 and 2013, under-5 mortality declined by 49%, from an estimated rate of 90 deaths per 1,000 live births to 46. The global rate of decline has also accelerated in recent years—from 1.2% per annum during 1990–1995 to 4.0% during 2005–2013.[2]

Vaccines are generally very safe, and serious adverse reactions are uncommon, which explains why they have become such an important component of national and international public health systems. They represent a low-risk, cost-effective intervention behind which there is a substantial history of safety and in which there has been built a great deal of trust. In this chapter, we examine the evidence, strategies, and challenges surrounding vaccine safety as new technologies and expanding

---

[1] Centers for Disease Control and Prevention, A CDC Framework for Preventing Infectious Disease, available at http://www.cdc.gov/oid/docs/ID-Framework.pdf.

[2] World Health Organization, Millennium Development Goals, available at http://www.who.int/mediacentre/factsheets/fs290/en/.

coverage introduce new factors to consider in maintaining the safety profile of current and new vaccines. While the fundamental principle behind vaccination (used interchangeably here with immunization) has remained constant over time—administration of agent-specific, but relatively harmless, antigenic components that in vaccinated individuals induce protective immunity against the corresponding infectious agent—the technologies behind antigenic components have evolved. After Edward Jenner and Benjamin Jesty observed that exposure to cowpox provided protection against smallpox disease–causing variola viruses, physicians and medical researchers discovered processes for inactivating whole bacteria, which could then be turned into vaccines, as well as bacterial toxins, the production of antitoxins, and the revelation that immune serum contained antibodies that rendered toxins harmless or interfered with bacterial replication. In the 1920s, researchers discovered that the addition of certain substances like aluminum compounds increased yields of serum antibodies, the origin of *adjuvants*, substances that can enhance and modulate the immunogenicity of the vaccine antigen.[3] Subunit vaccines contain pieces of the pathogens against which they are intended to promote an immune response, and a subcategory of these vaccines using recombinant genetic technology has provided some of the most important recent vaccine breakthroughs like hepatitis B, human papillomavirus (HPV), and candidate Ebola vaccines. In short, there are a number of methods by which vaccines have been developed to facilitate immunologic response, a growing number of technological advances across vaccine types, and therefore a corresponding growth in systems that must be adopted to monitor for adverse events related to these vaccines and related technologies. This chapter will first provide a general overview of how the regulatory process assures vaccine safety and efficacy through the development and licensure phases. While the vast majority of vaccines are developed and manufactured in high-resource jurisdictions, manufacturers in developing countries, especially India, have become a growing part of the global vaccine sector. Second, the chapter will review postlicensure vaccine safety and adverse event reporting systems at both the national and international levels. Finally, the chapter will assess weaknesses in the global system for adverse event monitoring, especially in light of advances in immunization coverage programs in low-income countries, and will propose some potential solutions to address those weaknesses.

Vaccine Development Stages and Regulatory Requirements for Safety and Efficacy

The vaccine development process may be understood as moving through five stages. In the first stage, researchers prioritize identification and isolation of the

[3] Nathalie Garcon et al., *Vaccine adjuvants*, 1(1) Perspectives in Vaccinology 89–113 (Aug. 2011).

relevant pathogen. This research is undertaken to understand, to the greatest extent possible, the biological mechanism or mechanisms that lead to disease.[4] The greater the degree of understanding of pathogenesis, the better researchers are able to identify correlates of protection or biological markers such as antibodies, as well as cellular-level response by the immune system. At this stage of vaccine development, researchers often work under an imperfect understanding of the biological mechanisms, even if they do achieve results that support the next stage of development: candidate design.[5]

In the second stage of development, vaccine candidates are developed using empirical approaches, historically the primary means by which candidates are constructed. The smallpox vaccine, for example, is a variant of the smallpox virus, vaccinia, obtained by passage through the cow, which, while not pathogenic to humans, nevertheless stimulates an immune response to the smallpox virus. While that candidate was found occurring in nature, other vaccines are developed by serial propagation through media that diminish their pathogenicity, or are killed or dissected after cultivation and used in relatively large doses, with adjuvants or in multiple doses to prompt immune response. "Reverse vaccinology" starts from genomic sequences and, by computer analysis, predicts those antigens that are most likely to be vaccine candidates. These techniques allow greater certainty for candidates given differences in what occurs in in vitro versus in vivo infection (or even pathogens that are not easily cultivable) and are less resource intensive than the cultivation process but depend on high computational power.[6]

In the third stage, candidates are tested in animals after developing models for testing immunogenicity and safety. Vaccine challenges are then administered to animals (under only rare circumstances to humans) to test for antibody response as well as adverse events. After animal testing, the vaccine sponsor applies for Investigational New Drug (IND) status from the US Food and Drug Administration (FDA), or an equivalent application and agency, which, technically speaking, authorizes the sponsor to undertake clinical trials on humans for safety, efficacy, and licensure. The first of these trials is designed to assess the safety, immunogenicity, and dose response of the vaccine in, typically, 20 to 100 healthy volunteers.

In the fourth stage, investigators expand the number of human subjects participating in clinical trials and extensively examine population-level data. In phase II, the sample size is increased to several hundred healthy volunteers, and investigators focus principally on safety as well as immunogenicity. In phase IIb

---

[4] Eduardo Groisman (ed.) Principles of Bacterial Pathogenesis (2001).

[5] Sylvia Yeh, *Pertussis: persistent pathogen, imperfect vaccines*, 2 Expert Review of Vaccines 113–127 (2003).

[6] Rino Rappuoli, *Reverse vaccinology, a genome based approach to vaccine development*, 19 Vaccine 2688–2691 (Mar. 2001).

"proof-of-concept" studies, dose ranges and vaccine components are confirmed before the investigators move to much larger phase III studies. In phase III vaccine trials, the sample size becomes usually up to thousands or tens of thousands of human subjects, and the focus is on efficacy and safety. Adverse events following immunization can be classified by frequency (common, rare), extent (local, systemic), severity (hospitalization, disability, death), causality, and preventability (intrinsic to vaccine, faulty production, faulty administration). Adverse events following immunizations may be either coincidental or the result of increased risk caused by the vaccine. Some adverse events following immunization may be due to the vaccine preparation itself and the individual response of the vaccinee, and would not have occurred without vaccination. Examples of such events are vaccine-associated paralytic poliomyelitis after oral polio vaccine or vaccine-strain measles viral infection in an immunodeficient recipient. Other health events may be precipitated by an immunization, such as a vaccine-associated fever precipitating a febrile seizure. Vaccine administration errors may lead to adverse events as well. However, many adverse events following immunization are coincidental; they are temporally related to immunization but occur by chance without a causal relationship. This scale of trial is important to detect sometimes rare adverse events. In 1998, for example, a rotavirus vaccine was licensed for use in the United States after phase III trials on approximately 10,000 infants showed safety and efficacy. However, when the vaccine was administered to a much larger population, an association between the vaccine and bowel obstruction was observed, resulting in the withdrawal of the vaccine from the market.[7] If larger phase III studies confirm safety and efficacy, the relevant national regulatory authority approves the vaccine for marketing after internal review of study data.

In the fifth stage, vaccines are subject to a wide range of postmarketing assessments intended to measure theretofore unknown side effects, longevity of protection against the targeted pathogen, and, to the extent possible, herd immunity conferred through widespread use of the vaccine. In high-resource settings, there are numerous channels through which physicians and other healthcare workers are advised on various aspects of these studies and evaluations. In the United States, the Advisory Committee on Immunization Practices (ACIP) of the Centers for Disease Control and Prevention (CDC) a group of medical and public health experts, develops recommendations on how to use vaccines to control diseases. The National Vaccine Advisory Committee under the US Department of Health and Human Services recommends ways to achieve optimal prevention of human infectious diseases through vaccine development and provides direction to prevent adverse reactions to vaccines. Other provider-specific organizations such as the

---

[7] Lone Simonsen et al., *More on RotaShield and intussusception: the role of age at the time of vaccination*, 192 J. Infect. Diseases S36–S43 (2004), available at http://jid.oxfordjournals.org/content/192/Supplement_1/S36.full.

American Academy of Pediatrics and other in-country committees play advisory and monitoring roles.

At the international level, the Strategic Advisory Group of Experts (SAGE) on Immunization was established by the Director General of the World Health Organization (WHO) in 1999 to provide guidance on WHO's work on immunization policy and programs. This group advises WHO on global policies and strategies, ranging from vaccines and technology, research and development, to delivery of immunization and its linkages with other health interventions. Recommendations from these organizations, on both the national and the international level, are informed by, but not necessarily constrained by, licensure decisions from national regulatory authorities. For example, at both the national and the international level, these organizations may recommend certain immunizations for pregnant women or adolescents, despite there being no subpopulation data that would otherwise be required for licensure or marketing authorization.

With respect to cost and time, the aforementioned process varies by vaccine, jurisdiction of licensure, and circumstances surrounding development (e.g., whether developed in an emergency context, tailored to a subpopulation particularly susceptible to an infectious agent, or other). Generally, the development of a human vaccine from concept to regulatory approval takes between 10 and 15 years, while "introduction plans for global deployment extend in most cases beyond 20 years, with coverage reaching no more than 80 per cent of the target population even in the best-case scenarios."[8] The expenditure for the development of one new vaccine generally requires investments ranging from "$500 million for the least complex to $1 billion or more for the most complex, including construction of facilities for manufacture."[9] Failure rates for vaccine candidates are also high. Approximately 7% of vaccine development projects that reach the preclinical development phase result in a licensed vaccine.[10]

Vaccine Safety and the Global Management of Infectious Diseases

The Public Health Relevance of Vaccine Risk and Perception of Vaccine Risk

Public confidence in immunizations and the systems that support them is a critical part of preventing the spread of infectious disease and the resurgence

---

[8] M. Bregu et al., *Accelerating vaccine development and deployment: report of a Royal Society satellite meeting*, 366 (1579) Philos Trans R Soc Lond B Biol Sci 2841–2849 (Oct. 12, 2011).

[9] Stanley A. Plotkin, Adel A. F. Mahmoud, and Jeremy Farrar, *Establishing a global vaccine development fund*, 373 N Engl J Med 297–300 (July 23, 2015).

[10] Esther S. Pronker et al., *Risk in vaccine research and development quantified*, 8(3) PLoS One (2013).

of those in retreat. Indeed, it is a paradox of the success of immunization that as the risk of disease is perceived to decline, individuals focus on the relatively adversarial context of vaccine administration. According to the CDC, "Today, vaccine-preventable diseases are at or near record lows. Many people no longer see reminders of the severity and potential life-threatening complications of these diseases. Recent outbreaks of vaccine-preventable diseases show that even vaccinated people are at risk for disease if there is not adequate vaccine coverage in the population."[11] Because vaccines are administered to otherwise healthy infants and adults, a higher standard of safety is expected. Perceptions of safety risk, even mild ones, may exert disproportionate effect on the willingness of individuals to accept vaccinations for themselves or to consent to immunizations for children. During the 1980s, for example, concerns about whole-cell pertussis vaccine led to the widespread adoption of an acellular alternative, which some evidence is beginning to suggest may confer shorter immunity.[12] Adding to public concern about vaccines is the fact that immunization is mandated by many state and local school entry requirements. Because of this widespread use, safety problems with vaccines can have a potential impact on large numbers of persons. This general lower risk tolerance means that researchers must undertake searches for rare adverse events that would not be necessary in the context of approval or acceptance for other kinds of pharmaceuticals.

In low-income countries, the risks to public confidence are even greater because those countries suffer from high background levels of morbidity and mortality, and coincidental deaths and injuries associated with vaccine administration may be wrongly associated with the vaccine or systems supporting immunization efforts.[13] In the context of Ebola, for example, the *Liberian Observer* published a column asserting a link between the outbreak and preexisting vaccination drives.[14]

Mechanisms to Ensure Vaccine Safety

There are potential improvements that might be made in the aforementioned stages of vaccine approval such as animal testing and prelicensure human studies. Researchers at the laboratory level, for example, may be able to better study variables in animals, such as diet, exposure to other pathogens, and other genetic

---

[11] CDC, Vaccination Safety, available at http://www.cdc.gov/vaccines/pubs/pinkbook/downloads/safety.pdf.

[12] Nicola P. Klein et al., *Waning protection after fifth dose of acellular pertussis vaccine in children*, 367 NEJM 1012–1019 (2012), available at http://www.nejm.org/doi/pdf/10.1056/NEJMoa1200850.

[13] Sam Halabi and John Monahan, *Sharing the burden of Ebola vaccine–related adverse events*, 24 Tulane Journal of International and Comparative Law 131 (2015).

[14] *The Ebola outbreak coincided with UN vaccine campaigns*, Liberian Observer, available at http://www.liberianobserver.com/commentaries/ebola-breakout-coincided-un-vaccine-campaigns.

susceptibilities that may be linked to adverse events that are now generally controlled.[15] In prelicensure human studies, phases I, II, and III of human trials are related. In any given context, researchers may more efficiently explore proof-of-concept factors at phase I, as well as improving identification of common reactions from trials at all phases. Increasing the number of participants during phase III trials, of course, is more likely to alert researchers to rare adverse events or side effects, although at both monetary and temporal costs.

The most promising channels for gains in ensuring vaccine safety, however, are likely to open through efforts at monitoring postlicensure events. Phase IV surveillance studies focus on identifying rare reactions, monitoring whether there are increases in known reactions, building complete lists of risk factors and signals, and closely monitoring vaccine lots with unusual rates or types of events. In the United States, the Vaccine Adverse Event Reporting System (VAERS) is a national vaccine safety surveillance program cosponsored by the CDC and the FDA. VAERS collects information about adverse events (possible side effects) that occur after the administration of vaccines licensed for use in the United States, providing a nationwide mechanism by which adverse events following immunization may be reported, analyzed, and made available to the public. Healthcare providers are required to report adverse events for certain routine childhood immunizations and are under professional obligations to report other health events. Patients and other caregivers and family members also submit reports through VAERS, with the system receiving up to 15,000 reports per year. Through VAERS, researchers detect new or rare events, identify increases in rates of known side effects, and enhance understanding of patient risk factors. Ordinarily, additional studies are required to confirm VAERS signals because all reports of adverse events are not necessarily causally related to the vaccine. There are limitations to the system, such as underreporting, stimulated reporting, or incomplete reports, and it cannot assess adverse event rates or determine causation.

The Vaccine Safety Datalink (VSD) is a collaborative project between the CDC's Immunization Safety Office and nine healthcare organizations. The VSD began in 1990 and continues today in order to monitor safety of vaccines and conduct studies on rare and serious adverse events following immunization. It uses electronic health data from each participating site, including information on vaccines—the kind of vaccine that is given to each patient, the date of vaccination, and other vaccinations given on the same day. The VSD also uses information on medical illnesses that have been diagnosed at physicians' offices, urgent care visits, emergency department visits, and hospital stays, and it conducts vaccine safety studies based on questions or concerns raised by the medical literature and reports made

---

[15] Helen McShane and Ann Williams, *A review of preclinical animal models utilised for TB vaccine evaluation in the context of recent human efficacy data*, 94(2) Tuberculosis 105–110 (Mar. 2014), available at http://www.ncbi.nlm.nih.gov/pmc/articles/PMC3969587/.

through VAERS. The VSD monitors safety of vaccines when new ones have been recommended for use in the United States or if there are changes in how a vaccine is recommended. Because VSD maintains nine databases and retains information regarding up to 2% of the US population, it enables performance of active surveillance by using data-mining processes. The CDC maintains these databases in the United States, and equivalent databases are maintained by health agencies in the United Kingdom and Canada.

Results from VAERS and VDS are also linked with larger databases like the CDC's Clinical Immunization Safety Assessment Network (CISA), which provides a clinical case evaluation service for US healthcare providers who have vaccine safety questions about a specific patient residing in the United States. CISA provides clinical expertise in various disciplines, including allergy, hematology, immunology, neurology, obstetrics, and pediatrics. It prioritizes research studies of influenza vaccine safety, vaccine safety in persons with autoimmune diseases, and vaccine safety in pregnant women. CISA complements other vaccine safety systems and focuses its efforts on scalable, prospective studies for US-licensed vaccines. Those studies are designed to address clinical vaccine safety questions in targeted or special populations that are often excluded from prelicensure clinical trials.

At the international level, the World Health Organization established the Global Advisory Committee on Vaccine Safety (GACVS) in 1999 in order to analyze and recommend action with respect to vaccine safety issues of potential global importance. GACVS primarily manages vaccine safety issues either referred to WHO by any government or drug regulatory authority or identified by the committee. Vaccine safety assessment in many low- and middle-income countries remains far less developed. Researchers have undertaken a small number of observational and experimental studies in these countries, but there are few mechanisms for ongoing assessment of vaccine safety, and in many cases, the regulatory review undertaken by an advanced regulatory authority like the FDA and subsequent prequalification by WHO are the exclusive means of addressing safety.

National and International Vaccine Injury Compensation Systems

Yet even with these advances, two aspects of immunization will always generate challenges with respect to vaccine hesitancy. First, it is not possible to eliminate all adverse events, even if many vaccines demonstrate only mild adverse events and severe adverse events occur in exceptionally rare circumstances. Second, incongruities persist between the perception of vaccine safety and the overall benefits that vaccination imparts to individuals and communities. For these reasons, we advocate the establishment of a global vaccine injury compensation system that would be modeled on aspects of current vaccine injury compensation schemes in place at national and provincial levels. There is a public health preparedness value in agreeing to compensate individuals through predefined legal mechanisms. In the vaccination context generally, the traditional argument is that the public health benefits of vaccination so far outweigh the risks that we, as a community, compensate individuals who pay the price in experiencing adverse events. While a global vaccine compensation scheme has heretofore been deemed practically unworkable, we set forth some aspects of a workable scheme, as well as some of the global public health benefits it would provide.

Vaccine injury compensation systems have existed at least since 1953, when the German Supreme Court ruled that people who were injured by compulsory vaccination were entitled to compensation.[16] Germany enacted a compensation program in 1961, and France implemented a similar scheme in the 1960s.[17] In the 1970s, concerns over adverse events related to diphtheria, tetanus and pertussis vaccination led to compensation regimes in five additional European countries, as well as in Japan and New Zealand. Finland, Quebec, Taiwan, and the United States followed. Italy, Norway, and the Republic of Korea adopted compensation policies in the 1990s.[18] While each system works under varying requirements for eligibility, administration, and funding, they share an origin in concerns that compensating victims of vaccine injury was both just and also an important component of maintaining public trust in immunization.

While we envision a binding international legal instrument as the ultimate conclusion to the proposal we outline here, the first steps would be simply to acknowledge a consensus among countries and international organizations that those suffering from vaccine-related injuries deserve compensation. First, there is a straightforward obligation based on principles of fairness and justice that those who suffer for the much broader good of public health protection should not be the ones paying for that protection.[19] Vaccine injuries may be severe and complex, and they are often suffered by children who require a lifetime of care and may not qualify for other benefits. Second, there is a public health rationale, with growing evidence supporting it, that compensation for those suffering from vaccine injury, especially where it is drawn from all responsible parties (governments that compel immunization and manufacturers that produce the vaccines), closes the gap between the perception of vaccine risk and the reality of disease protection and quite rare harm. Indeed, during the course of the Ebola outbreak and the scramble to develop a safe and efficacious vaccine, many participants in the global health community acknowledged the

---

[16] Clare Looker and Health Kelly, *No-fault compensation following adverse events attributed to vaccination: a review of international programmes*, 89 Bulletin of the World Health Organization 317-78 (2011).

[17] *Id.*

[18] *Id.*

[19] Michelle Mello, *Rationalizing vaccine-injury compensation*, 22 Bioethics. 32-42 (2008).

need to raise funds to compensate those potentially injured by a rapidly developed vaccine.

Once that consensus is formed, it would be possible to incrementally realize a global system for vaccine injury compensation. Those countries currently operating a vaccine injury compensation scheme would be exempted from regional or institutional-driven schemes, which could otherwise organize and implement compensation regimes. The PAHO Revolving Fund, for example, could add an excise tax to the price it currently pays for vaccine doses to fund a regional compensation fund. Gavi could require that finance ministries provide for at least a minimal compensation scheme for eligible countries, which would create a path for those schemes to persist after countries have graduated from Gavi support.[20] Europe and China are already moving toward regional and national compensation schemes, as are Australia, Canada, and Ireland. WHO and/or UNICEF would be well positioned to facilitate a compensation fund for those jurisdictions not covered by such programs.

While we leave specifics of administration and funding, eligibility, process and decision-making, standard of proof, elements of compensation, and litigation rights to work we have published elsewhere, we note that far more difficult problems have faced the global public health community, and they have been overcome through deliberation by stakeholders and effective use of limited resources.

Conclusion

Vaccines have contributed to global standards of quality of life never before seen in history, and medical and technological advances promise to expand the list of infectious diseases for which vaccines will continue to save millions or tens of millions of lives at relatively low cost. In this chapter, we have examined the key components of a system to strengthen vaccine availability, safety, and efficacy. Most important, we believe that a key aspect of that system—compensation for vaccine injury—is an important next step, especially for closing the growing gap between the perception of vaccine utility and the reality of the public health promotion vaccines provide.

References

Bregu, M., et al. *Accelerating vaccine development and deployment: report of a Royal Society satellite meeting*, 366 (1579) Philos Trans R Soc Lond B Biol Sci 2841–2849 (Oct. 12, 2011).
Centers for Disease Control and Prevention. A CDC Framework for Preventing Infectious Diseases. *Sustaining the Essentials and Innovating for the Future* (Oct. 2011).

---

[20] For elaborations on both the PAHO Revolving Fund and how Gavi works, see chapter 10 in this volume.

The Ebola outbreak coincided with UN vaccine campaigns. Liberian Observer. Available at http://www.liberianobserver.com/commentaries/ebola-breakout-coincided-un-vaccine-campaigns.

Garcon, N., et al. *Vaccine adjuvants.* 1(1) Perspectives in Vaccinology 89–113 (Aug. 2011).

Groisman, Eduardo A. (ed.) Principles of Bacterial Pathogenesis (2001).

Halabi, S., and John Monahan. *Sharing the burden of Ebola vaccine–related adverse events.* 24 Tulane J. Int'l. L. 131 (2015).

Immunology and Vaccine Preventable Diseases—Pink Book—Vaccination Safety. Available at http://www.cdc.gov/vaccines/pubs/pinkbook/downloads/safety.pdf.

Klein, Nicola P., Joan Bartlett, Ali Rowhani-Rahbar, Bruce Fireman, and Roger Baxter. *Waning protection after fifth dose of acellular pertussis vaccine in children.* 367 N Engl J Med 1012–1019 (2012).

Looker, Clare and Health Kelly, *No-fault compensation following adverse events attributed to vaccination: a review of international programmes,* 89 Bulletin of the World Health Organization 317–78 (2011).

McShane, Helen, and Ann Williams. *A review of preclinical animal models utilized for TB vaccine evaluation in the context of recent human efficacy data.* Available at http://www.ncbi.nlm.nih.gov/pmc/articles/PMC3969587/.

Mello MM. Rationalizing vaccine-injury compensation. Bioethics. 2008; 22:32-42.

Millennium Development Goals (MDGs). Fact sheet N290. Updated May 2015. Available at http://www.who.int/mediacentre/factsheets/fs290/en/.

Plotkin, Stanley, Adel Mahmoud, and Jeremy Farrar. *Establishing a global vaccine development fund.* 373 N Engl J Med 297–300 (2015).

Pronker E. S., et al. *Risk in vaccine research and development quantified.* 8(3) PLoS One (2013).

Rappuoli, R. *Reverse vaccinology, a genome based approach to vaccine development.* 19(17–19) Vaccine 2688–2691 (Mar. 21, 2001).

, L., C. Viboud, A. Elixhauser, R. J. Taylor, R. J., and A. Z. Kapikian. *More on RotaShield and intussusception: the role of age at the time of vaccination.* 192 J. Infect. Diseases S36–S43 (Sept. 1, 2004).

Yeh, S. *Pertussis: persistent pathogen, imperfect vaccines.* 2 Expert Review of Vaccines 113–127 (2003).

14

Global Access Considerations for HIV Vaccine Trials

MARY MAROVICH

Since the beginning of the HIV/AIDS epidemic, almost 78 million people have been infected with the virus, and approximately 39 million people have died of HIV. Globally, 35 million people were living with HIV at the end of 2013.[1] An estimated 0.8% of adults aged 15 to 49 years worldwide are living with HIV, although the burden of the epidemic continues to vary considerably between countries and regions.[2] Sub-Saharan Africa remains most severely affected, "with nearly 1 in every 20 adults living with HIV and accounting for nearly 71% of the people living with HIV worldwide."[3]

Historically, vaccines have been our best defense against deadly infectious diseases, including smallpox, polio, measles, and yellow fever. Unfortunately, we do not have a vaccine for HIV. The virus evades the human immune system's normal mechanisms, and experience so far suggests that the human body seems incapable of adapting an effective immune response against it. Consequently, medical researchers lack a clear approach to stimulate immunologic protection against HIV.[4]

Finding a safe, effective, and durable HIV vaccine remains a top priority for the US National Institute for Allergy and Infectious Diseases (NIAID). Through the Vaccine Research Center and the Division of AIDS, NIAID conducts and supports biomedical research that leads to increased knowledge about how HIV interacts with the human immune system and evaluation of the most promising vaccine candidates. While development of a vaccine to prevent HIV infection remains the

---

[1] World Health Organization, Global Health Observatory Data, available at http://www.who.int/gho/hiv/en/.

[2] Id.

[3] Id.

[4] National Institute for Allergy and Infectious Diseases, HIV Vaccine Research, available at http://www.niaid.nih.gov/topics/hivaids/research/vaccines/Pages/default.aspx.

ultimate objective, NIAID is also exploring alternate approaches to prevention of infection including monoclonal antibodies, that reduce the chance of becoming infected and may alter the course of disease and infectiousness of people already infected with HIV.

This chapter examines the first modestly successful HIV vaccine regimen, RV144, not only for the lessons learned about biomedical research and innovation aimed at a difficult medical problem, but the financing, logistic, and stakeholder aspects of the effort that illustrated the planning and foresight necessary to develop, finance, and then distribute a safe and efficacious HIV vaccine as well as the engagement with all constituencies as to the limits, if any, of that vaccine's mechanism of action. The RV144 Phase III HIV vaccine trials' data supported safety but was not sufficiently efficacious to proceed to licensure. However, in reviewing this large scale trial process, there are various considerations regarding vaccine access and challenges associated with the vaccine from a medical perspective that remain outstanding. The RV144 trial demonstrates the need for an effective approach to developing a global access plan.

This chapter discusses how the results of the RV144 phase III trial encouraged the formation of the Pox-Protein Public-Private Partnership (P5), which now includes the Bill and Melinda Gates Foundation, the HIV Vaccine Trials Network, Novartis Vaccines and Diagnostics/GSK, Sanofi Pasteur, the South African Medical Research Council, the US Military HIV Research Program, as well as NIAID's Division of AIDS, and the partnership's ensuing effort to build a successful and effective Global Vaccine Access Plan. The chapter examines how the P5 plans to build on the RV144 study, as well as what an effective Global Vaccine Access Plan must include.

Lessons Learned From RV144

RV144: The First Phase III Trial to Show That an HIV Vaccine Is Possible

The RV144 study is the first and only Phase III clinical trial of an HIV vaccine candidate to demonstrate protection from infection.[5] RV144 tested the "prime-boost" combination of two vaccines: ALVAC HIV vaccine and AIDSVAX B/E vaccine. The RV144 study was undertaken in Thailand with 16,000 HIV-negative adult volunteer participants. These volunteers were randomized into double-blind study groups, with those in the experimental group receiving the prime-boost combination. Eligibility criteria for participation in the study required that all volunteers be HIV-negative prior to enrollment in the study and be willing to participate in educational counseling intended to teach ways to reduce risk behavior associated with

---

[5] Supachai Rerks-Ngarm et al., *Vaccination with ALVAC and AIDSVAX to prevent HIV-1 infection in Thailand*, 161 New Eng. J. Med. 2209, 2210 (Dec. 3, 2009).

contracting HIV.[6] After vaccination, volunteers were asked to receive HIV testing every 6 months for 3 years, as well as receive additional risk-behavior counseling at every testing visit. The study was conducted through the Thai Ministry of Health, in collaboration with the US Military HIV Research Program and supported by NIAID. Vaccine products were provided by Sanofi Pasteur and Global Solutions for Infectious Diseases. The RV144 trial showed that after volunteers received the prime-boost regimen, the HIV infection rate was reduced by 31.2% three years after vaccination.[7] In a post hoc analysis, vaccine efficacy was as high as 60% at one year and then gradually waned over the ensuing years.[8] Overall, the RV144 trial yielded unprecedented scientific insight into the immunologic characteristics of an effective vaccine. These results re-energized the HIV vaccine field and led to the establishment of the P5

P5: A Public-Private Partnership to Build and Improve on RV 144

The P5 was established to build on the results of RV144 by testing RV144-like vaccine constructs in the Republic of South Africa to examine efficacy and durability of potential vaccines. The HIV Vaccine Trials Network (HVTN) plans to conduct clinical trials in heterosexual adults that will evaluate a prime-boost vaccine regimen similar to that used in RV144 adjusted to target the most common subtype of HIV in the region (subtype C).[9] A modified version of ALVAC, the pox vector vaccine used in RV144, will be used as the prime or first vaccination received by study participants. That prime will be followed by the boost vaccinations with the vector and bivalent gp120 proteins, two HIV envelope proteins that reflect the circulating virus in Southern Africa, subtype C.

Due to the HIV burden in South Africa, even modest vaccine efficacy (30% to 50%), coupled with other preventative strategies, could substantially alleviate the HIV epidemic. Planning for future access to a successful vaccine has heightened significance for the P5. As a result, the P5 will study the effect of an improved RV144 regimen, and the mode of testing will track the engagement with stakeholders accomplished in the RV144 trial. The objective of building and improving upon the

---

[6] Id.

[7] Press release, US Department of Health and Human Services, NIH Grantees Sharpen Understanding of Antibodies That May Cut Risk of HIV Infection (Mar. 19, 2014) (on file with author).

[8] Robb, Merlin L et al. Risk behaviour and time as covariates for efficacy of the HIV vaccine regimen ALVAC-HIV (vCP1521) and AIDSVAX B/E: a post-hoc analysis of the Thai phase 3 efficacy trial RV 144. The Lancet Infectious Diseases, Volume 12, Issue 7, 531 – 537.

[9] Global HIV Vaccine Enterprise, P5 Partnership, available at http://www.vaccineenterprise.org/content/P5Partnership.

RV144 study includes efforts to develop an effective Global Vaccine Access Plan should a safe and efficacious vaccine emerge.

A Global Vaccine Access Plan Provides a Roadmap

A Global Vaccine Access Plan is critical to committing partners to a clear, feasible, and effective public health strategy for development, manufacture, and distribution of a safe and effective HIV vaccine. This public health strategy is multifaceted and engages a wide range of stakeholders. First, the strategy must outline potential vaccine safety and efficacy scenarios. Second, it must determine the public health impact and target population(s) under those scenarios. Third, it must identify commercial, regulatory, manufacturing, policy, and deployment challenges. Fourth, this strategy must define conditions, processes, and provisions for access based on vaccine characteristics and public health objectives. The RV144 trial study revealed the importance of a well-thought-out strategy and also taught some lessons in how that strategy might be built and executed.

RV144: Precedent-Setting for HIV Vaccine Access Planning

The RV144 trial took place against a backdrop of reputational, regulatory, commercial, and cultural complexities that will inform any future campaign aimed at HIV vaccine development and distribution. Before the study commenced, a number of prominent HIV researchers publicly expressed skepticism of the scientific rationale because the two vaccine candidates alone had failed to elicit threshold immunologic responses.[10] After the RV144 results were released, some researchers questioned the method and timing by which the results and statistical evaluations were communicated, suggesting problems with transparency.[11] The government of Thailand had not previously served as a pioneering regulator over this precise kind of trial, raising questions about regulatory capacity generally. Relatedly, cultural norms by which decision-making and communication between partners were conducted differed from those in trials undertaken in high-resource contexts. The two vaccine components were provided by different manufacturers.

These aspects of the RV144 trial have informed future approaches, highlighting the need to plan trials considering three interdependent factors: (1) a contingency planning roadmap by which partners collaborate on a collective response to trial outcomes, (2) a regulatory capacity building plan under which competencies for vaccine licensure are part of the regulatory partnership, and (3) an access strategy

---

[10] Dennis R. Burton et al., *A sound rationale needed for phase III HIV-1 vaccine trials*, 303 Science 316 (Jan. 16, 2004).

[11] Olive Leavy, *HIV vaccine results in controversy*, 9 Nature Reviews Immunology, 755 (Nov. 2009).

for the study that defined access timelines and commitments under different efficacy scenarios. The planning process takes a tremendous amount of time and foresight, especially for outcomes that are aspirational or unlikely. Stakeholder engagement requires acknowledgment and management of diverse partner expectations, which must be mutually agreed upon and managed with well-defined and clear objectives. The RV144 experience informed the P5 access planning effort and facilitated a proactive, transparent, and collaborative access planning process for the phase IIb/III trial in South Africa.

The P5 Global Access Committee and Vaccine Access Plan

The P5 Global Access Committee studied the regulatory, cultural, and access-related factors that affected the perception and results following the RV144 when designing its Vaccine Access Plan. The experience gained from RV144 showed the essential role of mapping out strategies, planning ahead, and appropriately dividing access factors from one end of the supply chain to the other. Through a governance structure that included an executive committee, a management team, protocol teams, and working groups, P5 divided these factors into roughly five general issues.

Priority Populations and Targets

The risk profiles of populations and population subgroups necessarily differ between regions. Where it may make more sense to target higher-risk men-who-save-sex-with-men (MSM) groups in Thailand, target populations in South Africa are more likely to be higher-risk heterosexual groups. Priority populations and targets, in turn, affect decisions as to which protein boost will follow the initial ALVAC administration and what kind of placebo control will be used.

The HVTN (NIH funded HIV vaccines clinical trial network) 100 vaccine regimen, one of the RV144-adapted trials underway in South Africa, consists of two experimental vaccines: a canarypox-based vaccine called ALVAC-HIV and a bivalent gp120 protein subunit vaccine with an adjuvant that enhances the body's immune response.[12] Both ALVAC-HIV (supplied by Sanofi Pasteur) and the protein vaccine (supplied by Novartis Vaccines and Diagnostics/GSK) have been modified from RV144 to be specific to HIV subtype C. In addition, the protein vaccine in HVTN 100 is using a different adjuvant than did RV144 in the hope of generating a more robust and durable immune response. Finally, the HVTN 100 vaccine regimen will include booster shots at the 1-year mark in an effort to prolong the early protective effect observed in RV144. All study participants will receive a total of eight injections over the course of a year. The

---

[12] National Institute for Allergy and Infectious Diseases, NIH-Sponsored HIV Vaccine Trial Launches in South Africa: Early-Stage Trial Aims to Build on RV144 Results, available at http://www.niaid.nih.gov/news/newsreleases/2015/Pages/HVTN100.aspx

volunteers will be randomly assigned to receive either the investigational vaccine regimen (210 participants) or a placebo (42 participants).[13]

Market Conditions

Priority populations and targets, in turn, will shape the market conditions surrounding the development of a safe and efficacious vaccine. If the HVTN results are promising, that will affect what kind of demand may be expected from countries specially affected by HIV subtype C and what kinds of domestic and international financing mechanisms may be put in place for procurement. Costs related to every aspect of vaccine procurement, distribution, administration, and postvaccine surveillance will need to be assessed based on these funding mechanisms, manufacturer pricing, and related auxiliary materials.

Regulatory Requirements

Vaccine licensure and marketing approval requirements are specific to each region in which an applicant is seeking approval. Clinical trials in South Africa and Thailand are conducted under the national regulations applicable to both clinical trial and licensing regimes in those countries, including animal and toxicology studies, norms surrounding informed consent of trial volunteers, and required dossiers, which must support vaccine approval. Standards adopted by the US Food and Drug Administration (FDA) are often considered an international gold standard for medicines and vaccine approvals, but FDA requirements may be both over- and underinclusive depending on the region where the study is located or which region or national regulatory authority is reviewing licensure. Partners need to set out a regulatory strategy and implications for the study design, including, where necessary, specific personnel dedicated to understanding differences between the licensing environment experienced by a foreign researcher and in-country partners.

Technology Transfer

The public-private nature of the P5 necessarily means planning with respect to technology development, ownership rights, manufacturing capabilities with respect to any aspect of a safe and efficacious vaccine (including component proteins and adjuvants), and sharing expectations and what transfer agreements must be negotiated between manufacturers, governments, and stakeholders to support vaccine procurement and distribution. While "technology transfer" may be simply stated, it potentially implicates every aspect of a safe and efficacious vaccine, including

---

[13] *Id.*

transfer of skills, knowledge, technologies, methods of manufacturing, samples of manufacturing, and facilities, and therefore the legal environment under which transfer takes (or does not take) place. Technology transfer may occur to increase manufacturing capacity and access to products, share know-how and intellectual property, or lower the costs of goods, or it may take place because of a compelling legal mandate. Transfer agreements might be discrete and closed, like the transfer of some aspect of a manufacturing process, or they might be open-ended and necessarily continuing, like a component protein in which the manufacturer, under law, must monitor any use of the technology after transfer for potential safety or efficacy signals.

Manufacturing and Product Development

Similarly, for manufacturing and product development, a Vaccine Access Plan must identify funding commitments, manufacturing responsibility, and the volume and timing expectations for private sector suppliers. Just as with regulatory requirements and technology transfer agreements or understandings, manufacturers and developers of vaccine components including adjuvants necessarily make decisions based on market demandsand the opportunity costs from the diversion of resources from other potentially profitable activities that may occur as a result of participation in HIV vaccine collaborations. Also, potential liabilities related to the product supplied are part of a broader calculation as to the business wisdom of participation even if a safe and efficacious vaccine is developed. Manufacturers must be given the right set of incentives for participation to make short-, medium-, and long-term sense, and that set of incentives will typically be extended by both governments and funders. Overall, in the context of RV144 and the P5, aligning diverse partners around a single agenda requires concerted engagement, strong evidence, and management of expectations.

The P5's Three-Pronged Approach to the Access Plan

After analyzing priority populations and targets, market conditions, regulatory requirements, technology transfer factors, and manufacturing/private sector expectations, the P5's Global Access Committee developed a three-pronged approach to the access plan based on stakeholder engagement, public health impact modeling, and scenario planning.

Stakeholder Engagement

In South Africa, the Global Access Committee has clarified public health objectives and assumptions, identified barriers to access, and reached a consensus on the meaning of "sustainable commitment" critical to the wide range of stakeholders working on the trial. After extensive outreach to introduce the Global Access Committee and secure buy-in, our stakeholder engagement effort is focusing on gathering input and data critical to the modeling effort.

Public Health Impact Modeling

The Global Access Committee is working with the HIV Modeling Consortium to help identify target populations under different vaccine efficacy scenarios. This consortium brings together individuals from the Centers for Disease Control and Prevention; the Global Fund to Fight AIDS, Tuberculosis and Malaria; the National Institutes of Health; President's Emergency Plan for AIDS Relief; the World Bank; the World Health Organization; and UNAIDS, in addition to other model consumers and producers.[14] The consortium is able to model HIV epidemiology based on location and reach of antiretroviral access programs, the relationship between programs aimed at reducing mother-to-child transmission and programs aimed at reducing heterosexual transmission, HIV prevalence among subgroups like pregnant women, and other matrices that inform the likely public health impact of a safe and efficacious vaccine. Those models in turn help the Global Access Committee map out the health economics factors that would be used to calculate payer/cost considerations and how those costs would change based on priority populations and targets. HIV Modelling Consortium models also assist the committee in identifying potential barriers to implementation and uptake among specific subgroups even if those subgroups might otherwise look like priorities because of geographical or economic factors. The public health impact model sets the stage for deliberations around the future public health, regulatory, manufacturing, and technology-sharing strategy.

Scenario Planning

Stakeholder engagement and public health impact modeling inform the Global Access Committee's scenario planning for a safe and efficacious HIV vaccine. As P5 prepares for phase III trials in 2016, we are working together to identify conceivable safety, operational, and vaccine efficacy outcomes; to define commercial, scientific, operational, industrial, and communication strategies to manage and respond to these outcomes; and to coordinate all partners around a single, consensus-based agenda (Figure 14.1). Scenario planning compels partners to plan for success—and

---

[14] HIV Modelling Consortium, How the Consortium Works, http://www.hivmodelling.org/how-consortium-works.

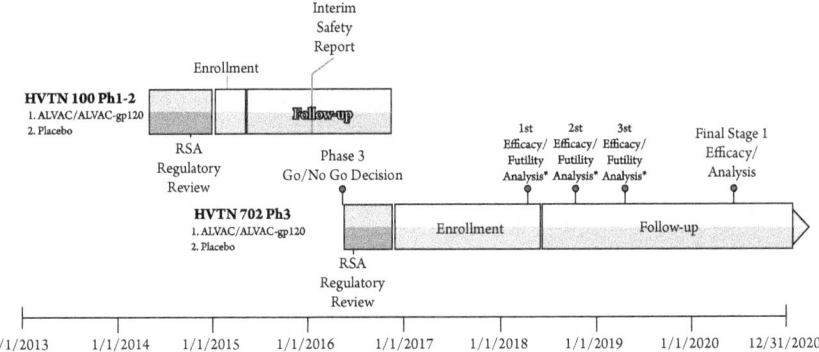

Figure 14.1 Projected Timelines for the P5 Phase III Program in RSA.

for crisis—and clarifies the conditions under which vaccine access provisions will be triggered.

Conclusion

The P5 partners are guided by four principles. First, the P5 understands there is a need for timely, sustainable access to an effective HIV vaccine. The group believes that vaccine access is a shared responsibility of the P5 partners and host countries. The P5 is committed to proactive stakeholder engagement. Finally, transparent and timely communication between those involved is a key value. The P5's commitment to building on the success of the RV144 experience is evident in the resources invested in assessing the regulatory, market demand, technology transfer, manufacturing, and pricing factors that will ultimately shape a plan for vaccine access. The product of this careful study, the Global Vaccine Access Plan, defines timelines, principles, activities, and provisions required for access, as well as securing sustainable commitments necessary for continued and expanded access to key populations.

The author acknowledges contributions from Nina Russell, Deputy Director HIV, Bill & Melinda Gates Foundation and Ryan Wiley, President, SHIFT Health.

References

Global HIV Vaccine Enterprise. P5 Partnership. Available at http://www.vaccineenterprise.org/content/P5Partnership.
HIV Modelling Consortium. How the Consortium Works. Available at http://www.hivmodelling.org/how-consortium-works.
Leavy, O. *HIV vaccine results in controversy*. 9 Nature Reviews Immunology 755 (Nov. 2009).

National Institute for Allergy and Infectious Diseases. HIV Vaccine Research. Available at http://www.niaid.nih.gov/topics/hivaids/research/vaccines/Pages/default.aspx.

———. NIH-Sponsored HIV Vaccine Trial Launches in South Africa: Early-Stage Trial Aims to Build on RV144 Results. Available at http://www.niaid.nih.gov/news/newsreleases/2015/Pages/HVTN100.aspx.

Rerks-Ngarm, Supachai, et al. *Vaccination with ALVAC and AIDSVAX to prevent HIV-1 infection in Thailand*, 161 New Eng. J. Med. 2209, 2210 (Dec. 3, 2009).

US Department of Health and Human Services. HIV Vaccine Regimen Demonstrates Modest Preventive Effect in Thailand Clinical Study (Sept. 24, 2009) (on file with author).

———. NIH Grantees Sharpen Understanding of Antibodies That May Cut Risk of HIV Infection (Mar. 19, 2014) (on file with author).

15

Isolation, Quarantine, and Infectious Disease Threats Arising From Global Migration

MARTIN CETRON

The Centers for Disease Control and Prevention (CDC) is responsible for the regulations and policies that are used to prevent the introduction, transmission, and interstate spread of communicable diseases into the United States.[1] Approximately 500,000 immigrants and refugees seek permanent residence in the United States per year.[2] Those seeking permanent residence receive overseas medical examinations that include testing for certain infectious diseases as part of their visa application process. In addition to those seeking permanent residence, approximately 300 people seek entry into the United States for temporary periods for every person seeking permanent residence. About 160 million of these temporary entrants enter the United States for work, school, business, or leisure. These applicants are not required to undergo the same medical screening as persons seeking permanent residence, such as immigrants and refugees, yet they represent just as much of a risk for the introduction and spread of infectious disease as those seeking to come to the United States permanently.[3]

Like many countries, the United States faces a continuing threat from infectious disease, most recently Ebola virus disease and pandemic influenza. These types of diseases can create serious problems for international and local public health authorities and health professionals. They may be highly contagious and lead to

---

[1] Centers for Disease Control and Prevention, Division of Global Migration and Quarantine, available at http://www.cdc.gov/ncezid/dgmq/.

[2] Department of Homeland Security, Yearbook of Immigration Statistics: 2012. Refugees and Asylees, available at http://www.dhs.gov/yearbook-immigration-statistics-2012-refugees-and-asylees.

[3] La'Marcus Wingate et al., *Cost-effectiveness of screening and treating foreign-born students for tuberculosis before entering the United States*, 10(4) PLoS ONE (2015).

death or serious illness. Infectious diseases levy substantial burdens on local and national economies. These concerns are often heightened where no proven vaccine or medical countermeasure is available to treat infected persons. Thus, the importance of containing these diseases before widespread transmission occurs becomes a priority for public health policy and planning.[4]

Because of the relationship between migration and disease, both federal and state governments have adopted laws and regulations aimed at preventing, detecting, and managing disease threats posed by the large and increasing migration of people into the United States. The purpose of this chapter is to analyze those statutory and regulatory mechanisms—with emphasis on isolation, quarantine, and alternatives—and, even where they are potentially applicable, understand the pragmatic and civil rights factors that may nevertheless influence their enforcement. The chapter assesses these mechanisms at the state, federal, and international levels.

Statutory and Regulatory Mechanisms to Control Infectious Disease Threats

Federal and state law delegate to various public health agencies and officials responsibility for determining not only when infectious diseases threaten individual and population health but also what measures to take to address those threats. When public health officials sign legal orders to execute the enforcement of these measures, they consider both the strict legal authorizations in place, as they must, and the normative and discretionary questions that, while not strictly required, play an important role in the legitimacy and proportionality lawmakers and the public expect with respect to balancing rights with public health protection. So public health officials must ask not only, "May I, or do I have the authority?" to issue an order but also "Is it possible for this order to be implemented in a proper, dignified way that, to the greatest extent possible, respects the rights of all parties? Are there adequate resources and capacity at our disposal to implement this order correctly?"

The "ought" part of public health decision-making is at least as relevant as the "may." The fact that legal authority and resource capacity exist sufficiently to adopt certain measures does not answer the question as to whether those measures *should* be taken. Especially when the question revolves around restricting individual rights, as public health law frequently contemplates, those restrictions must be the least restrictive possible so as to balance civil liberties and public health objectives. Decisions to isolate or quarantine illustrate both the difficult balance and the relevant questions public health officials must ask.

---

[4] RJ Blendon et al., *Attitudes toward the use of quarantine in a public health emergency in four countries*, Health Affairs (Millwood) (Jan. 2006).

Isolation and Quarantine

While blurred in common parlance, "isolation" and "quarantine" have specific meanings in the public health context. "Isolation" means to separate an ill person infected with a communicable disease from others in the community so as to prevent or reduce the spread of the disease.[5] "Quarantine" means the restriction of persons who are presumed to have been exposed to a contagious disease but are not ill. It may be applied at the individual, group, or community level and usually involves restriction to the home or designated facility. Quarantine may be voluntary or mandatory.[6] The purpose of quarantine is to aid individuals who are already infected or exposed and protect others from inadvertent exposure.[7]

Constitutional Allocation of Authority to Isolate and Quarantine

State Authority

Because states traditionally possessed responsibility for adopting laws to protect the health and safety of their citizens, state governments enjoy significant authority under the US Constitution to determine whether, and under what circumstances, persons will be isolated or quarantined as part of public health protection policies.[8] Federal authority to determine whether to isolate or quarantine ill or exposed persons is limited to those areas specifically allocated to the US government by the Constitution, for example, when the decision must be made with respect to a person entering the national borders of the United States.[9] The relative distribution of authority is reflected in the number of judicial decisions resolving questions as to the legality and scope of isolation and quarantine.[10] While there are few such decisions involving federal law or federal regulations, decisions involving state law are relatively common, especially for contagious diseases like tuberculosis.[11]

While the existence of 50 distinct legal approaches to isolation and quarantine has inevitably resulted in both minor and major variations, many states have

---

[5] Centers for Disease Control and Prevention, Legal Authorities for Isolation and Quarantine (2014); Marty Cetron and J. Landwirth, *Public health and ethical considerations in planning for quarantine*, 78 Yale Journal of Biology and Medicine 325 (2005).

[6] *Id.*

[7] *Id.*

[8] *Id.*

[9] James Misrahi et al., *HHS/CDC legal response to SARS outbreak*, 10 Emerg Infect Dis 353–355 (2004).

[10] David Fidler, Lawrence O. Gostin, and Howard Markel, *Through the quarantine looking glass: drug-resistant tuberculosis and public health governance, law and ethics*, 35 J. L. Med. & Ethics 616 (2007).

[11] Jared Cole, Federal and State Quarantine and Isolation Authority, Congressional Research Service Report (2004).

adopted provisions of the Model State Emergency Health Powers Act, a draft statute sponsored by the Centers for Disease Control and Prevention in the wake of the September 11, 2001, attacks and the anthrax-mail attacks that followed.[12] The model law was created in part because of the recognition of the great variation among state laws pertaining to public health emergencies, including laws authorizing isolation and quarantine. Sections of the act cover the degree of restriction to be used, due process, procedure, and standards for instituting isolation and quarantine. Although provisions of the model law apply only during officially declared public health emergencies, much of it has been incorporated into another model act that applies to both emergency and nonemergency contexts, the Turning Point Model State Public Health Act. Even before the model laws were drafted, many states showed a high degree of sensitivity to the balance between civil liberties and public health protection by adopting a "failure first policy" by which voluntary compliance with movement restrictions must be determined to have failed before state health authorities might impose more restrictive measures.

Federal Authority

Federal quarantine and isolation authority derives from the Commerce Clause of the US Constitution, which states that Congress shall have the power "to regulate Commerce with foreign Nations, and among the several states."[13] The Public Health Services Act (PHSA) enumerates the federal quarantine and isolation authority:

§ 264. Regulations to control communicable diseases

(a) Promulgation and enforcement by Surgeon General

The Surgeon General, with the approval of the Secretary, is authorized to make and enforce such regulations as . . . are necessary to prevent the . . . spread of communicable diseases from foreign countries into the States. . . .

(b) Apprehension, detention, or conditional release of individuals

Regulations prescribed under this section shall not provide for the apprehension . . . of individuals except for the purpose of preventing the . . . spread of such communicable diseases as may be specified from time to time in Executive orders of the President upon the recommendation of the Secretary, in consultation with the Surgeon General. . . .

---

[12] Frederic E. Shaw et al., Variation in Quarantine Powers Among the 10 Most Populous US States in 2004, available at http://www.ncbi.nlm.nih.gov/pmc/articles/PMC1854981/pdf/0970038.pdf.

[13] US Const. art. I, § 8, cl. 3.

(d) Apprehension and examination of persons reasonably believed to be infected
   (1) Regulations prescribed under this section may provide for the apprehension and examination of any individual reasonably believed to be infected with a communicable disease in a qualifying stage and (A) to be moving or about to move from a State to another State; or (B) to be a probable source of infection to individuals who, while infected with such disease in a qualifying stage, will be moving from a State to another State. Such regulations may provide that if upon examination any such individual is found to be infected, he may be detained for such time and in such manner as may be reasonably necessary. . . .
(e) Preemption
   Nothing in this section or section 266 of this title, or the regulations promulgated under such sections, may be construed as superseding any provision under State law . . . except to the extent that such a provision conflicts with an exercise of Federal authority.

Federal quarantine and isolation authority applied in terms of humans is restricted to nonspecified disease and is often executed by officials from the US Customs and Border Protection agency, the US Citizenship and Immigration Services, or the US Coast Guard, arms of the federal government not under the authority of the secretary of the Department of Health and Human Services (HHS).[14] A review may happen afterward (e.g., a postdetention review), but there is no explicit due process statute or regulation requiring such a review. In practice, there are many due process protections, including fair notification and an opportunity to appeal.

Section 361 of the Public Health Service Act gives the secretary of HHS the authority and responsibility to prevent the introduction, transmission, and spread of communicable diseases from outside of the United States and within the United States and it territories.[15] That authority has been delegated to the CDC, which may intervene both at the request of a state or if a determination is made that the state's efforts to control the disease locally are inadequate.[16] In practice, the CDC respects Section 264(e)'s protection of state law and has deferred to state and local health authorities in the primary use of their own separate "police power" quarantine authorities to restrict the movement of persons within their boundaries.

During the outbreak of severe acute respiratory syndrome (SARS), some states relied on their own legal authorities to control the movement of persons, so it was not necessary for the CDC to invoke federal quarantine power to compel the isolation or quarantine of a person within a state, but it undertook those actions parallel with a more inclusive approach that included state and local governments as

---

[14] US Centers for Disease Control and Prevention, *supra* note 5.
[15] *Id.*
[16] Cole, *supra* note 11.

key participants. The CDC established a series of telephone conferences, whereby federal, state, and local public health lawyers could discuss important legal issues arising under their isolation and quarantine provisions and exchange ideas about specific aspects of those legal issues. Those teleconferences were particularly useful in exchanging information concerning the interplay of quarantine authority at the federal, state, and local levels and discussion of procedural requirements involved in executing isolation or quarantine orders. The CDC followed a similar pattern during the peak of the monkeypox outbreak in 2003. Additionally, during that outbreak, the CDC developed a web-based clearinghouse where just-issued legal documents such as gubernatorial executive orders and state and local health department rules could be posted. These collaborative measures reduced the time required to identify relevant legal documents and disseminate them to public health lawyers on a "real-time" basis. Because of its long and successful history of collaboration with the states during public health emergencies, the CDC is likely to invoke federal quarantine power only rarely, such as at ports of entry or in other time-sensitive situations.[17]

While the CDC enjoys the broadest delegation of federal authority to adopt isolation and quarantine measures, the Department of Homeland Security and the Federal Aviation Agency are also authorized to isolate and quarantine under certain circumstances, including assisting the CDC in "the enforcement of quarantine rules and regulations."[18] Pilots of both interstate flights and flights to the United States are required to report certain illnesses they encounter during flight in advance of their arrival into the United States to the CDC Quarantine Station closest to their destination airport.[19]

World Health Organization Authority Under the International Health Regulations

In addition to state and federal authority for controlling infectious disease threats, the 1980s and early 1990s witnessed the emergence both of new infectious diseases such as HIV that quickly crossed international borders and of well-known diseases like cholera. The scope and magnitude of those threats made clear that an international

---

[17] Misrahi et al., *supra* note 9.

[18] Cole, *supra* note 11; 42 U.S.C. § 268. HHS also works closely with the Department of Homeland Security (DHS) and its agencies. HHS and DHS signed a memorandum of understanding in 2005 that sets forth specific cooperation mechanisms to implement their respective statutory responsibilities for quarantine and other public health measures, available at http://www.aclu.org/pdfs/privacy/hhs_dhs_mou.pdf. DHS has three agencies that may aid the CDC in its enforcement of quarantine rules and regulations pursuant to 42 U.S.C. § 268(b). They are the Customs and Border Patrol, US Immigration and Customs Enforcement (ICE), and the US Coast Guard. In addition to DHS, the CDC may also rely on other federal law enforcement agencies and state and local law enforcement agencies.

[19] 42 C.F.R. §§ 70.4, 71.21(b). It appears as though pilots would report illnesses to the Federal Aviation Administration (FAA) Air Traffic Services Unit, which would then communicate with the CDC Emergency Operations Center. See Press release, FAA Statement on Ebola (Oct. 3, 2014), available at http://www.faa.gov/news/press_releases/ news_story.cfm?newsId=17375.

coordinating mechanism was needed. In 1995, the World Health Assembly instructed the Director-General of the World Health Organization (WHO) to revisit the International Health Regulations (themselves an adaptation of the 1951 International Sanitary Regulations) because they neglected "the emergence of new infectious agents" and failed to provide for an adequate response of those that were covered.[20] The World Health Assembly attributed these failures to increased trade and migration of people. The outbreak of SARS in 2003 facilitated the 2005 revision process.

The IHR (2005) was revised to encompass the detection and prevention of all infectious diseases.[21] The regulations' scope was expanded to include any event that would constitute a public health emergency of international concern. As described by David Fidler and Lawrence Gostin:

> The Regulations now encompass public health risks whatever their origin or source (Article 1.1), including: (1) naturally occurring infectious diseases, whether of known or unknown etiological origin; (2) the potential international spread of non-communicable diseases caused by chemical or radiological agents in products moving in international commerce; and (3) suspected intentional or accidental releases of biological, chemical, or radiological substances.[22]

Acknowledging the importance of communication and cooperation to successful detection and prevention of communicable diseases, States Parties are obligated to "develop the means to detect, report, and respond to public health emergencies . . . [and] establish a National IHR Focal Point (NFP) for communication to and from WHO."[23] States Parties must inform WHO within 24 hours of an assessment of any event that could be considered a "public health risk to other States requiring a coordinated international response."[24]

---

[20] WHO, Revision Process of the International Health Regulations, available at http://www.who.int/ihr/revisionprocess/revision/en/index.html.

[21] The stated purpose is to "prevent, protect against, control and provide a public health response to the international spread of disease in ways that are commensurate with and restricted to public health risks, and which avoid unnecessary interference with international traffic and trade." World Health Organization, International Health Regulations (2005), 1 (2005).

[22] David Fidler and Lawrence O. Gostin, *The new International Health Regulations: an historic development for international law and public health*, 34 J. L. Med. & Ethics 85, 86–87 (2006).

[23] The NFP is a "national centre, established or designated by each State Party [and] must be accessible at all times for IHR (2005)-related communications with WHO." World Health Organization, International Health Regulations (2005): Toolkit for Implementation in National Legislation, 1, 7 (2009), available at http://www.who.int/ihr/NFP_Toolkit.pdf. As of July 2009, 99% of all states have established an NFP.

[24] Once an incident has been reported, WHO will then "coordinate communications across nations, provide technical assistance to responding nations, and work with international scientific experts to develop recommendations for mitigating the consequences of the event."

The drafters of the IHR (2005) included important limitations on the measures states could impose when facing a public health "event."[25] Isolation and quarantine, for example, impose significant restrictions on individual liberty. Under the IHR (2005):

> For a public health measure to restrict a civil and political right lawfully, the measure must (1) respond to a pressing public or social need; (2) pursue a legitimate aim; (3) be proportionate to the legitimate aim; and (4) be no more restrictive than is required to achieve the purpose sought by restricting the right. The rights-restricting measure must also be implemented in a non-discriminatory manner (International Covenant on Civil and Political Rights (ICCPR), Articles 2.1 and 26).[26]

The IHR created a floor rather than a ceiling for public health measures. States Parties may implement health measures that achieve the same or greater level of health protection as WHO recommendations, but they must be based on scientific principles, available scientific evidence, and relevant guidance or advice from WHO, and they cannot be more restrictive of international traffic or more invasive or intrusive to persons than reasonably available alternatives that would achieve the appropriate level of health protection.[27] Without such a justification, a state may face disputes at the World Trade Organization for adding unnecessary or overburdensome trade obstacles or international travel restrictions.

Under the IHR, within the specified time, the WHO director-general has the authority to declare a public health crisis of potentially global outbreaks.[28] For this to happen, the Director-General would convene an Emergency Committee to discuss whether the situation meets the criteria to be designated a public health emergency of international concern (PHEIC). Examples of recent PHEICs include the 2009 H1N1 pandemic and the 2014 Ebola outbreak. In contrast, the Middle East respiratory syndrome by coronavirus outbreak is not considered to be a PHEIC.

Under the PHEIC, WHO may issue recommendations regarding specific health measures, including vaccinations for traveling across the borders, isolation or quarantine measures, surveillance obligations, or even authorizing country governments to refuse entry or exit of certain types of persons.[29] The IHR further provides standards for humanitarian treatment of quarantine or isolation, such

---

[25] Fidler and Gostin, *supra* note 22, at 86–87.

[26] *Id.*

[27] World Health Assembly, Revision of the International Health Regulations, WHA58.3 (May 23, 2005).

[28] *Id.*

[29] *Id.*

as medical examination, vaccination, requirement of providing medical documents, and even providing financial support for those persons under quarantine or isolation.[30]

Application of State, Federal, and WHO Public Health Measures During the 2014 Ebola Outbreak

Ebola virus disease fatality rates exceed those of some of the most serious infectious disease threats of the last century, such as H5N1, SARS, and the 1918, 1957, and 1968 influenza pandemics. There is a high rate of infection by contact with containment patients, although the risk of transmission varies. In terms of a basic strategy for fighting the disease, it may be compared to firefighting in three zones: the middle of the hot zone is to identify the cases and contacts; the next zone is to stop the spread; the third zone is to increase preparedness of all other countries.

In the United States, the response to Ebola raised once again questions about the appropriate balance between measures that address the outbreak and the policies necessary to protect the US population. Although Ebola cases occurring in the United States were well managed, with only two fatalities, there were wide calls for isolation and quarantine, as well as majority support for suspension of air travel from "Ebola-stricken" countries. As the *Economist* noted, the question of protecting the US population was one of "bridges versus walls."[31] Indeed, during the outbreak, many African countries introduced flight bans.

While the sentiment behind a "walls" approach is understandable given the fear of the disease, the consensus in the public health community is that such an approach would magnify the problem. Shutting off the afflicted countries would create barriers for humanitarian and medical staff to treat patients and provide support, other, more hazardous travel routes would spring up, and the effect on the local economies would be severe. Using "bridges," it is possible to leave access to the countries open while allowing as many able healthcare workers as possible to assist in the response. For example, using exit screening in Guinea, Liberia, and Sierra Leone; assessing risk of exposure at airports; and screening for potential contact allowed aid and health agencies to marshal the necessary resources to bring new Ebola cases to zero in Liberia in May, with rapid decreases in new cases in Guinea and Sierra Leone as well.

For confirmed cases, WHO recommended that patients be isolated and treated. Those in contact with such patients should be monitored daily and restricted from traveling, unless a medical evacuation could be done safely. An international travel

---

[30] *Id.*
[31] *The spread of Ebola: bridges or walls*, Economist (Oct. 11, 2014).

ban was never recommended and, indeed, would have stymied the response. In short, the question used to frame the approach to this chapter: "May I? Should I?" was effectively implemented in the Ebola context. Although state, federal, and international regulatory structures might have authorized greater use of restrictions on exposed or infected persons, the decision was balanced with the approach necessary to control the spread of the disease.

Conclusion

Past experience has shown that voluntary cooperation and public trust are key ingredients of a successful response to a public health emergency. They may be important antidotes to individual fear and community panic that may be engendered by infectious disease outbreaks. Careful attention to the ethical values at stake in public health decision-making can help foster voluntary cooperation and public trust and should be a part of state and federal pandemic preparedness planning.

The growth in global migration will only increase as globalization creates more interconnectedness between peoples, goods, and services. Along with this movement will be greater risks for the spread of infectious disease. This chapter has illustrated that there are measures that can accommodate both large scale migration and the protection of public health from infectious disease emergencies.

References

Blendon RJ, DesRoches CM, Cetron MS, Benson JM, Meinhardt T, Pollard W. *Attitudes toward the use of quarantine in a public health emergency in four countries.* Health Affairs (Millwood) (Jan. 2006).

Centers for Disease Control and Prevention. Legal Authorities for Isolation and Quarantine. Available at http://www.cdc.gov/quarantine/aboutlawsregulationsquarantineisolation.html.

Cetron, M., and J. Landwirth. *Public health and ethical considerations in planning for quarantine.* 78 Yale Journal of Biology and Medicine 325 (2005).

Cole, Jared P. Federal and State Quarantine and Isolation Authority. Congressional Research Service Report (2004).

Department of Homeland Security. Yearbook of Immigration Statistics: 2012. Refugees and Asylees. Available at http://www.dhs.gov/yearbook-immigration-statistics-2012-refugees-and-asylees.

Fidler, David, and Lawrence O. Gostin. *The new International Health Regulations: an historic development for international law and public health.* 34 J. L. Med. & Ethics 85, 86–87 (2006).

Fidler, David, Lawrence O. Gostin, and Howard Markel. *Through the quarantine looking glass: drug-resistant tuberculosis and public health governance, law and ethics.* 35 J. L. Med. & Ethics 616 (2007).

Misrahi JJ, Foster JA, Shaw FE, Cetron MS. *HHS/CDC legal response to SARS outbreak.* 10 Emerg Infect Dis 353–355 (2004).

Shaw, F., Karen L. McKie, Clint A. Liveoak, Richard A. Goodman, and the State Public Health Counsel Review Team. Variation in Quarantine Powers Among the 10 Most Populous US States in 2004. Available at http://www.ncbi.nlm.nih.gov/pmc/articles/PMC1854981/pdf/0970038.pdf.

The spread of Ebola: bridges or walls. Economist (Oct. 11, 2014). Available at http://www.economist.com/news/international/21623711-panicky-response-west-may-worsen-conditions-west-africa-bridges-or-walls.

Wingate, La'Marcus T., et al. *Cost-effectiveness of screening and treating foreign-born students for tuberculosis before entering the United States.* 10(4) PLoS ONE (2015).

World Health Organization. International Health Regulations (IHR) (2005). Available at http://apps.who.int/iris/bitstream/10665/43883/1/9789241580410_eng.pdf.

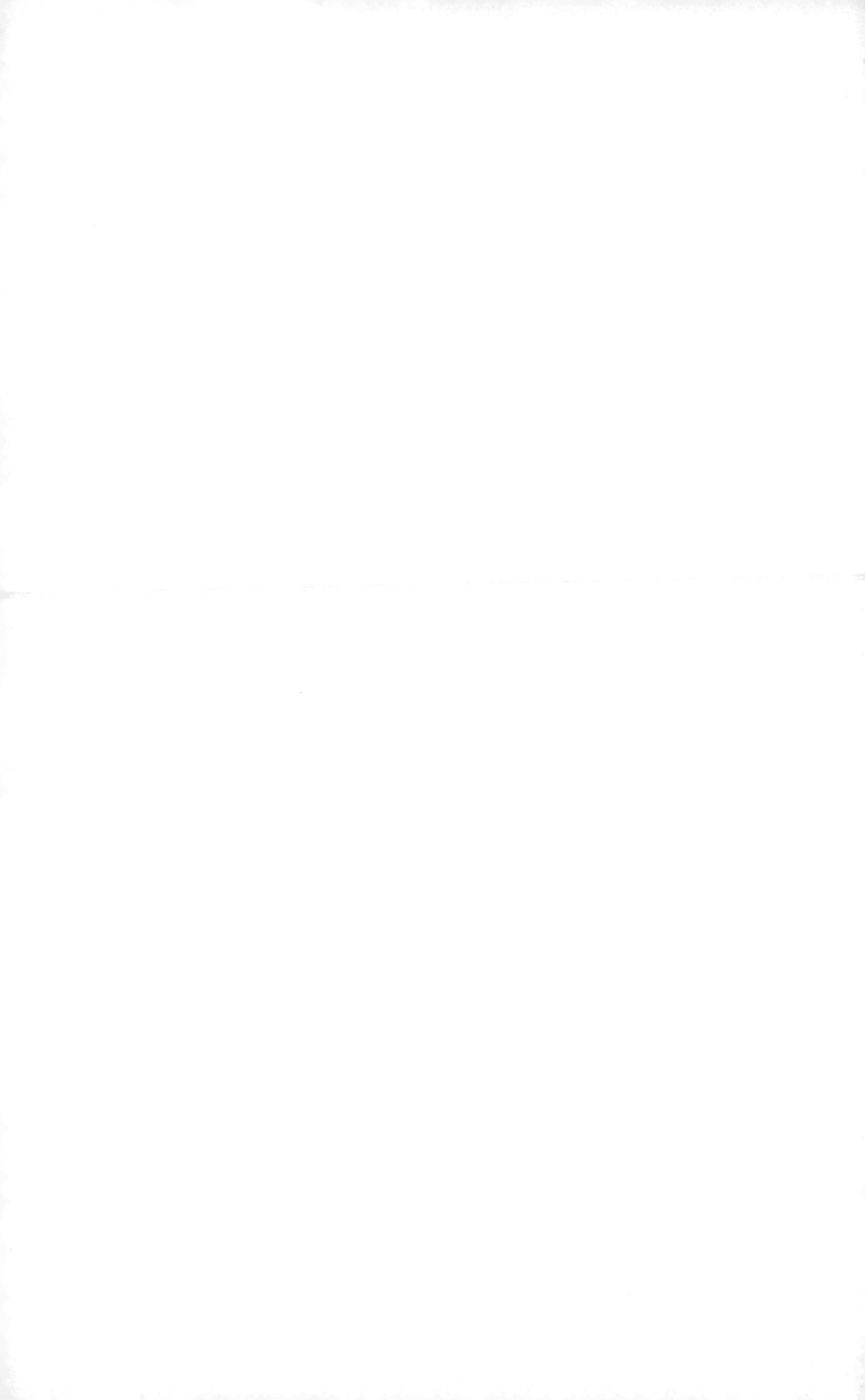

Epilogue

Plagues

Professional and Personal Reflections on Ebola, Polio, and Zika

RENÉE C. FOX

Since March 2014, when the world became aware of the severity of the outbreak of the hemorrhagic viral disease Ebola in West Africa, I have intently followed the trajectory of this lethal infectious disease of as yet unidentified origins. Although progress has been made, there remains no therapeutic drug or preventive vaccine for Ebola. When the outbreak occurred, it could not be diagnosed before a person incubating it became clinically ill, and the only way to stop its incidence was to break through the chains of transmission.

Ebola spread exponentially in three West African countries—Guinea, Liberia, and Sierra Leone—and became epidemic. According to the data issued by the US Centers for Disease Control and Prevention (CDC) in conjunction with the World Health Organization (WHO), by October 29, 2014, a total of 13,676 persons in these three countries had contracted Ebola, 4,910 of whom had died. By November 14, 2014, these figures were updated to a total of 14,383 cases, with 5,165 deaths. "Limited transmission" of Ebola had occurred in Nigeria (20 cases, with 1 death), in Spain (1 case, with no deaths), and in the United States (4 cases, with 1 death). There also had been 2 "travel-associated" cases—one in Mali and one in Senegal. The case in Mali was followed by 3 others, and all 4 were fatal. Concurrently with these outbreaks, but epidemiologically unrelated to them, a less virulent, more contained strain of the virus emerged in the equator region of the Democratic Republic of Congo. By late October, 38 laboratory-confirmed and 28 probable cases had been reported there, with a toll of 49 deaths. On October 17 and October 18, respectively, the outbreaks of Ebola in Nigeria and Senegal were declared over, when 42 days had elapsed in those locales since the last patient in isolation had become laboratory negative for the disease.

This was the 25th time that Ebola had occurred on the continent of Africa since its first known outbreak in Zaïre (now the Democratic Republic of Congo) in 1976. But the scope of the recent epidemic in West Africa, the rapidity with which it spread, and its mortality rate there were unprecedented. It was the biggest and deadliest Ebola outbreak on record. International recognition that this time the proportions that Ebola had developed constituted a public health emergency and humanitarian crisis of global import was belated—a delay that retrospectively was largely attributed to the shortsightedness and shortcomings of WHO.

The occurrence, spread, and effects of Ebola, and the reactions to it, have evocative personal meaning for me. To begin with, they are associated with two of the milieux in which I have conducted many years of firsthand sociological research: in Zaïre/the Democratic Republic of Congo; and inside of Doctors Without Borders /Médecins Sans Frontières (MSF), the international medical humanitarian organization that, since the inception of the Ebola outbreak in Guinea in March 2014, was on the ground in West Africa, providing most of the care of patients there stricken with the disease, while calling out to the world about the massive international mobilization of human and technical resources needed to cope with and curb an epidemic of this magnitude. MSF had some 3,400 staff dealing with Ebola in West Africa, where, as of the end of October 2014, it had treated more than 60% of all Ebola patients. It sent more than 700 international ("expatriate") staff members to the region, operated 15 Ebola management centers and transit centers in the three most affected countries, operating up to 8 simultaneously that provided approximately 600 beds in isolation units, and admitted more than 5,600 patients to these centers. Of these patients, 3,500 were diagnosed with Ebola, among whom 1,400 survived.

My own medical history also connects me with Ebola—most particularly through my experience as a patient with bulbar and spinal poliomyelitis in the mid-1940s, during a period in the United States when a polio epidemic occurred in some region of this country virtually every summer. There was no medicine to treat it, and no vaccine then existed to prevent it or produce immunity to it.

Another way in which I feel linked to the Ebola scene is a rather ironic one. It conjures up for me vivid memories of the three decades after World War II when the imminent worldwide "conquest" of infectious diseases was being hubristically heralded.

**

The media abounded in feature articles and programs about the Ebola epidemic.[1] I not only kept in touch with as many of these publications as I could, but because

---

[1] For example, *the New York Times* reported on December 6, 2014, that since late July, "more than 70 front-page Ebola stories have been published, carrying the bylines of nearly three dozen Times writers," and that the paper had "produced more than 350 articles about Ebola this year." Margaret Sullivan, *Journalism in the time of Ebola*, New York Times, Sunday Review Section 8 (December 7, 2014).

of the publication of my book about MSF,[2] I was interviewed a number of times by journalists about the attributes of MSF that I thought accounted for the fact that its provided the first responders to the Ebola crisis in West Africa and continued to be the primary medical aid group there on the front lines of battling the disease, its human ravages, and its epidemic spread. However, it was not via the media, but rather through MSF's websites—including its blogs, and the detailed Ebola response update document that it circulated every week to its headquarters, missions, and partner sections—and also the emails that I received from members of MSF whom I personally know, and from Suzanne Mikanda, my close friend and colleague in the Democratic Republic of Congo,[3] that I felt the most in touch with what healthcare workers, patients, and their families in Ebola-stricken African countries were experiencing.

Members of MSF described "the reality of the lives of people" in the three West African countries as "overwhelming". One described the situation as being like "nothing I have ever had to deal with in my life"; another referred to the "devastation, despair, and helplessness as whole families are wiped out"; and still others mentioned the especially heartbreaking deaths of so many children and the numbers of deaths that were occurring from other diseases that are normally treatable, like malaria, tuberculosis, and HIV/AIDS, due to the fact that the hospitals were filled with Ebola patients. All this, they said, was taking place in societies pervaded with poverty, whose pre-Ebola healthcare systems were rudimentary and barely functional to begin with—in Liberia and Sierra Leone, partly as a consequence of years of civil war. In their dispatches from the field, MSF staff depicted their "workload" as "enormous" and "extremely challenging, both physically and emotionally." They made reference to how intensely uncomfortable and depleting it was in high tropical temperatures for them to be encased in the personal protective gear that they were required to wear when they worked in the treatment centers—consisting of whole-body suits with safety goggles, breathing masks, three pairs of gloves, plastic aprons, and rubber boots—and how, regrettably, because they had to be careful to avoid hyperthermia and dehydration, this limited the intervals of time they could spend with Ebola patients. They expressed concern about whether in these circumstances they were giving patients optimal care. And they poignantly alluded to the fact that being swathed as they were restricted their ability to touch patients and to comfort them by holding their hands when frightened patients

---

[2] Renée C. Fox, Doctors Without Borders: Humanitarian Quests, Impossible Dreams of Médecins Sans Frontières (2014).

[3] For more details about Suzanne Mikanda, our relationship, and the sociological research we conducted together in the Congo, see Renée C. Fox, In the Field: A Sociologist's Journey 178–181, 183–186) and Renée C. Fox, In The Belgian Château: The Spirit And Culture Of A European Society In An Age Of Change 230–293 (1994). In my book *In the Belgian Château*, I gave Suzanne the pseudonym Sabine Mosabu to protect her identity at the time the book was published.

entreated them to do so.[4] Their own risk of contracting Ebola was mentioned in some of the MSF "voices from the field" dispatches, but it was not dramatized—even though 24 MSF workers had contracted Ebola, and 13 had died from it.[5] However, many said that MSF had been "stretched to its limits" in dealing with the velocity and scope of the disease's deadly trajectory, and they expressed how "anxious," "stressed," "angry," and "frustrated" they felt because of what they regarded as the inexcusable tardiness and inadequacy of the international community's response:

> How do we justify the global dragging of heels whilst thousands of persons die needlessly? . . . The angry frustration bubbling under my skin. International powers continue to remain limp in their response. Big statements, big ideas, but little feet on the ground. This epidemic never needed to explode, the fuse was in clear sight of everyone, slow motion and totally predictable.[6]

And yet, "amidst all the loss and suffering," an article posted on MSF South Africa's website affirmed, "There are stories of survival":

> Today, out of all the patients cared for in MSF's projects in Guinea, Sierra Leone, and Liberia, we celebrate the one thousandth survivor.[7]

A dispatch posted by an MSF physician working in Sierra Leone jubilantly reported that "a day of three miracles" had just occurred when "two of our sickest-ever patients were discharged, and a baby girl survived against all odds." She went on to describe the friendship group that had been formed by some of the women who had nearly recovered from Ebola and were waiting for a final negative test result before being discharged: "They take baths together, tell jokes, run races along the corridor to keep fit, and dance together." "I danced along with them in my protective suit," she exclaimed.[8]

---

[4] Hilde de Clerck, Struggling to Contain the Ebola Epidemic in West Africa (July 8, 2014), available at http://www.doctorswithoutborders.org/news-stories/voice-field/struggling-contain-ebola-epidemic-west-africa.

[5] David Gauthier Villars and Jeanne Whalen, *Ebola crisis stretches Doctors Without Borders' means*, Wall Street Journal, A6 (Nov. 29–30, 2014).

[6] Benjamin Black, May the forceps be with you, available at http://blogs.msf.org/en/staff/blogs/may-the-forceps-be-with-you. In recognition of how stressful it was to be dealing with Ebola under existing conditions, MSF rotated the expatriate medical staff whom they sent into the field in West Africa every 5 to 6 weeks rather than maintaining them there uninterruptedly for a longer period of time. Usually, MSF field assignments have a duration of at least 6 months.

[7] Alexander Kollie, *My son is MSF's 1000th survivor* (Oct. 21, 2014), available at http://www.msf.org/article/my-son-msf%E2%80%99s-1000th-ebola-survivor.

[8] Monica Arend-Trujillo, *Ebola: "Three Miracles" in Bo, Sierra Leone* (Nov. 20, 2014), available at http://www.doctorswithoutborders.org/article/ebola-three-miracles-bo-sierra-leone.

Furthermore, a physician who has been continually associated with MSF throughout most of his professional career and is currently working in South Africa informed me that MSF is "receiving an overwhelming number of candidates volunteering for Ebola fieldwork—many more than the number of postings we can provide." He attributed this in part to the fact that "everyone in the organization— even ones who had not worked for MSF in years felt compelled to contribute and volunteer to go [where] 'comrades' are involved." "Solidarity between volunteers" and "solidarity with people in need" account for it, he said. Notwithstanding the kind of solidarity that makes MSF a "movement" and "not just an organization," he assured me that they continue in their "typical MSF self-critical style" to debate such issues as whether they waited too long before speaking up about the need for an Ebola vaccine to control an epidemic of this magnitude, and if so, why.

* * *

I received news about the occurrence of Ebola in the Democratic Republic of Congo from Suzanne Mikanda. It was based on her observations in Kinshasa, where she lives, on the news conveyed to her by family members who resided in the Equator province where the Ebola cases were centered, and on information bulletins issued by the Kinshasa office of the UN Secretariat's Bureau of Coordination of Humanitarian Affairs.[9] In her emails, Suzanne addresses me as "Yaya" (which means "older sister" in Lingala) because we have remained closely tied to one another, in a kinship-like way, since we conducted sociological research together during the 1960s in the Congo.

She described the "panic" that ensued when the Congolese government first declared on August 24 that an outbreak of Ebola was occurring in the country—one that the UN bulletin stated was the seventh such outbreak to occur there since 1976 but was "unrelated" to the epidemic taking place in West Africa.

It was the Christian churches, more than the government, Suzanne related, that were protecting the members of their congregations—advising them to avoid shaking hands when greeting people, to wash their hands frequently with the medicinal soap Monganga, and to be careful not to buy food that had been exposed to flies. MSF responded immediately to the Ebola outbreak, she informed me, by sending in tons of relevant supplies and equipment and opening two treatment centers in Lakolia and Boende in the equator zone, where Ebola had erupted.[10] But, she reported, it had been difficult to convince some members of the local population

---

[9] Suzanne writes to me in French. I have translated the information and explanations she shared with me into English. When I thanked her for the research about Ebola in the Congo that she had conducted on my behalf, she replied: "I always like to do research, and to share with, and receive from others what I can. It always makes me happy, and helps me to move forward with what is presently happening in the world."

[10] This was facilitated by the fact that MSF has been working in the Democratic Republic of Congo since 1981 where, at the end of 2012, it had as many as 2,782 staff members; and that its so-called Pool d' Urgence Congo (Congo Emergency Pool) plays an epidemiological monitoring, evaluation, and intervention role in the country.

that because victims of Ebola are highly infectious when they die, and remain so for an indeterminate amount of time, it was imperative for their burial to be conducted quickly and in a way that did not transmit the virus to participants in the burial rituals. There are certain respects, Suzanne pointed out, in which traditional African cultural practices and the beliefs with which they are associated—most notably, the ritual washing of the deceased person's body by designated family members—run counter to the procedures for a safe burial. And so, "it has not always been easy," Suzanne wrote, "to isolate and deal with the deceased. There have been instances in which families have come and seized the bodies, washed them, and buried them according to custom." This is not only because it is the traditional way of respecting and honoring the dead, she explained, but also because they believe that "evil spirits and witchcraft" underlie the occurrence of Ebola, and that, therefore, if the traditional procedures and rites are not observed, these spirits will be angered and will cause even more "misfortune and perturbation" to befall the community.

On October 15, Suzanne informed me that a total of 66 cases of Ebola had been reported in the Democratic Republic of Congo, with 49 deaths. The physician in charge of dealing with Ebola in Boende had just announced over the national radio network, OKAPI, that no new cases of Ebola had occurred during the past 15 days, and that if this persisted over a period of 42 days, the country could be declared free of Ebola.

The next email that I received from Suzanne brought the news that on November 15, the national Minister of Health had announced the probable end of Ebola in the equator region. Nevertheless, he advised the population to continue to protect themselves by observing the prohibitions against touching when they greeted each other, and against eating animals "hunted and killed in the forest" and the meat of monkeys and bats. However, Suzanne reported, some people were ignoring the admonition about what foods were dangerous to eat because, they said, this has been our food since the time of our ancestors. Still, Suzanne concluded, with regard to the overall Ebola situation, "Light is beginning to appear."

On November 21, WHO officially declared that Ebola had been eradicated from the Democratic Republic of Congo, where there had been no Ebola cases in 42 days.

Suzanne's concerns about the health situation in the Congo were not confined to Ebola. With a mixture of dismay and indignation, she has written to me in the past about the deplorable physical state of the capital city of Kinshasa. Its pervasive filthy and unsanitary conditions, she says, its infestation by mosquitoes, and its poorly functioning healthcare system contribute to the high incidence of many forms of sickness among its population. In this connection, in her account to me about the Ebola situation, she mentioned that recently she had again been felled by an attack of malaria, which she attributed both to the fact that mosquitoes seem to "like me a lot" and to the overall "dirtiness" of Kinshasa.

* * *

On October 23, 2014, a chain of events brought me to the threshold of a new interlude in the way that medical professionals, public health experts, governmental and intergovernmental organizations, local and national US politicians, the media, and the American public were reacting to the Ebola epidemic. On that day, I was scheduled to be one of four participants in a live evening panel discussion in the auditorium of the public television station WHYY in Philadelphia—"Principles, Ethics and Dilemmas: Becoming Doctors Without Borders"—co-organized by Doctors Without Borders and the publisher of my book about them, the Johns Hopkins University Press. The chief panelist among us was expected to be Sophie Delaunay, who was then the executive director of Doctors Without Borders–USA. However, she did not make an appearance because, as the MSF public and internal events manager who had arranged the discussion quietly informed the other panelists, upon her arrival in Philadelphia she had immediately turned around and traveled back to her New York office when she received the news that an MSF physician, who had recently returned to that city from Guinea, where he had been taking care of Ebola patients, had tested positive for the Ebola virus and had been rushed to Bellevue Hospital. In a nonofficious way, the MSF events manager made it known to the panelists and to WHYY's behavioral health reporter who was the moderator for our discussion, that the reason for Sophie Delaunay's absence would not be given to the assembled audience.

Notwithstanding MSF's discretion about communicating what had happened, by 8:30 p.m., when I was back in my apartment, I turned on CNN television news, and the story of the MSF physician who had contracted Ebola was being dramatically telecast in a way that eclipsed all the other evening news. Since his arrival in New York on October 17, it was reported, this doctor—now identified as Craig Spencer, a 33-year-old emergency medicine physician associated with the New York–Presbyterian Hospital/Columbia University Medical Center—had been moving around in the city, jogging along the Hudson River, riding the subway, taking a cab, going bowling, frequenting a coffee stand, and eating at a meatball shop. On the morning of October 23, the newscasts recounted, he developed a temperature of 101.3, and it was not until then that he was transported to the special Ebola unit at Bellevue Hospital, where he was put in isolation. The stories about Dr. Spencer that were featured by television, radio, newspapers, and magazines during the days that followed criticized him for failing to quarantine himself upon his return from Guinea rather than "running around" the city while he was "sick" and thereby potentially exposing many others to Ebola. But, in fact, Dr. Spencer was not ill with Ebola or contagious until he developed fever; even then, his infecting others with the virus could have occurred only through their contact with his body fluids. Furthermore, upon his reentry to the United States, he had gone through a debriefing process in MSF-USA's New York office, following which he had adhered to MSF's guidelines for staff members returning from

Ebola-affected West Africa. Those guidelines included checking his temperature twice a day, finishing a regular course of malaria prophylaxis (because malaria symptoms can mimic those of Ebola), staying within 4 hours of a hospital with isolation facilities, being continually aware of relevant Ebola symptoms, and immediately contacting the MSF-USA office if any such symptoms developed. In addition, he was abiding by the MSF recommendation to returning staff not to resume their professional work for 21 days in order to regain their energy and protect their health after the challenging and exhausting work they had done in the field.

The dramatically critical way in which the media presented the story about Dr. Spencer, including the misinformation about his contagious state, had the immediate effect of raising public anxiety about the imminent danger of a widespread outbreak of Ebola in the United States. It also contributed to the entry of politics and politicians on the scene. MSF received a call from a high-ranking politician in Washington, DC, requesting that the organization limit further recruitment of volunteers to go to West Africa. And the day after Dr. Spencer was hospitalized, both New York governor Andrew Cuomo and New Jersey governor Chris Christie announced the establishment of a mandatory 21-day quarantine in their respective states for all healthcare workers returning from Ebola-affected countries in West Africa, whether or not they had symptoms of Ebola upon their arrival. The policies they instituted did not accord with those of the CDC or with the opinion of public health experts who opposed such mandatory quarantines on scientific and medical grounds. CDC and public health experts were also concerned that these overly cautious, restrictive measures of cordoning off those who had gone to West Africa to care for persons affected with Ebola, and the lack of recognition and esteem for them that this appeared to connote, might result in discouraging additional health professionals who were greatly needed to control the Ebola epidemic at its African epicenter (thereby also helping to keep Ebola from coming to our shores) from volunteering to do likewise.

Governors Cuomo and Christie's mandatory 21-day quarantine policy for all persons entering the country through the John F. Kennedy and the Newark Liberty airports who had had contact with Ebola patients in Guinea, Liberia, or Sierra Leone was immediately implemented when Kaci Hickox, a nurse who had been working with Doctors Without Borders caring for Ebola patients in Sierra Leone, landed at the Newark airport. There, immigration officials detained her for hours, subsequently took her temperature that they erroneously considered to be above normal, after which, accompanied by a police escort with sirens blaring, she was transported to University Hospital in Newark. When the physicians at the hospital took her temperature, it proved to be a normal 98.6 degrees. But despite her lack of fever or any other symptoms of Ebola, garbed in paper scrubs, she was put in an isolation tent on the hospital's grounds.

Kaci Hickox's experiences were even more histrionically reported by the media than Dr. Spencer's, partly because she chose to go public and "fight back"—deeming the way she had been treated "unacceptable," "inhumane," a "violation of [her] basic human rights," and a "big deterrent" to healthcare workers' willingness to go to West Africa to treat Ebola patients. She also hired a lawyer to represent her, who negotiated for her to be released from the hospital and permitted to travel home to Maine. Initially, Maine officials asked her to voluntarily quarantine herself in her house until November 10, when 21 days would have passed since her last contact with Ebola patients—an arrangement that would be involuntarily enforced if she resisted it. In the end, the chief judge for the Maine District Court lifted this measure on the grounds that Ms. Hickox did not show symptoms of Ebola and therefore was not infectious. However, the judge's order required her to submit to daily monitoring for symptoms, to coordinate her travel with state officials, and to notify them immediately if symptoms appeared—conditions to which she agreed. All these details of her case were closely followed and prominently reported by journalists.

Ms. Hickox refrained from moving about in the small town where she lives, though she and her partner took a morning bike ride on a trail near her house—followed by a Maine state trooper and members of the press, including photographers. She did not develop Ebola.

Dr. Craig Spencer recovered from Ebola and was discharged from Bellevue Hospital on November 11, 2014. "While my case has garnered international attention," he said in the public statement that he made at that time, "it is important to remember that my infection represents but a fraction of the more than 13,000 reported cases to date in West Africa—the center of the outbreak where families are being torn apart and communities destroyed." As he said in the public statement that he made at that time:

> It is for this reason that I volunteered to work in Guinea with Doctors Without Borders. For over five weeks, I worked in an Ebola treatment center in Guéckédou, the epicenter of the outbreak.
>
> During this time, I cried as I held children who were not strong enough to survive the virus. But, I also experienced immense joy when patients we treated were cured and invited me into their family as a brother upon discharge. Within a week of my diagnosis, many of those same patients called my personal phone to wish me well and ask if there was any way they could contribute to my care. Most incredibly, I watched my Guinean colleagues, who have been on the front lines since day one and saw friends and family members die, continue to fight to save their communities with so much compassion and dignity. They are the heroes that we are not talking about.
>
> Please join me in turning our attention back to West Africa, and ensuring that medical volunteers and other aid workers do not face stigma and

threats upon their return home. Volunteers need to be supported to help fight the outbreak at its source.[11]

* * *

By the end of October 2014, a veritable patchwork of different rules and procedures for quarantining doctors, nurses, and other healthcare professionals returning to the United States from Ebola-stricken West African countries had developed on the American scene. The US CDC held that mandatory quarantines for all medical workers coming back from Guinea, Liberia, and Sierra Leone were not scientifically based or justified. But it advised monitoring these individuals' health on a daily basis by taking their temperature and having them check in with a local health department official. To varying degrees, states such as Illinois and Florida, and also the District of Columbia, were following CDC guidelines. However, along with New Jersey and New York, California, Connecticut, Georgia, and Maine established stricter policies. And the Pentagon instituted the strictest policy of all: a mandatory 21-day quarantine on their home base for troops returning from the military's Ebola mission in West Africa.

Throughout the month of October, many incidents occurred in the United States associated with the widespread anxiety and fear about the imminent danger of contracting or transmitting Ebola. For example, a 7-year-old girl in Connecticut was barred from attending her elementary school because she had traveled to Nigeria with her parents to attend a family wedding.[12] The executive director of the Liberian Ministers Association of Minnesota reported that congregants in that network of some 50 churches were being "seen as a carrier of a virus . . . instead of being seen as a person," and that several church members who were healthcare workers had been "asked to go home from work after sneezing or coughing."[13] Researchers who had been in Guinea, Liberia, or Sierra Leone during the 3 weeks before the annual meeting of the American Society of Tropical Medicine and Hygiene took place in New Orleans were advised by the organization not to come to the meeting because the Louisiana health department would quarantine them by confining them to their hotel rooms.[14] And a Catholic bishop in Rochester, New York, forbade the priests in

---

[11] Statement from Dr. Craig Spencer (Nov. 11, 2014), available at http://www.doctorswithoutborders.org/article/statement-dr-craig-spencer.

[12] Ariel Kaminer, *Girl 7, barred from a Connecticut school over Ebola concerns goes back to class*, New York Times, A20 (Nov. 1, 2014).

[13] Jennifer Maloney, Scott Calvert, and Derek Kravitz, *For U.S. Liberians, stigma adds to Ebola's burden*, Wall Street Journal (Oct. 20, 2014), available at http://www.wsj.com/articles/for-u-s-liberians-stigma-adds-to-ebolas-burden-1413830673. Minnesota has the largest Liberian immigrant population in the United States.

[14] Jason Beaubien, *Ebola researchers banned from medical meeting in New Orleans*," NPR (Oct. 30, 2014), available at http://www.npr.org/sections/health-shots/2014/10/30/360179428/ebola-researchers-banned-from-medical-meeting-in-new-orleans.

his diocese to travel to West Africa or other countries in Africa because of the "seriousness of the Ebola epidemic" and out of "pastoral concern for the people of God here in Rochester."[15] Such anxiety and fear were also expressed through the way that some people working at Bellevue Hospital where Dr. Craig Spencer was being cared for in its Ebola unit were publicly shunned or discriminated against. Even within the hospital, nurses caring for him in that unit noticed that staff members who worked on other services tried to keep as much physical distance as possible from them in the hospital elevators.[16]

* * *

My absorption in the unfolding of the Ebola epidemic reawakened some of my memories of the polio epidemics in the United States during my youth, and of my personal experiences as a polio patient. Among them are recollections of how fearful parents became about the danger of their children contracting the disease with the approach of each summer—the season of the year when epidemic outbreaks usually occurred. Although the etiology of the disease and how it was transmitted were not yet fully understood, parents anxiously tried to protect their children from polio by keeping them out of public swimming pools and movie theaters, ice cream parlors, soda fountains, and restaurants that did not seem to be impeccably clean, and away from large public gatherings; by warning them not to use public toilets, public telephones, or drinking fountains and not to buy food from street vendors; and by taking precautionary measures to keep them from becoming overly tired. And on the assumption that, especially during the hot summer months, urban milieux were not as healthy as those outside of cities, parents who could afford to do so sent their children to camps in the mountains and/or on lakes in the countryside, or arranged long family vacations at the seashore, where they could benefit from what were regarded as the fortifying properties of "fresh" ocean air.

It was not only parents and members of the general public who reacted to the danger of polio with wariness and fear. So did some members of the medical profession and some hospitals. In connection with my own case, this took a rather dramatic form. On August 15, 1945, when our family physician made a home visit to the apartment where I lived with my parents in response to their alarmed call to him about how progressively ill I was becoming, he observed that in addition to

---

[15] David Andreatta, *New York bishop bans priest travel to West Africa*, Rochester (N.Y.) Democrat & Chronicle (Nov. 4, 2014), available at http://www.usatoday.com/story/news/nation/2014/11/04/bishop-ban-ebola-africa-travel/18461573/.

[16] Anemona Hartocollis and Nate Schweber, *Bellevue employees face Ebola at work, and stigma of it everywhere*, International New York Times (Oct. 29, 2014), available at http://www.nytimes.com/2014/10/30/nyregion/bellevue-workers-worn-out-from-treating-ebola-patient-face-stigma-outside-hospital.html?_r=0.

developing flaccid paralysis in my legs, I was having difficulty swallowing because the muscles in my throat did not seem to be functioning normally. His diagnosis was that I was succumbing to a life-threatening bulbospinal form of polio, which made it urgent to get me to a hospital as quickly as possible. August 15 was V-J Day, which marked Japan's surrender and the end of World War II. The throngs of celebrating people who filled the streets made it difficult for an ambulance to wend its way through the crowds and rapidly transport me to a hospital. But hospitalizing me involved an even more fundamental problem. What our physician encountered was the reluctance of the New York City hospitals that he contacted to admit an acutely ill, highly infectious polio patient. In the end, through negotiations that I was too sick to follow, Sydenham Hospital in Harlem agreed to admit me. Sydenham had been founded in 1892 as a black hospital with an all-white administration and staff of doctors and nurses. At the time that it agreed to admit me, although its patient population was still predominantly black, it had recently become the first US voluntary hospital to adopt a fully desegregated interracial policy, naming African Americans to its board of trustees and to its medical and nursing staffs. My inpatient emergency care was immediately taken in hand by the hospital's white superintendent and his wife and by a black nurse who, without donning protective masks or gloves, worked side by side to apply moist hot packs to my body that by this time was racked by muscle spasms. The same nurse kept vigil by my bedside all through the first night of my hospitalization. Putting her head beside mine on my pillow, she breathed every breath with me as my breathing and swallowing became more labored. It was because of her courageous willingness to expose herself to the contagiousness of polio in this way, and her extraordinary devotion to my care, that I survived that night.

When the National Foundation for Infantile Paralysis opened a special inpatient polio unit in Knickerbocker Hospital (located at 113th Street and Convent Avenue, not far from Sydenham), I was transferred there. I spent 4 months at that unit before I was discharged from the hospital to continue my convalescence in Florida with the home care of a physical therapist and a nurse. The term "quarantined" was never explicitly applied to the Knickerbocker polio unit, but, in fact, it consisted of an entire hospital floor whose occupants were all polio patients and the special team of health professionals recruited to care for and "rehabilitate" us. It was isolated from all the other services in the hospital. Through occasional anecdotes related to us by some of our nurses, we learned of incidents in which personnel from other floors tried to avoid contact with them. I don't know whether or not it was a formal policy, but the only visitors we had from the "outside-of-the-hospital world" were our parents. I have retained a poignant memory over the years of the one time that I saw my brother and sister during my long hospitalization, when they stood in the street directly below my hospital room, and with the help of my physical therapist, I was able to move close enough to its window to wave to them.

By the summer of 1946, I was reunited with my family. We vacationed together at Arrowhead Springs Hotel in San Bernardino, California, where my parents thought I might benefit from the dry, warm climate, its hot springs, and the hotel's outstanding swimming pool. It was a rather posh resort at the time, frequented by many Hollywood movie stars—a fact that delighted my young sister, who eagerly sought the autographs of those whom she recognized. I was still walking with the aid of crutches, and a number of the hotel guests seemed to know this was because I had had polio. That knowledge appeared to evoke as much anxiety as sympathy from some of them. The most notable encounter that my sister had in this connection occurred when she approached the table of a movie star who was breakfasting in the hotel's dining room and asked him for his autograph. He responded by drawing back in his chair, nervously inquiring whether I was "still contagious," and refusing to touch the autograph book and pen that my sister held out to him.

* * *

The other set of memories that my following of the 2014 Ebola epidemic evoked are antithetical to my lived experiences as a polio patient. They are recollections of the euphoric optimism that prevailed among Western physicians and medical scientists in the 1950s through 1970s about the progress that had been made toward eradicating every infectious disease that affected human beings. Key advances that were viewed as milestones toward reaching this victorious state were the discovery, development, and application of antibiotic drugs and of the Salk polio vaccine. Peter Piot, the co-discoverer of the Ebola virus, has described how in 1974, when he was about to complete his medical school studies, he "broached the idea of specializing in infectious diseases" with his teachers. "The unanimous verdict of my professors," Piot has recounted, "was that I would be a fool to do so." As he elaborated, "My professor of social medicine grabbed my shoulder firmly, to make sure I was paying attention. 'There's no future in infectious diseases,' he stated flatly, in a tone that bore no argument. 'They've all been solved.'"[17] The current era of "emerging," "new," and "re-emerging" or "resurging" "old" infectious diseases, in which Ebola has made its appearance, was inconceivable at that time.

HIV/AIDS, malaria, measles, tuberculosis, various strains of influenza, severe acute respiratory syndrome (SARS), Middle East respiratory syndrome (MERS), typhoid fever, West Nile virus, Lassa fever, Marburg virus (related to the Ebola virus), and, most recently, Zika virus are among the numerous infectious epidemic diseases presently occurring in the world to which human beings are susceptible. Along with biological and biomedical factors—such as the genetic mutation of the viruses involved, and the development of drug-resistant forms

---

[17] Peter Piot (with Ruth Marshall), No Time To Lose: A Life in Pursuit of Deadly Viruses 6 (2012). This footnote should read: Peter Piot (with Ruth Marshall), No Time to Lose: A Life in Pursuit of Deadly Viruses. New York and London: W.W. Norton & Company, 2012, p. 6.

of some of these diseases—climatic, economic, political, social, and cultural factors are contributing to their etiology and their spread. In addition, partly as a consequence of the overuse or misappropriate use of antibiotics, a significant increase in the incidence of serious, potentially fatal infections with a bacterium called *Clostridium difficile* (or *C. diff*) has been taking place in the United States. Furthermore, in the wake of the Ebola outbreak in Liberia, Guinea, and Sierra Leone and the extent to which the resources of those countries have been focused on responding to it at the expense of other health-relevant activities, there is an increased risk of the growing occurrence of measles, malaria, tuberculosis, and HIV/AIDS in those countries.

I am mindful of the enormous progress that has been made in medical scientific knowledge and clinical medicine since 1945 when I was a 17-year-old polio patient, And I am aware that "the global initiative to eliminate poliomyelitis through vaccination has helped to reduce the number of cases by more than 99% in 30 years."[18]

But polio is surging again in Pakistan, where, during the first week of October 2014, "the country reported 202 cases of paralysis, the first time in 14 years the figure topped 200." This accounted for 85% of the world's polio cases. Polio vaccination has not taken place for several years in the North Waziristan region of Pakistan, where it has been banned by the Taliban, who have "killed some fifty vaccinators or their police escorts" since 2012. And "as many as 350,000 unvaccinated children" who have been driven out of that area "now live in slums all over the country."[19] With its "ballooning polio case count," Pakistan also "constantly reinfects neighboring Afghanistan."[20] And the incidence of polio is reported to have risen once more in Syria, partly as a result of the breakdown in the medical and public health systems in that country.

In addition, researchers have discovered a new, "vaccine-resistant polio strain [whose] DNA sequence shows two mutations unknown until now of the proteins that form the 'shell' (capsid) of the virus"—an "evolution [that] complicates the task for the antibodies produced by the immune system of the vaccinated patient as they can no longer recognize the viral strain."[21] This accounted for the "exceptionally high mortality rate" that occurred in an outbreak of polio in 2010 in the Republic of Congo. Out of the 445 confirmed cases, 210 persons died. Researchers feared that other variants of the polio virus might emerge among populations immunized with the vaccine. And, indeed, in November 2014, this did occur. Two cases of "vaccine-derived polio paralysis" caused by

---

[18] Institut de Recherche pour le Développement (IRD), *Vaccine-resistant polio strain discovered*, Science Daily (Nov. 4, 2014), available at http://www.sciencedaily.com/releases/2014/11/141104111408.htm?.

[19] Donald G. McNeil Jr., *Polio on the rise again in Pakistan, officials say*, International New York Times (Oct. 13, 2014), available at http://www.nytimes.com/2014/10/14/health/-polio-on-the-rise-again-in-pakistan-officials-say.html.

[20] Leslie Roberts, *Just one poliovirus left to go?*, 346(6211) Science 795 (Nov. 14, 2014).

[21] IRD, *supra* note 18.

mutating polio vaccine were found in South Sudan, and one case was found in Madagascar.[22]

* * *

By late 2014, the number of cases of Ebola was decreasing. However, the transmission of the disease continued steadily into 2015, and it was not until August that the incidence declined to numbers as low as 3 cases per week. As of mid-August 2015, a total of nearly 28,000 cases had occurred,[23] with more than 11,000 deaths. Twenty-eight MSF staff members had become infected with the Ebola virus. Twenty-four of them were national staff, among whom 14 persons died from the disease.[24] The possibility that transmission of Ebola could reignite still existed, but tentatively promising results with the clinical trial of a potentially effective Ebola vaccine—the vesicular stomatitis virus-Ebola virus vaccine rVSV-EBOV—were reported. And a WHO-led endeavor, in which MSF was involved, was being undertaken to create a biobank and a data platform for the research and development of new anti-Ebola products and diagnostic tools.

As the 2014–2015 Ebola epidemic waned, what an article in the journal *Lancet* colorfully described as a "parade of global heath specialists" assembled in a series of meetings to consider what accounted for the failure of the WHO and the international community to appropriately and adequately respond to the outbreak of Ebola in West Africa, and how to better "prepare [for], detect, and respond to epidemic diseases in the future."[25]

On September 8, 2015, the Albert and Mary Lasker Foundation announced that its Lasker-Bloomberg Public Service Award would go to Médecins Sans Frontières/ Doctors Without Borders for the "monumental" role it had played in fighting Ebola in West Africa, and for the front-line work in which it has been engaged over the course of many years in dealing with medical emergencies throughout the world. It is notable that the award citation included a statement that MSF's bold response and leadership in responding to the Ebola outbreak was a "duty" that "rightfully" should have been filled by the international community.[26]

* * *

---

[22] Donald G. McNeil Jr., *Rare vaccine-derived polio discovered in 2 countries*, International New York Times (Nov. 14, 2014), available at http://www.nytimes.com/2014/11/15/world/africa/rare-vaccine-derived-polio-discovered-in-2-countries.html. The "vaccine-derived" form is created when the attenuated virus used in the trivalent oral polio vaccine reverts to its virulent, transmissible form.

[23] This figure includes probable and suspected cases, as well as confirmed ones.

[24] Deane Marchbein, *The response to Ebola—looking back and looking ahead. The 2015 Lasker-Bloomberg Public Service Award*, Vol. 314, No. 11, JAMA (2015), pp. 1115–1116.

[25] Richard Horton, *Offline: a pervasive failure to learn the lessons of Ebola*, 386(9998) Lancet 1024 (Sept. 12, 2015), available at http://thelancet.com/journals/lancet/article/PIIS0140-6736(15)00152-X/fulltext.

[26] Denise Grady, *Lasker Prizes given for discoveries in cancer and genetics, and for Ebola response*, New York Times, A26 (Sept. 9, 2015).

On January 14, 2016, WHO declared that the Ebola epidemic had ended. This was the date on which for the first time since the inception of the epidemic, Guinea, Liberia, and Sierra Leone had all reported zero cases of Ebola for at least 42 days (i.e., two, 21-day incubation cycles of the virus). The announcement was accompanied by a mixture of affirmations about the "monumental achievement" that this constituted and cautionary statements about not assuming that the work was done but to remain "vigilant" in order to prevent new outbreaks.

One day later, on January 15, a death from Ebola in Sierra Leone was reported. A 22-year-old woman had died on January 12 in Magburaka, a village in the Tonkolili district of northern Sierra Leone. A test for Ebola, which was carried out 2 days after her death, was confirmed positive on January 14, only a few hours after WHO had announced that the spread of Ebola had been halted in West Africa.

***

Zika Virus "Spreading Explosively" in Americas, W.H.O. Says[27]
Zika Virus a Global Health Emergency, W.H.O. Says[28]
Concern Over Zika Virus Grips the World[29]

While the Ebola epidemic was finally, though fitfully, ebbing away, these exclamatory headlines announced the emergence and epidemic spread of still another infectious disease—this one caused by the Zika virus that belongs to the Flaviviridae family of viruses associated with dengue, West Nile yellow fever, and Japanese encephalitis and is transmitted by the *Aedes aegypti* genus of mosquito. It was first isolated in 1947 from a rhesus monkey in the Zika forest of Uganda,[30] and for decades it mainly affected monkeys in a narrowly restricted area of equatorial Africa and Asia. However, by 2007, it had appeared in the Federated States of Micronesia, where 185 suspected cases of Zika affecting human beings were reported. Between 2013 and 2014, four other Pacific Island nations experienced large Zika outbreaks. In May 2015, the presence of Zika in the Americas was confirmed by WHO. By February 1, 2016, "the transmission of Zika virus [to human beings had] been reported in twenty-eight countries and territories, mainly in the Americas, including Brazil,

---

[27] Sabrina Tavernise, *Zika virus "spreading explosively" in Americas, W.H.O.*, International New York Times (Jan. 28, 2016).

[28] Sabrina Tavernise and Donald G. McNeil Jr., *Zika virus a global health emergency, W.H.O. Says*, International New York Times (Feb. 1, 2016).

[29] Udani Samarasekera and Marcia Triunfol, *Concern over the Zika virus grips the world*, Title of a Special Report, 387(10018) Lancet (Feb. 2, 2016), available at http://thelancet.com/journals/lancet/article/PIIS0140-6736(16)00257-9/fulltext.

[30] The first published communication about this "hitherto unrecorded virus" and how it was isolated is G. W. A. Dick, S. F. Kitchen, and A. J. Haddow, *Zika virus: isolations and serological specificity*, 46(5) Transactions of the Royal Society of Tropical Medicine and Hygiene 509–520 (Sept. 1952).

Colombia, Venezuela, Mexico, Haiti, and Barbados."[31] Dr. Anthony Fauci, director of the US National Institute of Allergy and Infectious Diseases, characterized the Zika epidemic as "an unfolding story." "As with Ebola," he said, "this virus is something that could exist for years under the radar, and we don't know until we get thousands of cases what it really does. With Zika, we're seeing new twists and turns every week."[32]

On January 28, 2016, in a meeting with the WHO Executive Board, Dr. Margaret Chan, stated that the Zika virus was "spreading explosively" in the Americas and that "the level of alarm [was] "extremely high," especially because although most people infected with Zika develop a mild form of the disease that lasts only several days to a week,[33] there was increasing concern (later confirmed) that there might be a causal relationship between infection by the Zika virus and the disturbing number of infants in Brazil being born with microcephaly—a medical condition in which the circumference of the baby's head is smaller than normal at birth due to underdevelopment of the cerebral cortex of the brain, which can result in physical deformities and grave, lifelong cognitive and motor disabilities.[34] Four days later, on February 1, 2016, WHO officially declared the Zika virus and its suspected link to birth defects to constitute a "public health emergency of international concern." It is "an extraordinary event and public health threat to other parts of the world," Dr. Chan stated in a press conference, that requires an "international response . . . to minimize the threat in infected countries and reduce risk of international spread."[35]

Just one day after that, on February 2, a case of Zika virus infection transmitted by semen through sexual relations, rather than by a mosquito bite, was discovered and reported in Texas, complicating still further the detection and prevention of Zika outbreaks and suggesting that safe-sex measures as well as mosquito control would be needed.[36]

* * *

"Less than a month ago, the world was celebrating the end of the Ebola outbreak. Now we are consumed by Zika," Victor Dzau, the president of the US National Academy of Medicine, stated in a letter that he sent to the academy's membership on February 5, 2016. "recommend reforms and measures to enable better preparedness

---

[31] Samarasekera and Triunfol, *supra* note 29.

[32] Quoted in Donald G. M. McNeil Jr., Simon Romero, and Sabrina Tavernise, *Medical mystery with a global reach*, New York Times, 1, 10 (Feb. 7, 2016).

[33] The mild symptoms of infection with the virus include headaches, fever, malaise, a maculopapular rash, conjunctivitis, and joint pains.

[34] Another neurological disorder, with which it began to be suspected Zika might be linked, was Guillain-Barré syndrome, which involves temporary whole-body paralysis in adults.

[35] Tavernise, *supra* note 27.

[36] Donald G. McNeil Jr. and Sabrina Tavernise, *Zika infection transmitted by sex reported in Texas*, International New York Times (Feb. 3, 2016).

and more effective governing and response to global health crises in the future – especially infectious disease crises and pandemic threats," he stated vehemently.[37]

* * *

Anthony Fauci has characterized "the ongoing struggle between microbes and humans [as] a challenge that is perpetual."[38] "Winning," in his view, "does not mean stamping out every last disease, but rather getting out ahead of the next one."[39]

My own perspective on infectious diseases is akin to Fauci's. It is symbolically expressed in the conclusion to Albert Camus's allegorical novel *The Plague*, which I have read and reread many times over the course of the years.

When the inhabitants of Oran, the Algerian coastal town where the novel takes place, begin to celebrate their liberation from a deadly plague and the quarantine into which it forced them. Dr. Bernard Rieux, a physician who has witnessed and chronicled what it has entailed, decides to write a final account "to say simply what it is that one learns in the midst of such tribulations":

> However, he knew that this chronicle could not be a story of definitive victory. It could only be the record of what had to be done, and what, no doubt, would have to be done again, against this terror and its indefatigable weapon, despite their own personal hardships, by all men who, while not being saints, but refusing to give way to the pestilence, do their best to be doctors.
>
> Indeed, as he listened to the cries of joy that rose above the town, Rieux recalled that this joy was always under threat. He knew that this happy crowd was unaware of something that one can read in books, which is that the plague bacillus never dies or vanishes entirely, that it can remain dormant for dozens of years in furniture or clothing, that it waits patiently in bedrooms, cellars, trunks, handkerchiefs, and old papers, and that perhaps the day will come when, for the instruction or the misfortune of mankind, the plague will rouse its rats and send them to die in some well-contented city.[40]

---

[37] In his letter, Dzau appealed to members to support the academy's Global Health Risk Framework for the Future, which has been launched to "recommend reforms and measures to enable better preparedness and more effective governing and financing in response to global health crises in the future—especially to infectious disease crises and pandemic threats."

[38] Anthony S. Fauci, Emerging and Re-emerging Infectious Diseases: The Perpetual Challenge (2005), Robert H. Ebert Memorial Lecture.

[39] David M. Morens and Anthony S. Fauci, *Emerging infectious diseases: threats to human health*, PLOS Pathogens (July 4, 2013), available at http://journals.plos.org/plospathogens/article?id=10.1371/journal.ppat.1003467.

[40] Albert Camus, *The Plague*, translated by Robin Buss, with an afterword by Tony Judt, pp. 237–238. *The Plague* was originally published in Paris, by Gallimard, in 1947, as *La Peste*. The edition from which I have extracted the quoted passage was published in Penguin Classics, Penguin Group (UK), London, 2013.

INDEX

Note: Page numbers followed by *f* or *t* denote figures or tables, respectively. Numbers followed by n indicate notes.

AbbVie, 204
Accenture Development Partnerships, 167–168
Access to treatments, 193–206
Access to vaccines
    availability of vaccines, 223–233
    benefits of, 188–189
    equitable, 186
    global, 179–190, 235–244
    for HIV vaccine trials, 235–244
    P5 approach, 241–243
Adaptive design, 196
Adaptive licensing, 198
Adjuvants, 224
AdVac EBOV + MVA Ebola vaccine regimen, 28–29
Advisory Group on Reform of WHO's Work in Outbreaks and Emergencies With Health and Humanitarian Consequences, 112*t*, 116–117
Advocacy, 199–202
Afghanistan, 108, 270
African Centres for Disease Control and Prevention, 68
African Union, 47
Agriculture, industrial, 89–90
Aid Transparency Index, 172
Aid workers, 38, 45. *See also* Health care workers (HCWs)
AIDS. *See* HIV/AIDS
AIDSVAX B/E vaccine, 236–237
Albert and Mary Lasker Foundation, 271
All-hazards strategy, 103
Althaus, Christian, 78
ALVAC HIV vaccine, 236–237, 239–240
American Academy of Pediatrics (AAP), 226–227

American Farm Bureau Federation, 95
American Health Institute, 95
American Society of Tropical Medicine and Hygiene, 266
Angola, 38n11
Animal health, 89–90, 95, 116
Animal testing, 225
Ankara, 28–29
Antibiotic resistance, 13, 87–97. *See also* Drug resistance
Antibiotics, 88
    development of, 92–93
    for food animals, 89–90, 95
    misuse of, 13, 88, 91
    overprescription of, 91
    as societal drugs, 93
Antimalarial tablets, 46
Antimicrobial resistance, 13, 88–89, 95–96. *See also* Drug resistance
Antiretroviral drugs, 196, 200–203
Antiviral agents, direct (DAAs), 203–204
Apple, 167
Aquaculture, 89
Artemisinin-based combination therapies (ACTs), 5
Australia, 232
Authority, 161
Avian influenza A (H5), 4
Avian influenza A (H5N1), 4, 115
Avian influenza A (H5N2), 4
Avian influenza A (H5N6), 4
Avian influenza A (H5N8), 4
Avian influenza A (H7N9), 4

275

276 INDEX

Bacteria
  antibiotic-resistant, 13, 87–97
  pneumococcal, 183–184
Bahrain, 76
Barbados, 272–273
Bavarian Nordic, 28–29
Bellevue Hospital, 263–265, 267
Benin, 171
BHP Billiton Sustainable Communities, 167
Bill and Melinda Gates Foundation, 16, 167–168, 170, 181–182, 188, 236
Biocontainment Patient Care Unit (Nebraska Medical Center), 26
Biological E, 170
Biomedical innovation, 27–30, 193–206
Boateng, Laud, 119
Bonds, vaccine, 178, 188
Botswana, 201
Branding, 167
Brazil, 109, 272–273
Brincidofovir, 49
Brundtland, Gro Harlem, 103
Bundibugyo ebolavirus, 21
Burials, 36–37
Burkina Faso, 185

California, 266
Cambodia, 197
Camus, Albert, 274n40
Canada
  health funding, 150–151, 152f
  response to Ebola outbreak, 48
  SARS outbreak, 79, 114
  vaccine development, 198–199
  vaccine injury compensation, 231–232
Cancer, cervical, 186
Center for Disease Control (CDC) (China), 187
Center for Global Health Preparedness and Response (WHO) (proposed), 115
Center of Excellence for Infectious Disease Control, 29–30
Centers for Disease Control and Prevention (CDC) (US), 30, 34, 170, 242, 245
  Advisory Committee on Immunization Practices (ACIP), 226
  authority to isolate and quarantine, 249–250, 250n18
  Clinical Immunization Safety Assessment Network (CISA), 230
  Emergency Operations Center, 250n19
  guidelines for medical workers returning from Guinea, Liberia, and Sierra Leone, 266
  guidelines for stewardship programs, 93
  Immunization Safety Office, 229–230
  Model State Emergency Health Powers Act, 247–248
  response to Ebola outbreak, 24, 36, 266
  response to Zika epidemic, 109
  staffing, 203
  teleconferences, 250
  Vaccine Safety Datalink (VSD), 229–230
Centers for Medicare and Medicaid Services (CMS) (US), 204
Cervical cancer, 186
Chad, 185
Chan, Margaret, 273
Chemical weapons, 110
Chevron, 167
Childhood immunization, 180–182
Children, 214–215
Children's Vaccine Initiative, 181
China
  Center for Disease Control (CDC), 187
  contributions to WHO Contingency Fund for Emergencies, 68, 68n73
  hepatitis B, 187
  hepatitis C, 202
  micronutrient deficiencies, 169
  response to Ebola outbreak, 47–48
  SARS outbreak, 103
  vaccine injury compensation, 232
Choi, Sugy, 82
Cholera, 102, 106, 110
Chowell, Gerardo, 82
Christie, Chris, 264
Citizenship and Immigration Services (US), 249
Civil society organizations (CSOs), 120, 127t
Civil war(s), 37
Clinical Immunization Safety Assessment Network (CISA), 230
Clinical laboratories, 29–30
Clinical research
  adaptive design, 196
  antibiotic, 92–93
  community engagement, 217–218
  ethical obligations, 219
  HIV vaccine trials, 235–244
  inclusions, 214–216
  informed consent for, 216–217
  phase I trials, 218, 229
  phase II trials, 218, 225–226, 229
  phase III trials, 218, 226, 229
  phase IV surveillance studies, 229
  postmarketing regulatory oversight, 196–197
  premarketing, 195
  proof-of-concept studies, 225–226
  randomized control trials (RCTs), 212–213
  RV144-adapted trials, 239–240
  trial designs, 213–214
  vaccine trials, 217–218
Clostridium difficile, 270
CNN, 263–264
Coca-Cola, 167–168

COFEPRIS (Mexico), 196
Co-financing, 183, 187
Colombia, 272–273
Commercial firms, 164, 165t
Commission on a Global Health Risk Framework for the Future, 112t, 133–134n2, 142–143
Commissions, 1–2. *See also specific organizations*
Commitment, sustainable, 241–242
Communication
 disease outbreak declarations, 39–42, 39n16
 media relations, 258–261, 258n1, 263–266, 272–273
 public health messages, 38–42
 "voices from the field" dispatches, 259–260
Community consent, 216, 218–219
Community engagement, 217–218
Community health programs, 64
Community health workers (CHWs), 63. *See also* Health care workers (HCWs)
Community mobilization, 48
Community-based services, 57–58
Conakry, Guinea, 36
Conference of the Parties (COP) (WHO), 120
Congo. *See* Democratic Republic of Congo
Congo Emergency Pool (Pool d' Urgence Congo) (MSF), 261n10
Connecticut, 266
Conspiracy theories, 38
Containment processes, 13. *See also* Isolation; Quarantine
Contingency Fund for Emergencies (WHO), 68, 68n73
Contraception outreach, 61
Convalescent plasma, 49
Corporate Champions Program (Global Fund), 167
Corporate Governance Code (UK), 163
Corporate law, 162–163
Corporations, 159. *See also specific corporations*
 articles of incorporation or organization, 162
 board of directors, 162–164, 173n94
 directors, 162, 162n30, 163
 finance and governance features of, 164, 165t
 for-profit, 162, 164, 165t
 governance systems, 162, 162n30
 independent directors, 163
 nonprofit, 159, 164, 165t, 173n94
 officers, 162
 Principles of Corporate Governance (OECD), 163
 shareholders, 162, 164
Corruption, 37
Cuba, 47
Cuomo, Andrew, 264
Current and emerging challenges, 21–97, 105f, 116, 269–271
Customs and Border Patrol (US), 250n18
Customs and Border Protection (US), 249

Dasabuvir, 203–204
Data collection, 200–201
Data management, 49
Data sharing, 218–219
Database and Creditor Reporting System (CRS) (OECD), 149–150
Declaration of Manhattan, 181
Delaunay, Sophie, 263
Democratic Republic of Congo
 Ebola outbreak, 33n2, 36, 257, 261–262
 filovirus outbreaks, 38n11
 health system, 262
 MSF activities in, 261–262, 261n10
 polio, 270–271
Diagnostics, 27–29, 198–199
Diphtheria, 180–181, 185
Diphtheria, tetanus, and pertussis (DTP3) vaccine, 181, 188–189, 231
Diplomacy, 14, 124, 133–147
Direct antiviral agents (DAAs), 203–204
Disease, 103, 116. *See also* Infectious disease
Disinfection kids, 46
Dispute Resolution procedures, 123
District of Columbia, 266
Doctors Without Borders. *See* Médecins Sans Frontières (MSF)
Donors, 164
Drug resistance, 269–270
 antibiotic resistance, 87–97
 evolution of, 13
 Global Action Plan on Antimicrobial Resistance (WHO), 13
 multidrug resistance, 5
 National Action Plan for Combating Antibiotic-Resistant Bacteria (Executive Order 13676) (US), 13, 94–96
Drug supply, 37
Drugs. *See also* Vaccines; *specific drugs*
 access to, 198–199
 antiretroviral, 196, 200–203
 development of, 207–221
 regulatory mechanisms, 195–199
 societal, 93
DTP3 (diphtheria, tetanus, and pertussis) vaccine, 181, 188–189, 231
Duncan, Thomas Eric, 26
Dzau, Victor, 273, 274n37

Ebola ça Suffit (Ebola that's enough), 124
Ebola Interim Assessment Panel (WHO), 112t, 117, 122, 136–137n11
Ebola management centers (EMCs), 34–40, 44–51, 45n43, 258
Ebola training centers, 44, 48
Ebola treatment units, 24
Ebola virus, 21–22

Ebola virus disease (EVD), 193
  case fatality rate, 207
  clinical course of, 22, 215
  diagnosis of, 27–28, 34
  disinfection kids, 46
  interventions for, 27–29, 208–212
  outbreaks, 34, 34n3, 37, 208
  Roadmap for Action on Ebola (WHO), 116–117
  symptoms of, 34
  vaccine candidates, 28–29, 194, 223–224
Ebola virus disease (EVD) epidemic (2013–), 1, 21–32, 33–53, 105f, 193–194, 252, 271–272
  economic effects, 61–62, 114
  fieldwork, 260–261
  guidelines for staff members returning from Ebola-affected West Africa, 263–264
  health care worker infections and deaths, 59–60, 64–66, 263–264, 271
  health outcomes and systems effects, 55–73
  Independent Panel on the Global Response to Ebola (Harvard-LSHTM), 1–2, 7–8, 112t, 134n2
  media coverage, 258–261, 258n1
  MSF response, 12, 12n37, 33–53, 33n2, 159, 258–260, 260n6, 271
  number of cases, 50n58
  origin and spread (2014-2015), 23–24, 24f
  outbreak in Guinea (2014), 23, 23f, 35–36
  outbreak in West Africa (2014-16), 34–36, 35f, 37, 55
  PHEIC designation, 108–109, 208
  professional and professional reflections on, 257–274
  response to, 1–2, 24, 27–28, 122, 133–134n2, 133–147, 208, 253–254, 260n6, 263–266
  Review Committee on the Role of the IHR in the Ebola Outbreak and Response (WHO), 112t, 117, 134n2
  scope, 257–258
  spread to US, 25–27, 245, 253–254, 263–267
  survivor clinics, 50
Ecuador, 169
Egypt, 202, 204
Eisenberg, Melvin, 163
Elderly, 214–215
Emergency and Review Committees (WHO), 121, 126t
Emergency pathways, 198
Emergency Response Framework (ERF) (WHO), 122
Emerging challenges, 21–97, 105f, 116, 269–271
Emerging threats, 153–154, 155f
Emory University Hospital Isolation Unit (Atlanta, GA), 26

Epidemic Intelligence Service (EIS) (Korea), 82–83
Equitable access to vaccines, 186
Ethical challenges, 49, 207–221
Ethical obligations, 193–254
Ethnic differences, 38
Europe, 231–232. *See also specific countries*
European Medicines Agency (EMA), 196–198
European Union (EU), 45, 47
European Union (EU) Institution, 150–151, 152f
Evacuations, 45
EVD. *See* Ebola virus disease
Executive Order 13676 (National Action Plan for Combating Antibiotic-Resistant Bacteria), 13, 94–96
Exit screening, 27, 253
Expanded Program on Immunization (EPI) (WHO), 180
Experimental interventions, 49, 212. *See also* Clinical research
Expertise
  mobilization of, 188
  public health experts, 264
  scientific, 121
Extensively drug-resistant tuberculosis (XDR-TB), 5

Failure first policy, 248
Falciparum malaria, 5
Family planning services, 58
Fauci, Anthony, 6–7, 17, 273–274
Favipiravir, 49
Federal Act on the Privileges, Immunities and Facilities and the Financial Subsidies granted by Switzerland as a Host State (Host State Act), 160–161
Federal Aviation Administration (FAA) (US), 250n19
Federal Aviation Agency (US), 250
Federated States of Micronesia, 272–273
Field Epidemiology Training Program (Korea), 82
Field hospitals, 46n44
Filovirus, 38n11
Filovirus, 21
Financing, 117, 119–120
  aid, 47, 149n2
  co-financing, 183, 187
  donor funding, 150–152
  future directions, 149–155
  official development assistance, 149–150n2
  recommendations for, 13, 126t
  soft loans, 149n2
  sustainable, 186–187
  vaccine bonds, 178, 188
  WHO budget, 138

INDEX 279

Finland, 231
Florida, 266
Foege, William, 181
Food and Agriculture Organization (FAO), 116, 123, 168
Food and Drug Administration (FDA) (US), 196, 198, 201, 225, 240
Food and Drug Administration Safety and Innovation Act (US), 198
Food animals, 89–90, 95
Food insecurity, 61–62
For-profit corporations, 162, 164, 165t
Forum for Collaborative HIV Research, 195, 197
Fox, Renée, 17, 257–274
Foya, Liberia, 36n6
Framework Convention Alliance, 120
Framework Convention on Tobacco Control, 120
France, 47–48, 67
French Polynesia, 109
French Red Cross, 48
Friedman, Eric A., 3
Fukuda, Keiji, 41
Fukushima nuclear disaster, 110
Future directions, 124
  for global financing, 149–155
  recommendations for IHR reform, 116–123

G7 Summit (2015), 101
Gabon, 38n11
GAIN (Global Alliance for Improved Nutrition), 14, 160–161, 168–169, 173–174
GAVI Fund, 174
Gavi Matching Fund, 170, 188
Gavi, the Vaccine Alliance, 6, 10, 14–15, 168–171, 181–183, 232
  board meetings, 174
  board of directors, 169–170, 174–175, 182–183
  co-financing for vaccines, 183, 187
  development and resource mobilization model, 186–188
  donor base, 188
  funding, 150–151, 152f, 153–154, 155f, 170, 188
  governance structure, 174–175
  HPV vaccine demonstration programs, 186
  incorporation of, 160–161
  market-shaping efforts, 187–188
  objective, 181
  priorities, 189
  private sector partners, 171, 188
  public sector partners, 170–171
Gene transfer, horizontal, 91–92
General Electric, 159
Genes, resistance, 91–92

Georgia, 202
Georgia (US), 266
Germany
  health funding, 68, 68n73, 150–151, 152f
  response to Ebola outbreak, 48, 67
  vaccine injury compensation system, 231
Ghana, 47
Gilead, 204
Global Action Plan on Antimicrobial Resistance (WHO), 13
Global Advisory Committee on Vaccine Safety (GACVS), 230
Global Alliance for Improved Nutrition (GAIN), 14, 160–161, 168–169, 173–174
Global Fund for Children's Vaccines, 174, 201–202
Global Fund to Fight AIDS, Tuberculosis, and Malaria, 6, 10, 14, 60–61, 119–120, 149–150, 165–168, 172–173, 242
  Corporate Champions Program, 167
  funding, 150–152, 152f, 153–154, 155f, 167
  Partnership Forum, 166
  Product Red program, 167
Global Health Reserve Workforce, 120
Global Health Risk Framework for the Future (NAM), 274n37
Global Health Security Agenda (GHSA), 13–14, 29, 68, 83, 118
  Action Packages, 119–120
  establishment of, 101–102, 105f, 139
  expansion of, 142
  High Level Meeting (September 2015), 83
  Steering Group (2017), 83
Global Healthcare Logistics Strategy Group, 171
Global Outbreak Alert and Response Network (GOARN) (WHO), 120, 136n9
Global Solutions for Infectious Diseases, 236–237
Global systems, 7–10, 101–190
Global Vaccine Access Plan, 236, 238, 245
Globalization, 83
Good faith efforts, 39n16
Gostin, Lawrence O., 3
Governance, 161
  private sector, 161–164, 165t
  public sector, 161–162
Governments, 164, 165t. See also specific governments
Grant, James, 180–181
Greater Mekong Subregion, 5
Gueckedou, Guinea, 49
"Guidelines for Response to MERS" (KCDC), 79
Guillain-Barré syndrome, 109–110, 144, 273n34
Guinea
  Ebola epidemic, 2–3, 23, 23f, 24, 24f, 33–43, 33n2, 48–49, 50n58, 55–73, 114, 139, 253, 257, 272

Guinea (*Cont.*)
  Ebola recovery plan, 3
  Ebola survivor clinics, 50
  Ebola vaccine candidates, 28–29
  economic losses, 61–62
  guidelines for medical workers returning from, 266
  health system, 55–73
  health workforce, 60
  HIV care, 58
  infectious diseases, 270
  Ministry of Health, 35–36
  MSF activities in, 34, 35*f*, 39–40, 42–43, 48
  national emergency, 42
  research network, 30
  rural health services, 63
  vaccination rates, 60–61
  vaccine development, 198–199

H1N1. *See* Influenza A
Haemophilus influenzae type b (Hib) vaccine, 182, 185
Haiti, 110, 272–273
Harvard Global Health Institute–London School of Hygiene and Tropical Medicine, 101, 115
  Independent Panel on the Global Response to Ebola, 1–2, 7–8, 112*t*, 134n2
Harvoni (ledipasvir and sofosbuvir), 203–204
HCV Drug Development Advisory group, 195
HCV TARGET, 203
Health care workers (HCWs), 5, 40
  EVD-related infections and deaths, 59–60, 64–66, 263–264, 271
  guidelines for medical workers returning from Guinea, Liberia, and Sierra Leone, 266
  protection and support for, 64–66
  recommendations for, 126*t*
  violence against, 38, 48–49
Health diplomacy, 14, 124, 133–147, 136*f*
Health facilities, 56–57, 59
Health funding
  donor funding, 150–152
  future directions, 149–155
  global financing, 149–155
  for infectious diseases, 151–152, 152*f*, 152*f*
  official development assistance for, 150, 151*f*
  US spending, 153–154, 154*f*, 155*f*
Health law, 157–158
Health partnerships, 164, 172
Health regulations. *See* International Health Regulations (IHR)
Health security, 51, 101–132, 135–136
Health services, 37, 57–58, 63–66
Health systems
  antibiotic misuse in, 91
  effects of Ebola virus disease on, 55–73

Healthcare infrastructures, 29–30, 37
Hemorrhagic diseases, 105*f*
Hemorrhagic fevers, 106
Hepatitis B, 185, 224
Hepatitis B vaccine, 182, 185, 187
Hepatitis C, 202–203
Hepatitis C virus (HCV), 4, 202–205
Hepatitis, viral, 4–5
Herd immunity, 184
Hickox, Kaci, 264–265
High-Level Panel on Global Response to Health Crises (UN), 8, 112*t*, 134n2, 142n34
High-resource settings, 75–85
HIV Modeling Consortium, 242
HIV vaccine, 223, 235–237, 239–240
HIV vaccine trials, 235–244
HIV Vaccine Trials Network (HVTN), 16, 236–237
HIV/AIDS, 4–5, 58, 103, 105*f*, 143, 199–202, 269–270
  burden of, 235
  drugs for, 196, 199–202
  financing for, 152, 152*f*, 153–154, 155*f*, 165–166
  Joint UN Programme on HIV/AIDS (UNAIDS), 137, 166, 242
  in South Africa, 237–238
Holy See, 103
Hong Kong, 78
Horizontal gene transfer, 91–92
Hospital infection prevention and control, 80
Human influenza, 106. *See also* Influenza
Human papillomavirus (HPV), 182, 185–186, 224
Human resources, 120
Human rights, 193–254
Human samples, 218–219
HVTN 100 vaccine regimen, 239–240

IeDEA, 200
Illinois, 266
Immigration and Customs Enforcement (ICE) (US), 250n18
Immunity, herd, 184
Immunization. *See also* Vaccines; *specific vaccines*
  adverse events after, 226
  benefits of, 182
  childhood, 180–182
  costs of, 188
  global mobilization of resources for, 181–183
  ring vaccination, 199
  vaccination rates, 60–61
  vaccine injury compensation systems, 230–232
Immunization programs, 179, 183–186
  Children's Vaccine Initiative, 181
  Expanded Program on Immunization (EPI) (WHO), 180

outreach-based services, 57–58
  universal childhood immunisation, 180–181
  vaccination trials, 214
Independent directors, 163, 182–183
Independent Panel on the Global Response to Ebola (Harvard-LSHTM), 1–2, 7–8, 112t, 134n2
India, 202
Indonesia, 115
Industrial agriculture, 89–90
Infection control, 56–57, 65–66, 80
Infectious disease, 274. *See also specific diseases*
  advances against, 269–271
  all-hazards strategy against, 103
  containment processes, 13
  current and emerging challenges, 21–97, 105f, 116, 269–271
  financing for, 149–155, 152f, 152f
  global management of, 2, 104–106, 107f, 227–228
  guidelines regarding response to, 81
  One Health approach to, 83
  outbreaks, 39–42, 39n16
  prevention and management of threats, 101–190
  statutory and regulatory mechanisms to control threats, 246–253
  threats from global migration, 245–254
  threats in high-resource settings, 75–85
  treatments for, 193–206
  zoonotic threats, 116
Influenza, 4, 269–270
  avian influenza A (H5), 4
  avian influenza A (H5N1), 4, 115
  avian influenza A (H5N2), 4
  avian influenza A (H5N6), 4
  avian influenza A (H5N8), 4
  avian influenza A (H7N9), 4
  funding for, 153–154, 155f
  human, 106
  Pandemic Influenza Preparedness (PIP) Framework (2011) (WHO), 13, 115, 122, 128t
Influenza A (H1N1) pandemic (2009), 1, 105f, 106–108, 114, 138, 245, 252
  response to, 121–123, 143
  Review Committee on the Functioning of IHR in Relation to the Pandemic (H1N1), 112t
  WHO Emergency Committee, 121
Informed consent, 216–219
Innovation(s), 49
  biomedical, 27–30, 193–206
  HIV, 199–202
  private sector–led, 202–205
International aid, 47, 149n2
International Court of Justice (ICJ), 123
International Federation of Pharmaceutical Wholesalers (IFPW), 171
International Finance Corporation, 169
International Finance Facility for Immunisation (IFFIm), 170, 188
International Health Regulations (IHR), 2, 9, 39n16, 101–132
  Annex 2, 106
  Article 43, "Additional Health Measures," 122–123
  compliance with, 110–111, 122–123, 127t, 143
  failure of, 114–115, 159, 271
  future directions, 116–124
  global governance of disease process, 104–106, 107f
  history of, 102, 104, 105f
  IHR Core Capacity Monitoring Framework, 104, 105t, 116
  IHR Monitoring Tool (IHRMT), 104, 112
  implementation of, 66–68, 83, 101–102, 111, 112f
  National IHR Focal Points (NFPs), 251, 251n23
  noncompliance with, 110–111, 143
  operationalization of, 110–111
  purpose, 9n31, 251n21
  recommendations for, 8–9, 13–14, 116–123, 125t–128t, 142n34
  reform, 123–124
  reform panels, committees, and reports, 111, 112t
  responsibilities for, 103
  Review Committee on the Functioning of IHR in Relation to the Pandemic (H1N1), 112t
  Review Committee on the Role of the IHR in the Ebola Outbreak and Response, 112t, 117, 134n2
  Review Conferences, 124
  scope, 103–106, 251
  standards for quarantine or isolation, 252–253
  State Parties, 103
  State Party core capacities, 103, 111, 117, 118f, 125t
  State Party self-assessments, 112–113, 118–119
  timeline, 104, 105f
  WHO authority to isolate and quarantine under, 250–253
International Monetary Fund (IMF), 47, 142
International organizations (IGOs), 159–162, 164, 165t, 172
International Organizations Immunities Act (IOIA) (US), 159
International public-private partnerships, 157–177
International Sanitary Conferences, 8
International Sanitary Convention (ISC), 8, 102
International Sanitary Regulations (ISR), 102
Invasive pneumococcal disease (IPD), 183–184
Ireland, 232

Isolation, 247, 252, 264
  authority to isolate, 247–253
  recommendations for, 253–254
  standards for, 252–253
Isolation units, 36n6
Isolation wards, 46n44
Italy, 231

Janssen, 28–29
Japan
  Fukushima nuclear disaster, 110
  health funding, 150–151, 152f
  vaccine injury compensation, 231
Japanese corporations, 163
Japanese encephalitis vaccine, 187
Jenner, Edward, 180, 224
Jesty, Benjamin, 180, 224
Job losses, 61–62
John F. Kennedy (JFK) International Airport, 27
John F. Kennedy (JFK) Medical Center (Monrovia, Liberia), 29–30
Johns Hopkins University Press, 263
Johnson & Johnson, 28–29
Joint External Evaluation (JEE) Tool, 118
Joint Republic of Korea-World Health Organization mission, 80–81
Joint statements, 123
Joint United Nations Programme on HIV/AIDS (UNAIDS), 137, 166, 242

Kenema Government Hospital, 40
Kenya
  HIV treatment, 201
  HPV vaccine, 186
  micronutrient deficiencies, 169
  PCV10 vaccine in, 183–184
Knickerbocker Hospital, 268
Knowledge, attitudes, and practices (KAP), 59
Koop, C. Everett, 199–200
Korea. *See* Republic of Korea
Korea Centers for Disease Control and Prevention (KCDC), 79–80, 83
Kraemer, John, 5–6
Kucharski, Adam, 78

Laboratories, 29–30
Laboratory workers, 59
Lactating women, 214–215
Lancet, 49, 269
Lasker Foundation, 271
Lasker-Bloomberg Public Service Award, 268
Lassa fever, 269–270
Law, 157–158, 162

Ledipasvir and sofosbuvir (Harvoni), 203–204
Lee, Jong-Koo, 80
Legal considerations, 157–177
Lenutrit, 169
Liberia
  civil war, 37
  Ebola epidemic, 2–3, 12n37, 23–25, 24f, 33, 33n2, 36n6, 38–48, 50n58, 55–73, 114, 139, 253, 257, 272
  Ebola recovery plan, 3
  Ebola survivor clinics, 50
  Ebola vaccine candidates, 28–29
  guidelines for medical workers returning from, 266
  health facilities, 56–59
  health system, 3, 55–73, 259–260
  health workforce, 5, 60
  infectious diseases in, 270
  maternal and child health services, 63
  Ministry of Health, 40–41
  MSF activities in, 12n37, 34, 35f, 39–41, 43–46
  rural health services, 63–64
  vaccination rates, 60–61
Liberian Institute for Biomedical Research (LIBR), 30
Licensing, adaptive, 198
Liechtenstein, 103
Liu, Joanne, 40, 46
Livestock, 89–90, 95
"Living document"-based guidelines, 200–201
London School of Hygiene and Tropical Medicine (LSHTM), 101, 115, 198–199
  Independent Panel on the Global Response to Ebola (Harvard-LSHTM), 1–2, 7–8, 112t, 134n2
Louisiana, 266

Macenta, Guinea, 48
Madagascar, 270–271
Maine, 265–266
Malaria, 5, 165–166, 223, 262, 269–270
Malaria control, 60–61
Malaria financing, 152–154, 152f, 155f, 165
Malawi, 186
Mali, 30, 33, 33n2, 257
Marburg virus, 21, 269–270
Markets for vaccines, 170, 187–188, 240
Maternal and child health services, 63
Measles, 60–61, 180, 269–270
Médecins Sans Frontières (MSF), 3, 261
  activities in Congo, 261–262, 261n10
  activities in Liberia, Sierra Leone & Guinea, 12n37, 34, 35f, 39–46, 48
  alerts, 40
  Ebola management centers (EMCs), 34, 36, 45–46, 45n43, 50–51, 258

Ebola training centers, 44, 48
field assignments, 260n6
guidelines for staff members returning from Ebola-affected West Africa, 263–264
Lasker-Bloomberg Public Service Award, 271
media relations, 45, 259–260
Pool d' Urgence Congo (Congo Emergency Pool), 261n10
"Principles, Ethics and Dilemmas: Becoming Doctors Without Borders" (WHYY Philadelphia), 263
response to Ebola outbreak, 12, 12n37, 33–53, 33n2, 159, 258–260, 260n6, 271
response to filovirus outbreaks, 38n11
roles and responsibilities, 12, 42–43, 50, 271
solidarity approach, 51
spending, 33n2
staff, 258, 261n6
staff infections and deaths, 33n2, 271
Supply Center, 48
treatment at home, 44–45
vaccine development, 198–199
"voices from the field" dispatches, 259–260
Media relations, 258–260, 258n1, 263–266, 272–273
Medicaid, 204
Medical diplomacy, 134
Medical evacuations, 45
Medical research, 196–197. *See also* Clinical research
Medical Stores Department of Tanzania, 167–168
Medical therapy. *See also* Clinical research; Vaccines
  advances in, 270
  antibiotics, 92–93
  antiretroviral drugs, 202–203
  development and deployment of, 207–221
  experimental interventions, 49, 212
  Model List of Essential Medicines (WHO), 204
  unregistered interventions, 208–210
  vaccine development, 198–199, 224–227
Meliandou, Guinea, 35–36
Meningitis A, 184–185
Meningitis A–specific vaccine, 184–185
Meningitis belt, 184–185
Merck, 28, 49, 198–199
Metrics, 112–113, 117–119, 125*t*
Mexico
  COFEPRIS, 196
  influenza (H1N1) pandemic, 106–108, 114
  Zika virus, 272–273
Microcephaly, 109–110, 144, 273
Micronutrient deficiencies, 169
Middle East respiratory syndrome (MERS), 75, 269–270

by coronavirus (MERS-CoV): outbreak (2015), 3–4, 13, 75–85, 77*f*, 105*f*, 110, 252
"Guidelines for Response to MERS" (KCDC), 79
2012-2013 outbreak, 81–82, 110
Midwives, 59
Migration, 245–254
Mikanda, Suzanne, 259, 261–262
Military HIV Research Program (US), 16, 236–237
Millennium Development Goals (MDG) (UN), 155, 223
Minnesota, 266
Model List of Essential Medicines (WHO), 204
Model State Emergency Health Powers Act (US), 247–248
Monkeypox outbreak (2003), 250
Monoclonal antibodies, 29
Monrovia, Liberia, 36n6, 45–46, 49, 58
Mozambique, 167, 186
MSF. *See* Médecins Sans Frontières
Multidrug resistance, 5
Muslims, 41

Naimah, Jackson K. P., 46–47
National Academy of Medicine (NAM) (US), 1–2, 101, 273–274, 274n37
  Commission on a Global Health Risk Framework for the Future, 112*t*, 133–134n2, 142–143
National Action Plan for Combating Antibiotic-Resistant Bacteria (Executive Order 13676) (US), 13, 94–96
National Foundation for Infantile Paralysis, 268
National IHR Focal Points (NFPs), 9, 9n33, 106, 251, 251n23
National Institute of Allergy and Infectious Diseases (NIAID) (US), 29, 200, 235–237
  Division of AIDS, 16
  NIAID/GSK cAd3 Ebola vaccine candidate, 28
  Vaccine Research Center (NIAID), 235–236
National Institutes of Health (NIH) (US), 24, 26, 30, 242
National Medical Center (Korea), 76
National Vaccine Advisory Committee (US), 226
Nebraska Medical Center, 26
The Neglected Dimension of Global Security: A Framework to Counter Infectious Disease Crises (Commission on a Global Health Risk Framework for the Future), 142–143
Neglected tropical diseases (NTDs), 153–154, 155*f*
Negotiation, 164
Neisseria meningitidis, 184–185

New Jersey, 27, 264, 266
New York, 27, 264, 266–267
New York Times, 258n1
New Zealand, 231
Newark Liberty Airport, 27
NewLink/Merck rVSV-EBOV Ebola vaccine candidate, 28, 49
Nigeria
  Ebola outbreak, 33, 33n2, 44, 44n36, 67, 257
  polio, 108
Nongovernmental organization (NGOs), 42, 48, 65
Nonprofit corporations, 159, 164, 165t, 173n94
Norway
  Institute of Public Health, 49
  vaccine development, 198–199
  vaccine injury compensation policy, 231
Novartis Vaccines and Diagnostics/GSK, 16, 28, 236, 239
Nurses, 59. *See also* Health care workers (HCWs)
Nutrition strategies, 169

Obama, Barack, 109
  Executive Order 13676 (National Action Plan for Combating Antibiotic-Resistant Bacteria), 13, 94–96
Office International d'Hygiène Publique (OIHP), 102
Official development assistance (ODA), 149–150n2
  for health, 150–152, 151f, 154
  for infectious diseases, 151–152, 152f
OIE (World Organization for Animal Health), 116, 118, 123
Ombitasvir, 203–204
One Health approach, 13, 83, 118, 128t
1000 Days Partnership, 169
Operational considerations, 157–177
Organization for Economic Cooperation and Development (OECD), 14, 149–150n2
  Database and Creditor Reporting System (CRS), 149–150
  Principles of Corporate Governance, 163
Outreach-based family planning services, 58
Outreach-based vaccination services, 57–58

P5. *See* Pox-Protein Public-Private Partnership
Pacific Island nations, 272–273
Pakistan, 108, 202, 270
Pan American Health Organization (PAHO), 109, 157, 180, 232
Pandemic Emergency Facility (PEF) (World Bank), 119–120

Pandemic Influenza and Other Emerging Threats program, 153–154, 155f
Pandemic Influenza Preparedness (PIP) Framework (WHO), 13, 115, 122, 128t
Paritaprevir, 203–204
Partners in Health (PIH), 26
Partnership for Research on Ebola Virus in Liberia (PREVAIL), 28, 30
Partnership Forum (Global Fund), 166
Partnerships
  global health partnerships, 164, 172
  international public-private partnerships, 157–177
  research partnerships, 29–30
Pasteur, Louis, 180
Patient-centered care, 15–16, 51
Pentavalent vaccine, 185, 188
Permanent Court of Arbitration Optional Rules for Arbitrating Disputes Between Two States, 123
Personal protective equipment (PPE), 56–57, 64–66
Personal reflections, 257–274
Pertussis (whooping cough), 180–181, 185
Pfizer, 159, 170
Physicians, 59. *See also* Health care workers (HCWs)
Piot, Peter, 269
Plague, 102
The Plague (Camus), 274n40
Planning
  family planning services, 58
  scenario, 242–243
Pneumococcal bacteria, 183–184
Pneumococcal conjugate vaccine, 183–184, 188
Pneumococcal disease, invasive, 183–184
Pneumococcal pneumonia, 182
Polio, 1, 105f, 108
  funding for, 153–154, 155f
  personal reflections on, 258, 267–269
  vaccination against, 180, 270
  vaccine-derived polio paralysis, 270–271, 271n22
  vaccine-resistant, 268–269
  wild poliomyelitis, 106
Political action, 42–46, 123–124
Politics, 39
Pool d' Urgence Congo (Congo Emergency Pool) (MSF), 261n10
Pox-Protein Public-Private Partnership (P5), 16, 236–238
  Global Access Committee, 239, 241–243
  guiding principles, 243
  Phase 3 Program, 242, 243f
  Vaccine Access Plan, 239, 241–243
Pre-exposure prophylaxis (PrEP), 201

Pregnancy, adolescent, 61
Pregnant women, 49, 214–215
President's Emergency Plan for AIDS Relief
 (PEPFAR) (US), 149–150, 153–154,
 201–202, 242
President's Malaria Initiative (PMI) (US), 150,
 153–154
Prevention. *See also* Vaccines
 bednets, 61
 global systems, 101–190
 pre-exposure prophylaxis (PrEP), 201
"Principles, Ethics and Dilemmas: Becoming
 Doctors Without Borders" (WHYY
 Philadelphia), 263
Principles of Corporate Governance (OECD), 163
Prioritization, 189, 211–212
Priority populations and targets, 239–240
Private actors, 158–161
Private resources, 164
Private sector governance, 161–164
Private sector–led innovation, 202–205
Product Red program (Global Fund), 167
Professional reflections, 257–274
Program for Monitoring Emerging Diseases
 (ProMED) website, 82
Proof-of-concept studies, 225–226
Public health
 ethical and human rights obligations in
  emergencies, 193–254
 exit screening, 17, 27, 253
 global management of infectious diseases, 2,
  104–106, 107f, 227–228
 impact modeling, 242
 response to antibiotic resistance
  epidemic, 93–95
 response to MERS-CoV outbreak, 79–80
 statutory and regulatory mechanisms to control
  infectious disease threats, 246–253
 vaccine risk, 227–228
Public health emergencies of international concern
 (PHEICs), 66–67, 252–253. *See also specific
 outbreaks or emergencies*
 criteria for, 43n35
 declarations, 1, 106–110, 122–123, 144, 252
 notifications, 106, 113–114, 113f
 recommendations for, 127t
 undeclared and potential PHEICs, 110
Public health experts, 264
Public health messages, 38–42
Public Health Services Act (PHSA) (US),
 248–249
Public opinion, 227–228, 266–269
Public resources, 164
Public sector governance, 161–162
Public-private partnerships, 158–161, 164
PVS Pathways, 13, 118

Qatar, 76
Quarantine, 247, 252
 authority to quarantine, 247–253
 enforcement of, 250
 fictional, 274
 mandatory, 27, 264, 266–267
 personal reflections on, 268
 rules and procedures for, 266–267
 standards for, 252–253

Randomized control trials (RCTs), 212–213
(PRODUCT)RED brand, 167
Red Cross, 36, 48
Redemption Hospital (Monrovia,
 Liberia), 29–30
Registration, 197
Regulatory requirements, 195–199, 224–227,
 240, 246–253. *See also* International Health
 Regulations (IHR)
Rehabilitation, 268
Relapsing fever, 102
Republic of Korea
 Epidemic Intelligence Service
  (EIS), 82–83
 Field Epidemiology Training Program, 82
 GHSA High Level Meeting (September
  2015), 83
 GHSA Steering Group (2017), 83
 guidelines and public health measures to
  combat infectious diseases, 75
 Joint Republic of Korea–World Health
  Organization mission, 80–81
 MERS-CoV outbreak, 3–4, 13,
  75–85, 110
 Ministry of Education, 82
 Ministry of Health and Welfare, 82
 vaccine injury compensation
  policy, 231
Republic of South Africa (RSA)
 HIV epidemic, 237–238
 HVTN 100 vaccine regimen, 239–240
 Medical Research Council, 16, 236
 micronutrient deficiencies, 169
 PCV7 vaccine, 184
 PCV13 vaccine, 184
 regulatory review and approval, 197
 RV144-like vaccine construct testing, 237–238,
  241–242, 243f
Research and development, 49, 207–221. *See also*
 Clinical research
 antibiotic, 92–93
 antiretroviral drug, 202–203
 experimental interventions, 212
 medical research, 196–197
 vaccine development, 198–199, 224–227

Research partnerships, 29–30
Resistance genes, 91–92
Resources
  allocation of, 211–212
  combination of, 164
  human, 120
  mobilization of, 164, 181–183, 186–188
Reston ebolavirus, 22
Reverse vaccinology, 225
Review Committee on the Functioning of IHR in Relation to the Pandemic (H1N1) (WHO), 112t
Review Committee on the Role of the IHR in the Ebola Outbreak and Response (WHO), 112t, 117, 134n2
Review Conferences, 124
Reybanpac, 169
Ribavirin, 202
Ring vaccination, 199
Ritonavir, 203–204
Roadmap for Action on Ebola (WHO), 112t, 116–117
Rome Agreement, 102
Rotavirus, 182, 188, 226
Rural health services, 63–64
Russia, 47
RV144, 16, 236–239
RV144-adapted trials, 239–240
RV144-like vaccine construct testing, 237–238, 241–242, 243f
Rwanda, 171, 186

Safety
  burial, 36–37
  regulatory requirements for, 224–227
  vaccine, 223–233
Samaritan's Purse, 44
Sample sharing, 115–116
Samples, human, 218–219
Samsung Medical Center (Seoul, Korea), 76
Sanitary Conferences, 102
Sanofi Pasteur, 16, 236–237, 239
Saudi Arabia, 4, 76, 78, 81–82, 110
Scenario planning, 242–243
School closures, 82
Scientific expertise, 121
Screening, 17, 27, 253
Security, 142–143
  health, 51, 101–132, 135–136
  national, 51
Senegal, 33, 33n2, 257
Serum Institute, 184–185
Severe acute respiratory syndrome (SARS), 103, 106, 269–270

Severe acute respiratory syndrome (SARS) outbreak (2003), 81–82, 105f, 114, 249–251
  global response to, 137–138, 143
  public health measures against, 79
  superspreading events, 78n7
Shareholders, 162, 164
Sharing data, 218–219
Sharing samples, 115–116
Siedner, Mark, 5–6
Sierra Leone
  civil war, 37
  Ebola epidemic, 2–3, 23–24, 24f, 33, 33n2, 38–44, 48–49, 50n58, 55–73, 114, 139, 253, 257, 260, 272
  Ebola recovery plan, 3
  Ebola survivor clinics, 50
  Ebola vaccine candidates, 28–29
  guidelines for medical workers returning from, 266
  health facilities, 57–58
  health system, 55–73, 259–260
  health workforce, 60
  infectious diseases, 270
  MSF activities in, 34, 35f, 39–40, 257, 260
  research network, 30
  rural health services, 63
  vaccination rates, 60–61
Smallpox, 102, 106, 225
Smart global health diplomacy, 124
SN Brussels Airlines, 45
Social mobilization, 37
Societal drugs, 93
Sofosbuvir (Sovaldi), 203
Sofosbuvir and ledipasvir (Harvoni), 203–204
Soft loans, 149n2
South Africa. See Republic of South Africa (RSA)
South Sudan, 185, 270–271
Sovaldi (sofosbuvir), 203
Spain, 257
Special Clinical Studies Unit (NIH Clinical Center), 26
Spencer, Craig, 263–266
Staff shortages, 37
Stakeholders, 241–242
Starbucks, 167
Statutory mechanisms, 246–253
Stewardship, 93
Strategic Advisory Group of Experts (SAGE) on Immunization, 227
Sub-Saharan Africa. See also specific countries
  HIV/AIDS, 5, 200
  infection control, 65
  meningitis belt, 184–185
Sudan ebolavirus, 21
Supari, Siti Fadila, 115
Superbugs, 88

Superspreaders, 78n7
Superspreading, 13, 78–79, 78n7
Sustainability, financial, 186–187
Sustainable commitment, 241–242
Sustainable Development Goals (SDG) (UN), 119, 142n34, 155
Switzerland, 160–161
Sydenham Hospital (Harlem), 268
Syria, 110, 270

Taï Forest ebolavirus, 22
Taiwan, 231
Taliban, 270
Task Force for Child Survival, 181
Technology transfer, 240–241
Teleconferences, 250
Terminology, 88
Tetanus, 180–181, 185
Texas, 273
Texas Health Presbyterian Hospital, 26
Thailand, 236–238
Therapeutics, 29
Tobacco control reforms, 120
Transparency, 121, 126t, 172
Travel and trade restrictions, 45, 106–109, 113–114, 122–123, 253–254
  exit screening, 17, 27, 253
Treatments. *See also* Medical therapy
  access to, 193–206
  guidelines for, 200–201, 203
Tropical diseases. *See also specific diseases*
  neglected (NTDs), 153–154
Tuberculosis, 165–166, 223, 269–270
  extensively drug-resistant (XDR-TB), 5
  funding for, 152, 152f, 153–154, 155f, 165
  multi-drug-resistant (MDR-TB), 5
  vaccination against, 180
Turning Point Model State Public Health Act (US), 248
Typhoid fever, 269–270
Typhus, 102

UNAIDS (Joint United Nations Programme on HIV/AIDS), 137, 166, 242
UNICEF (United Nations Children's Fund), 36–37, 170–171, 180–182, 232
United Arab Emirates, 76
United Kingdom
  Corporate Governance Code, 163
  Department for International Development (DFID), 171, 188
  health funding, 150–151, 152f, 188
  response to Ebola outbreak, 47–48, 67
United Nations, 1–2, 42, 46, 101
  General Assembly, 142
  Millennium Development Goals (MDG), 155, 223
  Mission for Ebola Emergency Response, 14
  Office for the Coordination of Humanitarian Affairs (OCHA)., 47
  panels, committees, and reports related to IHR reform, 112t
  Resolution 2177, 47
  response to Ebola outbreak, 24, 109
  Secretary General High-Level Panel on Global Response to Health Crises, 8, 112t, 134n2, 142n34
  Security Council, 46–47, 109, 137, 142
  Sustainable Development Goals (SDG), 119, 142n34, 155
United Nations Children's Fund (UNICEF), 36–37, 170–171, 180–182, 232
United Nations Mission for Ebola Emergency Response (UNMEER), 47, 109, 137
United States
  authority to isolate and quarantine, 247–250, 250n18
  Citizenship and Immigration Services, 249
  Constitution, 247–248
  corporations, 162–163, 173n94
  Customs and Border Patrol, 250n18
  Customs and Border Protection, 249
  Department of Health and Human Services (HHS), 194, 200–201, 203, 226, 249–250, 250n18
  Department of Homeland Security (DHS), 250n18
  Ebola outbreak, 24–27, 47–48, 67, 109, 153–154, 194, 245, 255–257, 263–267
  Federal Aviation Agency, 250
  Global Health Security Agenda (GHSA), 101
  health spending, 67, 150–154, 152f, 154f, 155f, 170, 194
  hepatitis C, 202
  Immigration and Customs Enforcement (ICE), 250n18
  influenza (H1N1) pandemic, 106–108, 114, 245
  International Organizations Immunities Act (IOIA), 159
  mechanisms to control infectious disease threats, 246–253
  migration into, 245
  Military HIV Research Program, 16, 236–237
  Model State Emergency Health Powers Act, 247–248
  monkeypox outbreak, 250
  National Action Plan for Combating Antibiotic-Resistant Bacteria (Executive Order 13676), 13, 94–96

United States (*Cont.*)
  polio epidemic, 258, 267–269
  President's Emergency Plan for AIDS Relief (PEPFAR), 149–150, 153–154, 201–202, 242
  President's Malaria Initiative (PMI), 150, 153–154
  Public Health Services Act (PHSA), 248–249
  quarantine policy, 266
  quarantine rules and procedures, 266–267
  Reagan administration, 199–200
  SARS outbreak, 249–250
  Turning Point Model State Public Health Act, 248
  vaccine injury compensation, 231
United States Army Medical Research Institute for Infectious Diseases, 30
United States Coast Guard, 249, 250n18
United States Surgeon General, 248
Universal childhood immunisation, 180–181
Universal Health Coverage (UHC), 119
University Hospital (Newark, NJ), 264
Unregistered interventions, 208–210
UPS, 171
Urgent care, 50
USAID, 171

Vaccine Adverse Event Reporting System (VAERS), 229–230
Vaccine bonds, 170, 188
Vaccine Fund, 174
Vaccine injury compensation systems, 230–232
Vaccine Research Center (NIAID), 235–236
Vaccine risk, 227–228
Vaccine Safety Datalink (VSD), 229–230
Vaccine trials
  community engagement in, 217–218
  Ebola ça Suffit (Ebola that's enough), 124
  HIV vaccine trials, 235–244
  informed consent for, 216–217
  phase II, 225–226
  phase III, 226
Vaccine-derived polio paralysis, 270–271, 271n22
Vaccines, 5–6, 28–29. *See also* Immunization; *specific vaccines*
  access to, 179–190, 198–199, 223–233, 235–244
  availability, efficacy, and safety of, 223–233
  co-financing for, 183
  deployment of, 207–221
  development of, 198–199, 207–221, 224–227, 241
  economic benefits of, 182
  Gavi-supported, 183
  health benefits of, 184, 223

  Investigational New Drug (IND) status, 225
  manufacturing of, 241
  markets for, 170, 187–188, 240
  mechanisms to ensure safety, 228–230
  meningitis A-specific, 184–185
  outreach-based services, 57–58
  pentavalent (five-in-one), 185, 188
  prices, 187
  regulatory requirements, 195–199, 224–227, 240
  reverse vaccinology, 225
Venezuela, 272–273
Vesicular stomatitis virus-Ebola virus vaccine (VSV-ZEBOV or rVSV-ZEBOV), 28, 49, 198–199, 271
Viekira Pak (ombitasvir, paritaprevir, and ritonavir tablets, and dasabuvir tablets), 203–204
Vietnam, 202
Violence against health workers, 38, 48–49
Viral hemorrhagic fevers, 106
Viral hepatitis, 4–5
Vodafone, 171
"Voices from the field" dispatches, 259–260

Walter, Carol, 181
Watson, Bill, 181
Wellcome Trust, 198–199
West Africa. *See specific countries*
West Nile virus, 269–270
Whooping cough (pertussis), 180–181, 185
WHYY Philadelphia, 263
Wild poliomyelitis, 106
Witchcraft, 262
Women
  job losses, 61–62
  lactating, 214–215
  pregnant, 49, 214–215
Working conditions, 64–65
World Bank, 68, 142, 182, 188
  definition of governance, 161
  health funding, 150–151, 152f
  Pandemic Emergency Facility (PEF), 119–120, 122
  partnership with Gavi, 170
  public health impact modeling, 242
  response to Ebola outbreak, 47, 67
World Food Program, 169
World Health Assembly (WHA), 101–103, 122, 141, 161–162, 251
World Health Organization (WHO), 1–2, 8–9, 34–36, 41, 142, 169, 182
  Advisory Group on Reform of WHO's Work in Outbreaks and Emergencies With Health and Humanitarian Consequences, 112t, 116–117

authority, 114, 161, 250–253, 251n24
budget, 138
Center for Global Health Preparedness and Response (proposed), 115
Conference of the Parties (COP), 120
Constitution, 9–10, 102, 161
Contingency Fund for Emergencies, 68, 68n73, 122
declaration of Ebola outbreak PHEIC, 24, 43–44
declaration of influenza H1N1 pandemic outbreak PHEIC, 106–108
declaration of Zika epidemic PHEIC, 1, 273
Department of Immunizations, Vaccines and Biologicals, 171
diplomatic activities, 140
Director-General, 145
Dispute Resolution procedures, 123
Ebola Interim Assessment Panel, 108, 112t, 122, 134n2, 136–137n11
Emergency and Review Committees, 121–123, 126t
emergency fund, 67
emergency response capabilities, 141
Emergency Response Framework (ERF), 122
establishment of, 157
Expanded Program on Immunization (EPI), 180
failures, 114–115, 159, 271
funding, 3, 67, 150–151, 152f
Global Action Plan on Antimicrobial Resistance, 13
Global Advisory Committee on Vaccine Safety (GACVS), 230
Global Outbreak Alert and Response Network (GOARN), 120, 136n9
governance, 114–115, 161–162
and IHR, 101
IHR Core Capacity Monitoring Framework, 104, 105t, 116
IHR Emergency Committee, 113
IHR Monitoring Tool (IHRMT), 104, 112
IHR reform panels, committees, and reports, 111, 112t, 115
Joint Republic of Korea-World Health Organization mission, 80–81

leadership, 41–42, 67, 137
member states, 114
Model List of Essential Medicines, 204
Office International d'Hygiène Publique (OIHP), 102
Pandemic Influenza Preparedness (PIP) Framework (2011), 13, 115, 122, 128t
partnership with Gavi, 170–171
PHEIC declarations, 66–67
prequalification services, 196–197
public health impact modeling, 242
recommendations for, 8–9, 13–14
recommendations for isolation, 253–254
Regional Office for Africa, 114
resources, 114
response to Ebola outbreak, 2, 24, 39–40, 47, 208
responsibilities, 103, 251n24
Review Committee on the Functioning of IHR in Relation to the Pandemic (H1N1), 112t
Review Committee on the Role of the IHR in the Ebola Outbreak and Response, 112t, 117, 134n2
Roadmap for Action on Ebola, 112t, 116–117
role, 123, 137
staffing, 138, 203
Strategic Advisory Group of Experts (SAGE) on Immunization, 227
temporary recommendations, 122–123
vaccine development, 198–199
vaccine injury compensation, 232
World Organization for Animal Health (OIE), 116, 118, 123
World Summit for Children, 181
World Trade Organization (WTO), 123

Yellow fever, 102, 106

Zaire ebolavirus, 21–22
Zambia, 186
Zika epidemic, 1, 109–110, 144, 272–273
Zika virus, 1, 269–270, 272–273, 273n33
ZMapp, 29, 211–212
Zoonotic threats, 116

www.ingramcontent.com/pod-product-compliance
Ingram Content Group UK Ltd.
Pitfield, Milton Keynes, MK11 3LW, UK
UKHW021051260426
12049UKWH00034B/63